NCLEX-RN® 101: How to Pass!

Eleventh Edition

LORETTA MANNING, MSN, RN, GNP
President, I CAN Publishing®, Inc.

SYLVIA RAYFIELD, MN, RN, CNS
Sylvia Rayfield & Associates, Inc.

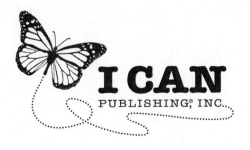

I CAN Publishing®, Inc. ♦ Duluth, GA
www.icanpublishing.com

Technical Assistance: Erica Manning, Suwanee, GA; Jennifer Robinson, Duluth, GA

Editorial Support: Erica Manning, Suwanee, GA

Cartoon Illustrations: C. J. Miller, BSN, RN, Iowa City, IA

Cover Design/Image Illustrations: Teresa Davidson, Greensboro, NC

Quotes from Michael Dooley or tut are from Totally Unique Thoughts. You can visit their website—http://www.tut.com—where all the latest, totally unique graphics and thoughts can be found.

© 2023 by I CAN Publishing®, Inc.

All rights reserved. No part of this book may be used or reproduced or transmitted in any form or by any means, electronic or mechanical, including photocopying, recording, or by an information storage and retrieval system without written permission from I CAN Publishing®, Inc., except for the inclusion of brief quotations in a review.

ISBN: 978-1-7334977-4-9
Library of Congress Control Number: 2023936315

Printed in the United States of America

Nursing procedures and/or practice described in this book should be applied by the nurse, or health care practitioner, under appropriate supervision according to established professional standards of care. These standards should be used with regard to the unique circumstances that apply in each practice situation. Every effort has been taken to validate and confirm the accuracy of information presented and to describe generally accepted practices. However, the authors, editors, and publisher cannot accept any responsibility for errors or omissions or for consequences from application of the information in this book and make no warranty, express or implied, with respect to the contents of this book.

Every effort has been exerted by the authors and publisher to ensure that drug selection and dosage set forth in this text are in accord with current recommendations and practice at the time of publication. However, in view of ongoing research, the constant flow of information relating to government regulations, drug therapy, and drug reactions, the reader is urged to check the manufacturer's information on the package insert of each drug for any change in indications and dosage and for added warnings and precautions. This is particularly important when the recommended agent is a new or infrequently used drug.

This book is written to be used as a test question review book for the NCLEX-RN® examination. It is not intended for use as a primary resource for procedures, treatments, medications, or to serve as a complete textbook for nursing care.

NCLEX-RN® is a registered trademark of the National Council of State Boards of Nursing, Inc. (NCSBN).

Copies of this book may be obtained directly from:

I CAN Publishing®, Inc.
2650 Main Street N.W., Suite 100
Duluth, GA 30097
770.495.2488

www.icanpublishing.com

THE BIG DIFFERENCE FOR THIS BOOK

You will learn how to "THINK"!

T   Think about Clinical Decision-Making/Judgment Strategies

H   Helps you master how to answer NCLEX®-style questions

I   Incorrect and correct answers have rationales

N   Next Generation NCLEX® discussed in the first chapter

K   Know we care and want you to be successful!

Contents

Contributors... vii
Acknowledgments... ix
Prelude... xiii
"SAFETY"... xv
Clinical Decision-Making/Test-Taking Strategies... 1
Guidelines for NCLEX® Success!... 11
Prioritization: New Strategies for Success!... 12
Clinical Decision-Making Strategies for Prioritizing... 13
Structure for Prioritizing Management and Safety Standards... 14
Structure for Answering Pharmacology Questions... 15

1. **Next Generation NCLEX®**... **17**
   Section 1: A Step-by-Step Approach to the NCSBN Cinical Judgment Model... 17
   Section 2: Linking Clinical Judgment to Stand-Alone Cases... 57

2. **Prioritization**... **65**
   Nursing Activities and Questions... 65
   Answers & Rationales... 76

3. **Alternate-Item Format Questions**... **95**
   Nursing Activities and Questions... 95
   Answers & Rationales... 108

4. **Pretest**... **123**
   Questions... 124
   Answers & Rationales... 132

5. **Management of Care**... **143**
   Nursing Activities and Questions... 143
   Answers & Rationales... 154

6. **Safety and Infection Control**... **162**
   Nursing Activities and Questions... 162
   Answers & Rationales... 172

CONTENTS

7. **Health Promotion and Maintenance** 181
   Nursing Activities and Questions 181
   Answers & Rationales 190

8. **Psychosocial Integrity** .198
   Nursing Activities and Questions 198
   Answers & Rationales 207

9. **Physiological Adaptation** 216
   Nursing Activities and Questions 216
   Answers & Rationales 226

10. **Reduction of Risk Potential**. 235
    Nursing Activities and Questions 235
    Answers & Rationales 244

11. **Basic Care and Comfort** 253
    Nursing Activities and Questions 253
    Answers & Rationales 262

12. **Pharmacological and Parenteral Therapies** 271
    Nursing Activities and Questions 271
    Answers & Rationales 280

13. **Post-Test #1** 290
    Questions 290
    Answers & Rationales 300

14. **Post-Test #2** 310
    Questions 310
    Answers & Rationales 319

15. **Post-Test #3** 328
    Questions 328
    Answers & Rationales 337

16. **Practice Exam** 348
    Questions 348
    Answers & Rationales 363

Normal Reference Ranges for Lab Tests 378

References. 379

Contributors

Patti Akins, MSN, RN
Adjunct Clinical Faculty
Northwestern State University College of Nursing and School of Allied Health
Education Consultant
I CAN Publishing®, Inc.
Shreveport, Louisiana

Karen E. Alexander, PhD, RN, CNOR
Director of Nursing and Associate Professor
University of Houston–Clear Lake
Houston, Texas

Carol Anne Baker, MBA/HM, BSN, RN
Director of Compliance and Risk for Advantage Behavioral Health
Athens, Georgia

Linda Delunas, PhD, RN, CNE
Professor of Nursing
Indiana University Northwest
Gary, Indiana

Judy J. Duvall, PhD, EdD, RN
Education Consultant
Sylvia Rayfield and Associates
Dahlonega, GA

Darlene Franklin, MSN, RN
Assistant Professor of Nursing Emeritus
Whitson-Hester School of Nursing
Tennessee Technological University
Cookeville, Tennessee

Kathy Gallun, MSN, RN
Education Consultant
Sylvia Rayfield and Associates
I CAN Publishing®, Inc.
Tampa, Florida

Sandra Galura, PhD, RN
Assistant Professor
Director, Master in Nursing Leadership and Management Program
Department of Nursing Systems
University of Central Florida
Orlando, Florida

Melissa J. Geist, EdD, FNP-BC, PPCNP-BC, CNE
Professor of Nursing
Whitson-Hester School of Nursing
Tennessee Technological University
Education Consultant
I CAN Publishing®, Inc.
Cookeville, Tennessee

Annette M. Guy, DNP, BSN, RN
Dean of Nursing
Spartanburg Community College
Spartanburg, South Carolina

Sylvia McDonald, RN, MEd, MSN
Education Consultant
I CAN Publishing®, Inc.
Duluth, Georgia
Sylvia Rayfield & Associates, Inc.®
Dahlonega, Georgia

Kimi McMahan Walker, RN, MSN-Ed
Hospice, RN Support
Four Seasons Center for Life
Flat Rock, North Carolina

C. J. Miller, BSN, RN
Illustrator
Iowa City, Iowa

Tina Rayfield, MSN, RN, BS, PA-C
President
Sylvia Rayfield & Associates, Inc.®
Dahlonega, Georgia

Continued on next page

Susan Snell, MSN, RN, FNP
Education Consultant
I CAN Publishing®, Inc.
Shreveport, Louisiana

Deb Bagnasco Stanford, MSN-Ed, RN
Clinical Assistant Professor
University of North Carolina-Greensboro
Greensboro, North Carolina

Linda J. Stirk, MS, RN, CNE
Associate Professor of Nursing
North Park University
Chicago, Illinois

Mayola L. Villarruel, DNP, ANP-BC, NEA-BC
Consultant
Community Hospital
Munster, Indiana

Larry Zager, MSN, BSN
Leadership and Education Consultant
Hendersonville, Tennessee

Lydia R. Zager, MSN, RN, NEA-BC
Co-Executive Director
Leading Learning, LLC
Educational Consultant
Hendersonville, Tennessee

Acknowledgments

We wish to express our love and appreciation to our families, associates, and good friends who have offered their support during the preparation of this book.

Loretta's husband, Randy Manning, what can I say? Your support, tolerance, wit, and love during this project as well as during my busy professional life keep me inspired and motivated! Thank you!

Loretta's daughter, Erica Manning, for her continuing support and love as we were writing, rewriting, and editing over and over again to create a book that will make a difference in the lives of nursing students.

Jennifer Robinson, our administrative director, who was always willing to jump through a hoop to meet our deadlines. Her never-ending humor and love reminded us daily what was really important in life! A very special thank you for keeping our projects organized as well as our business running smoothly.

Teresa Davidson, our dear friend and artist, who was willing to create and work with us through the end with unexpected requests.

Sylvia McDonald, for her friendship, love, and support. Thank you for keeping life in perspective for me as we work on major projects and throughout our life.

Thank you to Sylvia Rayfield & Associates who assist nursing graduates across the country to use this book and achieve successful outcomes on the NCLEX-RN®.

Thank you to all of you nursing students, graduates, and faculty who continue to read and study our books! Without each of you, we would not be writing any of these acknowledgments!

Our sincere appreciation to Dr. Phoebe K. Helm, who developed some of the test-taking strategies we have included in this book.

NCLEX-RN® 101: How to Pass!

11th EDITION

This eleventh edition is current and streamlined with questions to help you develop NCLEX® standard mastery and continue developing clinical decision making and judgment skills. The exam items in this book are written to mimic the computer adaptive test. The latest information on the NCLEX-RN® and Next Generation NCLEX® have been included in this book to assist you in achieving success by passing the NCLEX®. The exam, as reflected by the test plan published by the National Council of State Boards of Nursing has been updated and will go into effect April 2023. Chapter One will introduce the Next Generation NCLEX® (NGN) and discuss a step-by-step approach to the NCSBN Clinical Judgment Measurement Model. An example of an unfolding case with NGN style questions and rationales will be included in this chapter. Section II in the first chapter will also include information on linking clinical judgment to stand-alone cases. This first chapter will provide an example of an NGN Bow-Tie item including answers and rationales.

Due to the changes both in clinical practice and the NCLEX-RN®, we have included one chapter with the focus on prioritization; however, prioritization will be included throughout the book as well. The chapters have been organized with the Client Need Categories except for the Alternate-Item Format Questions, the Pretest and Post-tests. Alternate-Item Format Questions will also be integrated throughout the book.

As a result of the research from the National Council of State Boards of Nursing, it is imperative to transform the traditional strategies used for answering exam items into new and current clinical decision-making and clinical judgment strategies. The first chapter introducing the Next Generation NCLEX® will review the new exam items and how they will be organized. Each cognitive thinking skill will provide you with some new techniques for developing your clinical decision making/judgment necessary for NCLEX® success.

Remember to keep this in perspective! The agenda for the NCLEX-RN® is to evaluate current and entry-level practice and be fair and comprehensive. Your key to success is to FOCUS on questions evaluating the NCLEX-RN® nursing activities! Let's get started in learning how to prepare for this BIG EXAM!

For an extensive review of unfolding case studies and stand-alone cases, we recommend the book, *A Step-by-Step Approach to Developing Clinical Judgment for the Next Generation NCLEX® and Clinical Success*, by Manning, L., Akins, P. & Brocato, C. (2022), I CAN Publishing, Inc. Duluth, GA. 30097, www.icanpublishing.com; 770.495.2488. The answers and rationales will provide you with an excellent approach to develop clinical decision making and judgment mastery.

Loretta Manning and Sylvia Rayfield

Prelude

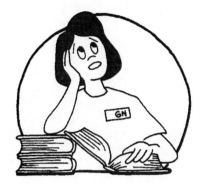

✔ What if you've just graduated from nursing school?

✔ What if you've just applied to take the NCLEX® exam?

✔ What if you have 50,000 pages of notes, tape recordings and nursing books and you don't have a clue as to where to start?

✔ What if you just need help?

Then …

Read on …

What if you knew—

✔ How to focus—not freak out?

✔ Proven NCLEX® clinical decision-making (test-taking) strategies?

✔ How the NCLEX® is organized?

✔ How to determine your own study needs?

✔ What the questions look like on the computer exam?

✔ That test questions in this book are organized around the most current NCLEX-RN® Test Plan?

The Priority for the NCLEX® is always "SAFETY."

This acronym is organized around the priority NCLEX-RN® activities and provides a structure to organize thinking.

S System-Specific Pathophysiology, Assessments, Labs, and Diagnostic Procedures

A Analysis of Concepts

F First-Do Priority Nursing Plans/Interventions
First-Do Medications

E Evaluation of Expected Outcomes

T Trend for Potential Complications

Y You Must Manage Care to Prevent "RISK" to the Client

Adapted from: © National Council of State Boards of Nursing, Inc. (NCSBN). (2022). 2021 *RN Practice Analysis: Linking the NCLEX-RN® Examination to Practice*. Chicago: Author.
Organized into "**SAFETY**" by I CAN Publishing®, Inc., 2023.

Surround yourself with people who respect you and treat you well.

—Claudia Black

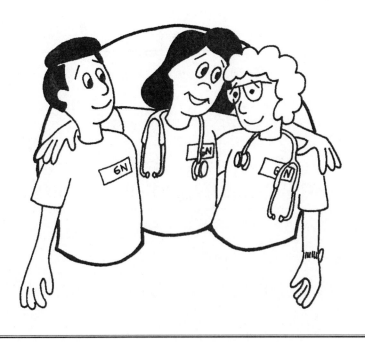

*Supportive people give you strength.
It's hard to think with people
putting you down.*

Remember ...

If you think you can do it—you CAN!

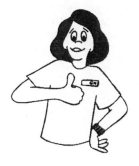
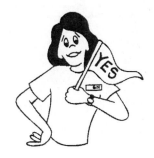

Yes! You CAN do it!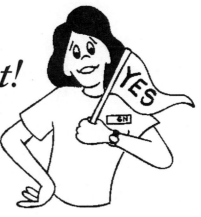

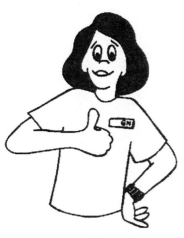 *Now, let's get started on how you can be successful on the NCLEX-RN®!*

CLINICAL DECISION-MAKING/TEST-TAKING STRATEGIES

Our passion is to assist you in being successful at passing this exam. We have conducted hundreds of NCLEX® reviews and pharmacology workshops and have more than seventy years total experience in helping new graduates obtain their licenses.

PASS THE NCLEX®!

Let's look at how this exam is organized. Here is the "bottom line."

➢ The National Council of State Boards of Nursing (NCSBN) (the organization that provides the exam to the local state board office), conducts periodic research on new graduates to determine what kinds of "nursing activities and roles" the new graduates perform most frequently in their work setting and which of these activities have the highest priority for client safety.

➢ After the research is completed, the "nursing activities" become the "backbone" of the NCLEX-RN® exam. These nursing activities are divided into four areas of client needs which are:

- ➢ Safe and Effective Care Environment
  - Management of Care   15–21%
  - Safety and Infection Control   10–16%
- ➢ Health Promotion and Maintenance   6–12%
- ➢ Psychosocial Integrity   6–12%
- ➢ Physiological Integrity
  - Basic Care and Comfort   6–12%
  - Pharmacological and Parenteral Therapies   13–19%
  - Reduction of Risk Potential   9–15%
  - Physiological Adaption   11–17%

YOU MAY RECOGNIZE THIS TERMINOLOGY—particularly if you have taken some sort of diagnostic pretest for NCLEX®. Many of the pretests use these words to indicate your strong and weak areas.

The Nursing Process is also used as a way to approach the exam. If you are like most new grads, you know the nursing process because you have been trying to figure out which instructor wants which thing in which column of your care plans/concept maps for at least the last two years.

You will find a list of the nursing activities at the beginning of each chapter, except the Pretest, Post-tests, and Practice Exam. These nursing activities are from the National Council of State Boards of Nursing, Inc. Refer below to reference.

Adapted from: © National Council of State Boards of Nursing, Inc. (NCSBN). (2022). 2021 *RN Practice Analysis: Linking the NCLEX-RN® Examination to Practice.* Chicago: Author.

First, let's look at techniques that will improve your pass rate!

Question Types:
The NCSBN has operationalized the use of "alternate item format" questions. These items will be in addition to the multiple choice format that has been used in the past. These questions may include:

- ✳ Fill in the blank (type numbers in a calculation item)
- ✳ Multiple-response items (select two or more responses)
- ✳ Hot spot items (identify one or more areas on a graphic or picture)
- ✳ Graphics (instead of text, the answer will be a graphic)
- ✳ Ordered response ("Drag and Drop" items to rank order)
- ✳ Charts or Exhibit Format
- ✳ Videos
- ✳ Audio

Any item formats, including standard multiple-choice items, could include multimedia, charts, tables, or graphic images.

The NCLEX-RN® 101: How to Pass includes examples of these types of items for your practice.

A Step-by-Step Approach to Clinical Decision Making (Test-Taking)

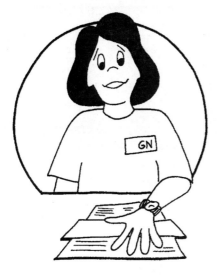

Step 1

Cover the Distractors.

➢ Did you know that in educational jargon, the question part of a multiple-choice question is called the stem and the options are called DISTRACTORS????

➢ Did you know that instructors stay up nights WRITING DISTRACTORS????

➢ We do not want you to be DISTRACTED—so cover the DISTRACTORS with your hand, a 5x7 card, a leftover Lotto ticket, your shirttail, or anything!!!

➢ YOU CAN'T BE DISTRACTED IF THEY ARE COVERED.

➢ Read the Stem (Question).

➢ Answer the question in your head. USE YOUR BRAIN. IT'S THE ONLY THING YOU CAN TRUST!!!

Step 2

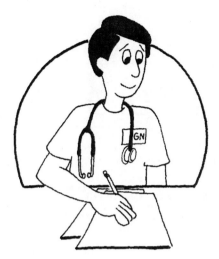

After thinking, "What does it mean?" and "Where do I begin?" Create a pool of answers (generate solutions/first-do plan).

*W*here were you on September 1, 2016?

Did you raise your palms to heaven and say, "How am I supposed to know that?"

That's exactly what some people do when they see an NCLEX-RN® question.

The brain thinks first in large chunks of material, then smaller chunks. Like this...

*T*hink—how old was I in 2016? Married, single, in school???

Most of you at least know where you were in September 2016.

First of school year? Near an anniversary, birthday, or holiday?

*D*on't worry about what you don't know. Think about what you do know!

*N*ow think, "Where do I begin?" (Prioritize data)

Step 3

Uncover the distractors and make your decisions— one by one (Take-action) and Evaluate your response (Evaluate outcomes).

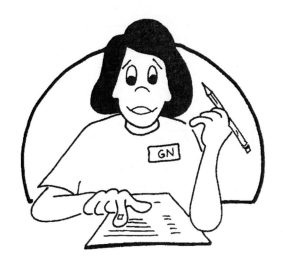

> ➤ After creating a pool of answers, uncover the first distractor.
>
> Is it a *yes or no?*
>
> **MAKE A DECISION.**
>
> ➤ Next, uncover the second distractor. *Is it a yes or no?* GET THE DRIFT?
>
> ➤ Uncover Distractor 3. *Yes or No?* BE SURE, and uncover Distractor 4. Even though you may have found a good answer in 1, 2, or 3, the last one might be the highest priority!
>
> ➤ Remember—these options are written to distract—so make a decision on **each** before continuing.

Step 4

Commit one hour per day to answering questions.

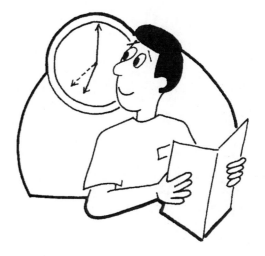

> ➢ Our experience has documented that the more questions practiced, the better success rate on NCLEX®!!!
>
> ➢ The people who wrote this book have over 75 years of collective successful experience in preparing graduates to PASS the NCLEX®. We have put together a team of experts in item writing and have given them specific guidelines that reflect the NCLEX-RN® Test Plan and the "nursing activities" that are the basis of the NCLEX-RN® exam.
>
> ➢ This book has been divided into sections of 65 items.

Don't major in a minor activity.

Each question is worth one-two minutes of your time.

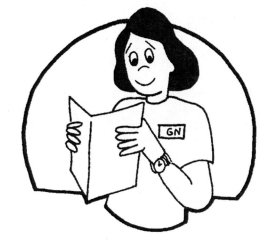

> ➤ **DO NOT**—repeat—**DO NOT** look at the end of the chapter for the answers.
>
> ➤ Forget "instant gratification" until the entire test is completed. Then determine which questions were missed and why.
>
> ➤ Looking at the answers after each question encourages memorization, and **WE DON'T WANT YOU TO MEMORIZE! Why? Because we doubt if any question in this book or any other question/review book on the market will be exactly as it is on NCLEX®.**

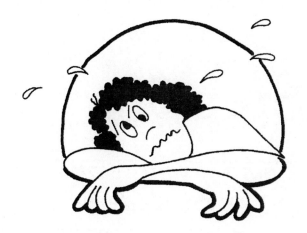

I thought we'd never take a break!

Take a break between Steps 4 and 5.

You deserve it!

All work and no play is no fun.

Step 5

Commit your second hour per day to studying what you don't know!

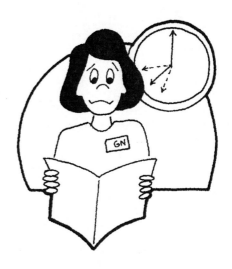

Our experience has taught us that new graduates like to study the material they are the most comfortable with. You want to forget the stuff you don't know because it gives you butterflies!

Here are some ways to use this book:

➢ Figure out which questions you got correct. FORGET THEM! Don't say, "Oh, that was just a lucky guess." You had some basis for choosing the correct answer. Let them go!

➢ Now, WHICH ONES DID YOU MISS? Were they on Management, Safety & Infection Control, Health Promotion, Psychosocial Integrity, Basic Care and Comfort, Physiological Adaptation, Pharmacology, and/or Reduction of Risk Potential? Use the Test Worksheet, Content Analysis page, and Table of Contents to help guide your studying.

➢ Once you have determined your study needs, use a good review book to refresh your memory on the facts. To help you with easy, fun ways to remember, we recommend *Nursing Made Insanely Easy* and *Pharmacology Made Insanely Easy* by Loretta Manning and Sylvia Rayfield, I CAN Publishing®, Inc. (icanpublishing.com)

HOT TIPS to Decrease Stress and Improve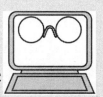

You can take the test in any state and practice in the state where you have applied for license. You will have choices of dates, times, and test centers. You will be FINISHED WITHIN HOURS! The NCSBN currently contracts with Pearson Vue for administration of the NCLEX®. Pearson Vue has over 200 testing sites that administer the NCLEX®.

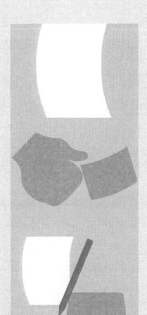

- ❤ You will get an authorization to test from your state board office. It's like American Express—"Don't leave home without it!"

- ❤ Don't leave home without your finger either because you will be fingerprinted and have your picture taken. You will need your signature and your picture identification for the testing center.

- ❤ You may be provided with lockers for your "stuff."

- ❤ You will be given a computer practice period with help on the equipment. There will be someone to help you get started on your computer—a warm-up time.

- ❤ The testing center will provide note boards and markers as you will not be allowed to take in any paper, books, food, drinks, purses, wallets, beepers, cell phones, guns, knives. *Security is very serious*.

- ❤ There will be a drop-down calculator for math calculations and a mouse for your use.

- There are a minimum of 85 questions and a maximum of 150. DO NOT PANIC if you hit question #86! It means you have more time to demonstrate your clinical decision-making skills. Refer to chapter 1, Next Generation NCLEX®.

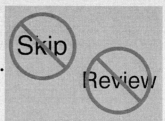

- You will have five (5) hours to complete the NCLEX-RN®. This is from start to finish, including warm-up time.

- You will not be able to skip a question or go back and review questions once they have left the screen. This is an advantage since many "changed" answers are wrong.

- There is no time limit per question, BUT DO NOT SIT ON A QUESTION FOR MORE THAN TWO (2) MINUTES or you may not have enough time in the five-hour limitation to answer enough questions to pass.

- If you don't have a clue as to the answer, pick any one.
    Which response represents the best guess?
    1. *Alright!*
    2. *Boy Howdy!*
    3. *Cool!*
    4. *Delightful!*

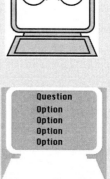

- The questions in this book look similar to the ones you will see on the computer screen.

- The computer offers you break times. Take time for breaks!

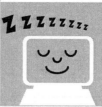

YES!

Guideline "STANDARDS" for NCLEX® Success

S — "SAFETY" for the client is priority! Organize studying around the "SAFETY" Structure!

T — Therapeutic Communication, Teaching and Learning, Trends (Pay attention to assessment changes)

M **A** — Slow's (Maslow's) Hierarchy of Needs

N — Nursing Process

D — Determine relevant facts in both question and distractors

A — Alternate-Item Format Questions

R — Remember the 6 P's: Pathophysiology, Physical assessment, Prioritizing, Pharmacology, Protect client from complication(s), and Protect from falls

D — Delegation/Documentation

S — Study using Strategies for clinical decision-making! Stay CALM and believe in yourself! You can be SUCCESSFUL!

PRIORITIZATION: New Strategies for Success!

Due to the continuous changes in health care from the complexity of nursing care to multiple system involvement with both acute and chronic medical conditions, the aging population, the multiple medications clients use, and the list goes on, it has become imperative for the nursing student to learn how to be skillful in clinical decision making, clinical judgment, and prioritization of nursing care. Nursing students must learn how to prioritize all aspects of health care including (i.e., assessments, which client to see first due to either potential or actual complications, nursing interventions, medication administration, clients who are presenting with changes in the clinical presentation, and this list also goes on).

In the past, nursing students had to learn how to identify and recognize basic signs and symptoms of hemorrhaging, pain, fluid and electrolyte imbalance, etc. Today, it is of paramount importance for the nursing student to learn how to assess and recognize early versus late clinical findings for complications. The skill of prioritizing is developed by comparing, contrasting, and trending clinical assessment findings. Based on the analysis of the clinical findings, the student must learn how to prioritize the plan of care and determine what intervention should be implemented. This competency requires a new approach to learning, thinking, and processing clinical data. Today, the student needs to know more about the interpretations of the clinical assessment findings of bleeding such as if the client is presenting with early signs of shock versus late signs of shock than simply learning the signs and symptoms of bleeding.

Our focus for Chapter 2 is to provide you with practice questions focusing on how to prioritize. We have included a new approach and structure to assist you in learning the process of prioritization. This new approach, as outlined in the mnemonic on the following page, requires you to expand the basic assessments to include the critical elements (i.e., client history, medications, equipment, etc.) that may impact these findings. Refer to the book *Nursing Made Insanely Easy* for further description. The outcome of these expanded assessments will facilitate prioritizing the plan of care. Prior to being able to initiate this process as an RN, we understand your initial goal is NCLEX® SUCCESS!!!!

Of course, you must have an excellent understanding of nursing in order to learn how to prioritize. Many of the traditional test-taking strategies do not work with the process of prioritizing, so we are going to assist you in learning new clinical-decision making strategies with this new approach to prioritization. The clinical-decision making strategies have been developed within the framework of the NCLEX® standards.

If you continue to feel overwhelmed with information from Medical Surgical Nursing, we recommend the book, *Medical Surgical Nursing Concepts Made Insanely Easy: A New Approach to the Next Generation NCLEX®* by Manning & Zager. This book includes an additional chapter dedicated to learning how to prioritize. This can be purchased from I CAN Publishing, Inc. at www.icanpublishing.com. The Insanely Easy book package is also very popular and helpful as you continue to perfect this process. These other two books include, *Nursing Made Insanely Easy* and *Pharmacology Made Insanely Easy*, Manning & Rayfield.

Our hope for you is that after reviewing this chapter and book, you will progress from saying, "How can I prioritize care when it seems that all of the clients are a priority to see" to saying "I understand how to prioritize nursing care based on the specific strategy for the clinical situation!"

We wish you much success on your journey with learning prioritization! Remember, every journey begins with the first step. Of course, the first step is for you to believe in yourself, and know you CAN be SUCCESSFUL!

Manning, L. and Zager, L. (2019). *Medical Surgical Nursing Concepts Made Insanely Easy! A New Approach to the Next Generation NCLEX®!* Duluth, GA: I CAN Publishing®, Inc.

Clinical Decision-Making Strategies for Prioritizing

P — Prioritize: Assess, the first step in the nursing process

R — Review if Maslow's Hierarchy of basic needs is the priority; review ABC's

I — Identify the client who is unstable or highest risk for developing complications

O — Organize priority nursing interventions based on the key concepts

R — Remember to think about what the expected outcome is from the care, med, etc. Evaluation is an ongoing process

I — Identify standard of practice (i.e., scope of practice, verify if order is wrong, drug interactions)

T — Trends, compare, and contrast client's vital signs, clinical presentation, etc.

Y — You must manage care to prevent "RISK" to the client (Refer to next page for description)

Structure for Prioritizing Management and Safety Standards

R   Recognize professional leadership (i.e., scope of practice for delegation). Recognize appropriate code of ethics for registered nurses

I   Infection prevention. Improvement quality. Interdisciplinary Team Collaboration (i.e., know how to prepare for transfer). Integrate culture, spirituality, and communication

S   Structure care with evidence-based practice (Standards of Practice). Safe Practices (i.e., Security/Disaster Plan, Safe equipment, Safe client handling—ergonomic principles, fall prevention, restraint safety, patient identification, room assignments). Supportive communication (i.e., positive conflict resolution, receive or give report, identify accuracy of orders, documentation, informed consent, maintain confidentiality)

K   Know how to incorporate health-promotion standards (i.e., teach, growth, and development)

Adapted from: © National Council of State Boards of Nursing, Inc. (NCSBN). (2022). 2021 *RN Practice Analysis: Linking the NCLEX-RN® Examination to Practice.* Chicago: Author.
Organized: Manning, L. and Zager, L. (2019). *Medical Surgical Nursing Concepts Made Insanely Easy! A New Approach to the Next Generation NCLEX!* (p. 5), Duluth, GA: I CAN Publishing®, Inc.

Structure for Answering Pharmacology Questions Organized With the NCLEX® Pharmacology Standards

A
- Action of medication
- Administration of medication; blood product and dosage ordered; How to administer
- Assessment
- Adverse Effects. List significant ones
- Accuracy/Appropriateness of order; Is it indicated based on client's condition, known allergies, drug-drug or drug-food interactions? If not, what action did you take?

I
- Interactions (Drug-Drug, Food-Drug, Disease-Drug, Dye-Drug)
- Identify priority plan prior to giving drug (i.e., vital signs, labs, allergies, etc.)
- Identify priority plan after giving drug

D
- Desired outcomes of the drug
- Discharge teaching—Administration considerations for client and family
- Documentation

E
- Educate client about medication(s)
- Evaluate client's response to medication/blood product

S
- Safety (client identification, risk for falls, vital sign assessments)
- Safe and controlled environment for handling and/or administering controlled substances within regulatory guidelines
- Safe medication reconciliation process

Adapted from: © National Council of State Boards of Nursing, Inc. (NCSBN). (2022). *2021 RN Practice Analysis: Linking the NCLEX-RN® Examination to Practice*. Chicago: Author.

Notes

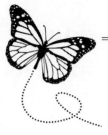

CHAPTER 1, SECTION 1
Next Generation NCLEX®

> If we're growing, we're always going to be out of our comfort zone.
> — JOHN MAXWELL

A Step-by-Step Approach to the NCSBN Clinical Judgment Measurement Model

You Can Do This! Yes, success can be achieved on the new NGN exam!

The big question you may be asking yourself is, "Why is the National Council of State Boards of Nursing (NCSBN) moving forward with the Next Generation NCLEX® (NGN)? Why is there a need to focus on clinical judgment?" The answer is the NCSBN research (NCSBN, 2018) shows the following:

- 50 percent of novice nurses were involved in errors in some way.
- 65 percent of those errors were attributed to poor clinical decision-making skills.
- Only 20 percent of employers are satisfied with clinical decision-making skills of novice nurses.

There is a need to focus on clinical judgment because the research also demonstrates that to practice successful clinical judgment the nurse must have the underlying clinical knowledge; however, this does not necessarily occur in reverse. Nurses can have underlying clinical knowledge, but it may not result in successful clinical judgment.

This brings us to the purpose of this book - to make sure you have what you need to be successful!

The learning outcomes for Chapter 1 are:

- Review the National Council of State Boards of Nursing (NCSBN) Clinical Judgment Measurement Model.
- Discuss the application of the six cognitive skills to a case study.
- Review clinical judgment strategies for success when making clinical decisions with the six cognitive skills in answering multiple NGN-style test items.
- Practice NGN case study and questions.
- Discuss how to become a self-directed learner!

This chapter will be organized in a question-and-answer format.

Question: You keep referring to the National Council of State Boards of Nursing (NCSBN) Clinical Judgment Measurement Model (NCJMM). What does this mean?

Answer: The Clinical Judgment Measurement Model is a multilayered model based on Dickison, et. al. (2019):

- Nursing observation
- Cognitive skills
- Contextual factors

Layer 1: First layer of clinical judgment is observation. During nursing care, nurses observe or make many system-specific assessments in which safe clinical decisions need to be made. These clinical decisions occur in many different contexts, (i.e., environmental, personalized cues and needs, etc.).

Layers 2 and 3: The six cognitive thinking skills used by nurses as a result of the observations are represented in these very important layers of the model.

Layer 4: Contextual factors are included in layer 4. These include both individual and environmental factors that can have an impact on the effective clinical judgment by the nurse.

Question: What are the cognitive thinking skills?
Answer: The cognitive thinking skills are imperative for safe clinical judgment and consist of mental (thinking) processes. These cognitive skills include:

- ☐ Recognize Cues
- ☐ Analyze Cues
- ☐ Prioritize Hypotheses
- ☐ Generate Solutions
- ☐ Take-action
- ☐ Evaluate Outcomes

Question: Wow, this seems overwhelming! What does this mean to me as a student?
Answer: The chart below compares the cognitive skills to what you know and have practiced since you started nursing school. You should understand the new terminology, but do not let it intimidate you or make you doubt what you know!

The Cognitive Skills	Nursing Process with Applying Clinical Judgment Questions to Yourself
Recognize Cues	What are your observations and assessments?
Analyze Cues	What are your observations and assessments telling you (i.e., are there concerns with oxygenation and breathing, does the client have mobility issues, etc.)?
Prioritize Hypotheses	What is the concept ranking based on priority? (Do NOT let the word "hypotheses" intimidate you!) Perhaps you prioritize oxygenation from a case because respirations increased to 25 breaths/min & SaO_2 decreased to 93% versus the client has difficulty with getting up from a chair because of osteoarthritis.
Generate Solutions	What is the plan of care that will assist in meeting expected outcomes? What are possible interventions that can be done to help with oxygenation (i.e., performing an incentive spirometer, coughing and deep breathing, etc.)?
Take-action	What interventions should be implemented?
Evaluate Outcomes	Did the client achieve the expected outcomes? Did the nursing care help? Did the SaO_2 increase, respiratory rate decrease after the nebulizer treatment, was sputum expectorated, breath sounds clear, etc.?

The hypotheses may represent the concept(s) and need to be ranked based on priority. Ask the question "Where do I start?"

Let's start by introducing a case study to assist in guiding you with how to apply clinical knowledge into practicing clinical decision making and judgment with complex client contexts. It is much easier to apply as we review this process. The great news is that nursing graduates have told us for years, *"If only the NCLEX® tested more like clinical practice, then I would not be so anxious!"* The NGN is all about safe clinical practice! You CAN do this and do it well!

Question: How will the case study be placed in respect to the question?
Answer: The case will be on the left side of the screen and question on the right side. This book will illustrate the NCSBN question and case placement. The only variation from the NCSBN is that we will have several questions on the right page in order to optimize space on the page.

The Information outlined below may be included in the cases and is organized within the mnemonic "**CASE**".

CASE

C Central concepts contextual (pertinent background, physical assessments)

A Appropriate clinical data: vital signs, laboratory results, history, physical, nurses' notes, MAR

S Signs and symptoms of specific concept(s)/medical condition

E Environmental and time pressure cues
Expected physiological and psychosocial changes with aging

Question: Will there be a different case with each question?
Answer: No, there will be **6 questions per case**. The information in the case study may change (unfold) with different questions. You will manage each question as if this was your client in the hospital or specific health care setting and focus on detailed assessment findings (cues) that may require specific revisions in the plan of care or nursing actions. The questions in the book, *A Step-by-Step Approach to Developing Clinical Judgment for the Next Generation NCLEX® and Clinical Success!*, by Manning, Akins, & Brocato, will provide you with substantial amount of practice with the cases and experience how clients change in condition will require a revision in the priority of care. In some cases, as in this first case, the data will be given to you, and this will be consistent throughout the question. The case will be provided for you with each set of questions, so you do not have to recall all of the details. This is also what you can expect from the NCLEX®.

Question: Will each case include all the information included in the mnemonic "**CASE**"?
Answer: Each case will not include all the information outlined in the mnemonic "**CASE**". As you work through the book, you will experience some questions, include more contextual information than others while some questions only present minimal laboratory results, etc. You can expect the same experience when you take the NGN. Let's review an actual case.

Clinical Judgment Application Exercise
Case study: (Oxygenation) Pneumonia

The case study will be presented on the left page in this chapter.

Nurses' Notes: 0830: The nurse is caring for a 38-year-old male in the Emergency Department (ED). The client was brought to the ED by his wife due to an increase in a frequent wet cough and shortness of breath. Client is presenting with general muscle aches throughout his body. Admitting vital signs, laboratory test results, and clinical assessment findings are below.

Vital Signs (Admission)	
Temperature	101.8° F (38.8° C)
Heart rate (HR)	114 bpm (Sinus Tachycardia w/o ectopy)
Respiratory rate (RR)	32 breaths/min
Blood pressure (BP)	110/76 mm Hg
Weight	187 lbs. (80 kg)

Clinical Assessment Findings	
Neurological	Oriented but somewhat lethargic. Responds to verbal stimuli and follows commands.
Cardiovascular	$S_1 S_2$ w/o murmurs, rubs, or gallops (MRG); peripheral pulses 1+ bilaterally. 2+ pretibial edema. Denies chest pain.
Pulmonary	Breath sounds with coarse rales bilaterally; diminished in bases.

Skin is pale, moist. Client is sitting in high Fowler's position. Frequent wet cough productive of thick greenish-yellow secretions. Social History: Client admits to smoking approximately two packs of cigarettes per day and drinking "a few beers on weekends".
O_2 at 4L/min per nasal prongs initiated after laboratory test results completed.

Laboratory Test Results			
SaO_2	92% on room air	Hematocrit	48%
pH	7.47	Platelets	245,000 mm³ (245 x 10⁹/L)
PaO_2	80% mm Hg	Sodium	142 mEq/L (142 mmol/L)
$PaCO_2$	34 mm Hg	Potassium	4.5 mEq/L (4.5 mmol/L)
HCO_3	22 mEq/L (22 mmol/L)	BUN	12 mg/dL (4.29 mmol/L)
WBC Count	16,000 mm³ (16 x 10⁹/L) with 83% seg count	Creatinine	0.9 mg/dL (79.58 μmol/L)
Hemoglobin	12.8 g/dL (7.94 mmol/L)	Blood Glucose	182 mg/dL (10.1 mmol/L)

Cognitive Skill — Recognize Cues

Begin each case study by asking yourself, "What matters most? What is most important?" You will be using the first cognitive skill for the NCSBN CJMM — **Recognize Cues.** Recognizing cues requires you to know and recognize what cues are most important to the client for the case being presented.

You will find the questions for each case on the right page in this chapter.

---

1. Case Question for Student: RECOGNIZE CUES

Highlight or place an x next to the assessment findings for this client presenting with shortness of breath that will require follow up by the nurse.
- ☐ Muscle aches
- ☐ Heart rate (HR)
- ☐ Respiratory rate (RR)
- ☐ Breath sounds
- ☐ Sodium level
- ☐ Potassium level
- ☐ Temperature
- ☐ WBC Count
- ☐ SaO₂

Question: What relevant cues did you select?
Answer: In applying your knowledge to this case, you may have selected the following cues that are either trending down or up, relevant to the case, present an immediate concern, or findings are abnormal. These include the following:

Selected Cues
- ☐ Heart rate (HR)
- ☐ Respiratory rate (RR)
- ☐ Breath sounds
- ☐ Temperature
- ☐ WBC Count
- ☐ SaO$_2$

Question: When the question, like this one, requires highlighting, how many options can I expect?
Answer: Great question! This question type will have a maximum of 10 options formally referred to as **Enhanced Hot Spot (Highlighting)**.

Enhanced Hot Spot Items allow you to select the answer by highlighting (or in this book you could also place an x by) pre-defined words or phrases. When you are taking the NCLEX®, you will be able to select and deselect the highlighted parts by clicking on the words or phrases.

You can breathe a sigh of relief! This NGN is all about making safe judgments, so nursing graduates are providing safe and effective care. We are confident that as we move forward you are going to realize that you CAN do this!

I CAN Thinking TIP!

A strategy for answering this first cognitive skill, **Recognize Cues**, is to observe the assessment findings (cues) that are most relevant and are most concerning to the nurse. Ask yourself, "What matters most?" "**TRIP**" will assist you in organizing this tip!

Ask the following questions to help you make the appropriate clinical decisions:

1. Is there any evidence of any vital signs, lab values, etc. **Trending down or up** indicating an immediate concern to the client?
2. What are **Relevant** assessment findings (cues) to this case?
3. What clinical data presents an **Immediate** concern for the client?
4. Is there any **Presentation** of abnormal clinical data that would be most concerning for the client? Why is this client presenting with these specific assessments (cues)?

T Trending

R Relevant cues to case

I Immediate concern

P Presentation is abnormal

Question: Are you saying that the **I CAN Thinking TIP** will guide me in answering any question on the NGN testing the first cognitive skill, **Recognize Cues**?

Answer: Yes, you are correct! The questions outlined with the **I CAN Thinking Tip** will guide your thinking as you review the clinical data that matters most and is most concerning to the nurse. The key to success is to know the questions to ask yourself about newly learned concepts, so you can become a self-directed critical thinker. Questions have been developed to assist you in mastering each of the 6 cognitive skills to become skillful in clinical decision making and judgment. It is a step-by-step approach.

Did you struggle with any of the clinical data presented in the case? Remember, the first step in developing clinical judgment is to master information. Refer to the next page for the mnemonic from the book, *Medical Surgical Nursing Concepts Made Insanely Easy: A New Approach to the Next Generation NCLEX®*. "**DYSPNEA**" will assist in remembering the system-specific assessments (cues) to any medical condition resulting in hypoxia. You do not have to memorize the mnemonic in chronological order. This is simply a structure for organizing volumes of information representing assessment findings (cues) for many different medical conditions that can result in altered oxygenation (i.e., pneumonia, bronchitis, etc.).

DYSPNEA: Memory Tool for System-Specific Assessments (Cues): Concept Oxygenation

Dyspnea, orthopnea & nocturnal

Yes, early signs: (↑T, ↑RR, ↑HR, ↑BP); restlessness; skin & mucous membranes pale; late signs: ↑VS, cyanosis, ↓LOC, lethargy, lightheadedness.
(Geriatric clients: acute confusion is early sign.)

Secretions altered, productive cough (color, consistency, tenacity, & odor). Pulmonary edema: pink-tinged, frothy sputum; Signs of infection (i.e., ↑temp, ↑WBC, yellow secretions, etc.).

Precipitating factors: infection, immobility, allergens, stress trauma, post-op complications, pleurisy.

Note characteristics of the cough (i.e., dry, moist, productive) alleviating or aggravating factors → discomfort with breathing; symptoms with cough such as fever or shortness of breath.

Evaluate SaO$_2$ < 95% or arterial blood gases (ABGs), pulse oximetry < 92%.

Adventitious breath sounds (wheezes, crackles, atelectasis after post-op); immobility; dysrhythmias; use of accessory muscles; asymmetrical chest expansion; activity intolerance.

<small>Manning, L., and Zager, L. 2019. *Medical Surgical Nursing Concepts Made Insanely Easy: A New Approach to the Next Generation NCLEX®.* I CAN Publishing, Inc. Duluth, GA. p. 125.</small>

Summary for the first cognitive skill, Recognize Cues

"**TRIP**" will guide you as to how you know what cues are relevant for the concept (s) presented in the case.

T Trending

R Relevant cues to case

I Immediate concern

P Presentation is abnormal

There are questions you will consistently ask as you learn to master this first cognitive skill, **Recognize Cues**. The bottom line for this skill is "What matters most and what clinical data presents an immediate concern to the nurse?"

Cognitive Skill – Analysis of Cues

Question: What is the second cognitive skill in the Clinical Judgment Measurement Model?
Answer: The second cognitive skill is **Analysis of Cues**. To assist in analysis of cues for this case, review if client findings (cues) support client condition (s).

Clinical Judgment Application Exercise
Case study: (Oxygenation) Pneumonia

Nurses' Notes: 0830: The nurse is caring for a 38-year-old male in the Emergency Department (ED). The client was brought to the ED by his wife due to an increase in a frequent wet cough and shortness of breath. Client is presenting with general muscle aches throughout his body. Admitting vital signs, laboratory test results, and clinical assessment findings are below.

Vital Signs (Admission)	
Temperature	101.8° F (38.8° C)
Heart rate (HR)	114 bpm (Sinus Tachycardia w/o ectopy)
Respiratory rate (RR)	32 breaths/min
Blood pressure (BP)	110/76 mm Hg
Weight	187 lbs. (80 kg)

Clinical Assessment Findings	
Neurological	Oriented but somewhat lethargic. Responds to verbal stimuli and follows commands.
Cardiovascular	S_1S_2 w/o murmurs, rubs, or gallops (MRG); peripheral pulses 1+ bilaterally. 2+ pretibial edema. Denies chest pain.
Pulmonary	Breath sounds with coarse rales bilaterally; diminished in bases.

Skin is pale, moist. Client is sitting in high Fowler's position. Frequent wet cough productive of thick greenish-yellow secretions. Social History: Client admits to smoking approximately two packs of cigarettes per day and drinking "a few beers on weekends".
O_2 at 4L/min per nasal prongs initiated after laboratory test results completed.

Laboratory Test Results			
SaO$_2$	92% on room air	**Hematocrit**	48%
pH	7.47	**Platelets**	245,000 mm^3 (245 x 10^9/L)
PaO$_2$	80% mm Hg	**Sodium**	142 mEq/L (142 mmol/L)
PaCO$_2$	34 mm Hg	**Potassium**	4.5 mEq/L (4.5 mmol/L)
HCO$_3$	22 mEq/L (22 mmol/L)	**BUN**	12 mg/dL (4.29 mmol/L)
WBC Count	16,000 mm^3 (16 x 10^9/L) with 83% seg count	**Creatinine**	0.9 mg/dL (79.58 µmol/L)
Hemoglobin	12.8 g/dL (7.94 mmol/L)	**Blood Glucose**	182 mg/dL (10.1 mmol/L)

It is important for the nurse not to just identify priority information, but to interpret the information. In this second question, the nurse needs to relate the clinical findings to specific medical conditions.

2. Case Question for Student: ANALYSIS OF CUES

For each client finding below, use an x to specify if the finding is consistent with pneumonia, COPD, and/or influenza. Each finding may support more than 1 medical condition.

Client Finding	Pneumonia	COPD	Influenza
Generalized muscle aches	X	X	X
Frequent wet cough productive of thick greenish-yellow secretions	X	☐	☐
Breath sounds with coarse rales bilaterally; diminished in bases	X	☐	☐
Temperature	X	X	X
Sinus tachycardia without ectopy	X	X	☐

As you interpreted the client findings in the question above, you most likely noticed that several of these can occur in each of the medical conditions. The question will clearly guide you, so that you understand there may be more than one condition for each finding. Remember, this skill takes time to practice and develop and requires knowledge of the condition and the concept.

Question: What type of NGN test item format is this question that we just reviewed for the second cognitive skill, Analysis of Cues?
Answer: This is referred to as a **Matrix Multiple Response** test item.
Scoring: Remember, the National Council of State Boards of Nursing wants you to be successful! We want you to be successful! The decision has been made by the National Council of State Boards of Nursing that you will receive partial credit, so you do not miss all the available points if you miss a few of these options!

Question: What are the maximum potential options that could be included with this test item format?
Answer: The columns are exactly what you see in this sample, 2–3, and there could be 4–10 options or in other words 4-10 rows of client findings. This Matrix test item format allows you to select one or more answer options for each row and/or column. This test item format can be used in measuring multiple aspects of the clinical judgment measurement model with a single item. In the example above, each of the five rows will need to have one of the three option choices selected.

Strategies are always helpful when learning something new. Let's use the mnemonic "**CAFÉ**" for the second cognitive skill, **Analysis of Cues**.

> **I CAN Thinking TIP!**
>
> A strategy for answering this second cognitive skill, **Analysis of Cues**, is to determine client conditions/concepts consistent with the client findings (cues). Ask the question "What could it mean?" Use "**CAFÉ**" to guide you!
>
> Ask the following questions to help you make the appropriate clinical decisions:
>
> 1. What **Conditions (medical)/concepts** are consistent with clinical data (cues)?
> 2. What clinical **Assessments (cues)** are priority for a specific condition (medical)/concept?
> 3. Are there any assessment **Findings (cues)** that support or contradict any specific client conditions?
> 4. What other clinical assessment findings will assist in **Establishing significance** of assessments (cues) for priority concepts?
>
> **C** Conditions (medical)/concepts are consistent with clinical data (cues)
>
> **A** Assessments (cues) priority for condition (medical)/concept
>
> **F** Findings (cues) that support or contradict any medical condition
>
> **E** Establish significance of assessments (cues) for priority medical condition/concept

These inquiry questions will guide you in mastering this second cognitive skill in the CJMM. "Repetition is the mother of learning." As you answer the questions, use the questions outlined in the I CAN Thinking Tips to assist you. For example, with this second cognitive skill, we recommend starting with conditions/concepts that are consistent with clinical data (cues) and assessments (cues) that are priority for the condition/concept. The strategy of repetitively asking and answering questions within each of the cognitive skills will help move the information into your long-term memory. As a self-directed learner, the repetition of questions will help determine where to focus your review.

> **Summary** for the second cognitive skill, **Analysis of Cues**
>
> "**CAFÉ**" will guide you in organizing **Analysis of Cues** to determine client conditions/concepts consistent with the clinical findings (cues). The key questions, "What could this mean?"
>
> **C** Conditions (medical)/concepts are consistent with clinical data (cues)
>
> **A** Assessments (cues) priority for condition (medical)/concept
>
> **F** Findings (cues) that support or contradict any medical condition
>
> **E** Establish significance of assessments (cues) for priority concept

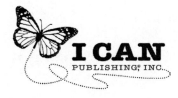

Let us never consider ourselves
finished nurses... we must be
learning all our lives.

— Florence Nightingale

Cognitive Skill – Prioritize Hypotheses

The focus is to proceed to illustrate the third cognitive skill, **Prioritize Hypotheses**.

Clinical Judgment Application Exercise
Case study: (Oxygenation) Pneumonia

Nurses' Notes: 0830: The nurse is caring for a 38-year-old male in the Emergency Department (ED). The client was brought to the ED by his wife due to an increase in a frequent wet cough and shortness of breath. Client is presenting with general muscle aches throughout his body. Admitting vital signs, laboratory test results, and clinical assessment findings are below.

Vital Signs (Admission)	
Temperature	101.8° F (38.8° C)
Heart rate (HR)	114 bpm (Sinus Tachycardia w/o ectopy)
Respiratory rate (RR)	32 breaths/min
Blood pressure (BP)	110/76 mm Hg
Weight	187 lbs. (80 kg)

Clinical Assessment Findings	
Neurological	Oriented but somewhat lethargic. Responds to verbal stimuli and follows commands.
Cardiovascular	S_1S_2 w/o murmurs, rubs, or gallops (MRG); peripheral pulses 1+ bilaterally. 2+ pretibial edema. Denies chest pain.
Pulmonary	Breath sounds with coarse rales bilaterally; diminished in bases.

Skin is pale, moist. Client is sitting in high Fowler's position. Frequent wet cough productive of thick greenish-yellow secretions. Social History: Client admits to smoking approximately two packs of cigarettes per day and drinking "a few beers on weekends".
O_2 at 4L/min per nasal prongs initiated after laboratory test results completed.

Laboratory Test Results			
SaO_2	92% on room air	Hematocrit	48%
pH	7.47	Platelets	245,000 mm³ (245 x 10⁹/L)
PaO_2	80% mm Hg	Sodium	142 mEq/L (142 mmol/L)
$PaCO_2$	34 mm Hg	Potassium	4.5 mEq/L (4.5 mmol/L)
HCO_3	22 mEq/L (22 mmol/L)	BUN	12 mg/dL (4.29 mmol/L)
WBC Count	16,000 mm³ (16 x 10⁹/L) with 83% seg count	Creatinine	0.9 mg/dL (79.58 μmol/L)
Hemoglobin	12.8 g/dL (7.94 mmol/L)	Blood Glucose	182 mg/dL (10.1 mmol/L)

Based on the analysis of cues, prioritize the hypotheses. The hypotheses may represent the concept(s) or medical conditions and need to be ranked based on priority. Do not let the word "hypotheses" intimidate you! You are simply making a decision where to start your care!

3. Case Question for Student: PRIORITIZE HYPOTHESES

Complete the following sentences by choosing from the list of options.

The client is at risk for developing _____ as evidenced by the client's _____.

Select (Options 1) ▼
dysrhythmias
hypoxia
deep vein thrombosis
cerebrovascular accident

Select (Options 2) ▼
cardiovascular assessment
neurological assessment
neurovascular assessment
respiratory assessment

Answer: You most likely selected hypoxia and respiratory assessment.

The decrease in oxygenation is due to an impairment of gas exchange from the inflammatory exudates in the lungs. The lungs are attempting to compensate by increasing the respiratory rate. As breathing becomes labored from the secretions becoming more consolidated and difficult to expectorate, the result will be hypoxia as evidenced by the increase in the Heart rate (HR), Respiratory rate (RR), coarse and diminished breath sounds, and decrease in the SaO_2 (**respiratory assessment**).

Question: What type of NGN test item format is this question that we just reviewed for the third cognitive skill, **Prioritize Hypotheses**?

Answer: This is referred to as a **Cloze (Drop-Down)** test item. Cloze (Drop-Down) test items will have statements about the presented client case that require completion. With each blank, you will have one or more lists of options for selection of answers. These drop-down lists can be used as words or phrases within a sentence, table and/or chart. In the example above, you prioritize from the case that the clinical presentation presents a concern with the client developing hypoxia. Most of this clinical data is from the respiratory assessment. This test item format can also evaluate analysis of cues.

Question: Will we always just have 2 drop-down menus?

Answer: No, you can have between 2–5 drop-down menus presented in each paragraph or item with 3-5 choices in each drop-down menu.

> ### I CAN Thinking TIP!
>
> A strategy for answering this third cognitive skill, **Prioritize Hypotheses**, is based on the analysis of cues to prioritize the hypotheses. The hypotheses may represent the concept(s) and need to be ranked based on priority. Ask the question "Where do I start?" "RISK" will guide you in organizing the tip for prioritizing hypotheses. In developing your skill in becoming a *"self-directed thinker"*, ask yourself the following questions:
>
> 1. What are the possible **Risks** that may be occurring with the client and what are the most likely explanations?
> 2. What is the most likely **Identified concern** for this client?
> 3. Are there any **Safety** risks involved with this client?
> 4. Is there any **Knowledge** that I have learned from the case that creates a sense of **Urgency**? Why?
>
> **R** Risk
> **I** Identified Concern
> **S** Safety
> **K** Knowledge of urgency

At this point, you probably are thinking that this is beginning to make sense. I am sure, however, you still have some concerns and feel that it is all very new and different from how you have been tested in the past with the new test item formats.

Practice is the key to mastery, and Mastery is the first step in becoming a self-directed critical thinker! Continue to remain focused and review the summary for the third cognitive skill.

> ### Summary for the third cognitive skill, **Prioritize Hypotheses**
>
> "RISK" will guide you in organizing **Prioritize Hypotheses**. The hypotheses may represent the concept(s) or medical conditions and need to be ranked based on priority.
>
> **R** Risk
> **I** Identified concern
> **S** Safety
> **K** Knowledge of urgency
>
> There are questions you will consistently ask yourself when learning to master this third cognitive skill, **Prioritize Hypotheses**. The bottom line for this skill is "Where do I start?"

You now have the first three cognitive skills and the sample questions to assist in answering the questions. You also have three easy mnemonics to jog your memory as to what is important for each skill.

Think of the three mnemonics as a travel story!

> *- First, before the "TRIP", you need to know what matters most in how to get to the destination (Recognize Cues). You are not interested in irrelevant facts!*

- *Second, during the "TRIP", you must take a break at the "CAFÉ" to analyze what could this mean (Analysis of Cues).*

- *Third, you need to determine what will present the highest "RISK" to you on the "TRIP" (Prioritize Hypotheses).*

Believe that I CAN do this! Now on to the fourth cognitive skill.

Cognitive Skill - Generate Solutions that will meet the client outcomes.

We will only review a question here, but it does refer to the same case that has been outlined on the left page for the previous 3 questions. The cases or specific clinical data will typically be outlined on the left page with the question(s) on the right page. The purpose of this next step is to review the strategies for the cognitive skill, **Generate Solutions**, and the new test item format.

4. Case Question for Student: GENERATE SOLUTIONS

The nurse has reviewed the Nurses' Note entries and is planning care for this client who is experiencing shortness of breath. For each potential nursing intervention, click or fill in the circle to specify whether the intervention is indicted or contraindicated for the client.

Potential Intervention	Indicated	Contraindicated
Increase supplemental oxygen per order.	●	○
Restrict oral intake.	○	●
Maintain O₂ saturation > 92 %	●	○
Obtain sputum sample by oral expectoration for culture and sensitivity.	●	○
Insert an intravenous peripheral line.	●	○

Note: Each column must have at least 1 response option selected.

Question: What type of NGN test item format is this question that we just reviewed for the fourth cognitive skill, Generate Solutions? It looks like the Matrix that we reviewed with the second question.
Answer: This is referred to as a **Matrix Multiple Choice** test item; however, with this question there is only one correct answer per row or per potential intervention. Each column must have at least one response option selected. This question is evaluating whether the plan is indicated or contraindicated.

Question: Are the maximum potential options that could be included with the test item format the same as you indicated with the second question?
Answer: Yes, the columns are exactly what you see in this sample, 2–3, and there could be 4–10 options or in other words 4–10 rows of potential interventions. As we reviewed previously, this test item formal can be used in measuring multiple aspects of the clinical judgment measurement model with a single item. With this example, each of the five rows will need to have one of the two option choices selected.

Question: What is the strategy for this fourth cognitive skill, **Generate Solutions**?
Answer: The key here is to "**SOLVE**" the client's problems by determining "*What can I do?*"

> ### I CAN Thinking TIP!
>
> A strategy for answering this fourth cognitive skill, **Generate Solutions**, is to observe the solutions that will meet expected client outcomes. Ask the question, "What can I do?" "**SOLVE**" will assist you in organizing this tip! Ask yourself the following questions:
>
> 1. If I plan to implement this action (**Solution**) for my client experiencing symptoms of respiratory distress, then what will be the outcome?
> 2. What are the expected **Outcome(s)** for this client?
> 3. What **Plan(s)** based on the hypotheses should be included, avoided, or contraindicated?
> 4. What **Variety** of interventions from multiple concepts should be included to meet expected outcomes?
> 5. What **Evidence-based plans** should be included to meet expected outcomes?
>
> **S** Solutions
>
> **O** Outcomes
>
> **L** List plans of care; review what should be included, avoided, or contraindicated
>
> **V** Variety of interventions from multiple concepts to meet expected outcomes
>
> **E** Evidence-based plans to meet expected outcomes

Question: How can I remember the expected outcomes for this client who is experiencing respiratory distress?
Answer: This is EASY! Do you recall the list for the cues (system-specific assessments) for clients experiencing hypoxia (respiratory distress)?

Question: Is the answer "**DYSPNEA**"?
Answer: Congratulations! It is outlined below. Do you see, it is exactly what we were assessing in "Recognizing Cues"! When you have a structure to organize information, thinking is simplified!!

> ### DYSPNEA: Memory Tool for Expected Outcomes to Guide Plan of Care
>
> The desired outcomes in this case are that the client will:
> Have adequate oxygenation and present with "No **DYSPNEA**":
>
> **D**yspnea will not be present
>
> **Y**es, vital signs will be within the defined range
>
> **S**ecretions, sputum, color clear
>
> **P**recipitating factors NONE
>
> **N**o cough
>
> **E**valuation of SaO_2 > 95% on ABGs, O_2 saturation > 92%
>
> **A**dventitious breath sounds – NONE

Did you struggle with this cognitive skill, **Generate Solutions** (First-Do Priority Plans)? Remember, the first step to learning clinical judgment is to master information. Refer to the mnemonic from the book, *Medical Surgical Nursing Concepts Made Insanely Easy: A New Approach to the Next Generation NCLEX®*.

"**BREATHE**" will assist in remembering the evidence-based plans of care for generating solutions for this client who is experiencing hypoxia. You do not have to memorize the mnemonic in chronological order. This is simply a structure for organizing evidence-based actions representing the cognitive skill, Generate Solutions (First-Do Priority Plans), for many different medical conditions that can result in altered oxygenation.

BREATHE: Memory Tool to Generate Solutions/Take-action (First-Do Priority Plans/Interventions): Concept Oxygenation

Breath sounds, SaO_2, vital signs, DYSPNEA assess and monitor (trend); O_2 as needed, assess dysrhythmias; lightheadedness.

Reposition to facilitate ventilation and perfusion, (i.e., HOB ↑, up in chair, ambulate, particularly after surgery).

Evaluate airway status; prepare for oxygen supplement, (i.e., ambu bag); initiate EMERGENCY management as needed, (i.e., CPR, mechanical ventilation).

Assess and document ABG values, sputum color, consistency and amount, good oral care every 2 hours.

The airway needs to be suctioned PRN to maintain patency. Chest physiotherapy & postural drainage per protocol, bronchodilators, and handheld nebulizers as prescribed.

Hand washing, wear appropriate PPE, apply infection control standards (i.e., room placement, assignment, etc.); obtain cultures before antibiotics.

Encourage deep breathing and coughing, incentive spirometer, evaluate outcome of medications.
Educate/emotional support, encourage fluids based on clinical presentation.

Manning, L., and Zager, L. 2019. *Medical Surgical Nursing Concepts Made Insanely Easy: A New Approach to the Next Generation NCLEX®*. I CAN Publishing, Inc. Duluth, GA. pp. 129-130.

Summary for the fourth cognitive skill, **Generate Solutions**

"**SOLVE**" will guide you in organizing **Generate Solutions**. The solutions will be selected for the plan of care that will meet expected client outcomes.

S Solutions

O Outcomes

L List plans of care; review what should be included, avoided, or contraindicated

V Variety of interventions from multiple concepts to meet expected outcomes

E Evidence-based plans to meet expected outcomes

There are questions you will consistently ask yourself as you learn to master this fourth skill, **Generate Solutions**. The bottom line for this skill is "What can I do?"

Question: Prior to moving to the next cognitive skill, let me reflect over what I think I understand about Generate Solutions. I need to consider evidence-based plans that will "**SOLVE**" the client needs and meet the expected outcomes for this client. Is this correct?

Answer: This is partially correct. The other part of this cognitive skill is to review which plans should be avoided or contraindicated for the case. Fluid intake should not be restricted for this client. Restricting oral intake would be contraindicated, since fluid will assist in decreasing the viscosity of the secretions.

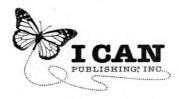

Nothing great or new can be done without enthusiasm. Enthusiasm is the fly-wheel which carries your saw throughout the knots in the log. A certain excessiveness seems a necessary element in all greatness.

— Dr. Harvey Cushing

Clinical Judgment Application Exercise
Case study: (Oxygenation) Pneumonia
Unfolding

Nurses' Notes: 0830: The nurse is caring for a 38-year-old male in the Emergency Department (ED). The client was brought to the ED by his wife due to an increase in a frequent wet cough and shortness of breath. Admitting vital signs, laboratory test results, and clinical assessment findings are below.

Nurses' Notes: 0900: Client is restless, less alert, can only talk in brief monosyllabic responses; diaphoretic, prominent use of accessory muscles. HOB at 30 degrees. States "I can't get enough air".

ADMITTED TO MICU: PNEUMONIA WITH RESPIRATORY COMPROMISE

Vital Signs	0900	1100
Temperature	101.7° F (38.7° C)	101.9° F (38.8° C)
Heart rate (HR)	120 bpm	128 bpm
Respiratory rate (RR)	32 breaths/min	38 breaths/min
Blood pressure (BP)	110/76 mm Hg	102/58 mm Hg

Clinical Assessment Findings	0900	1100
Gastrointestinal	Bowel sound hypoactive X 4 quadrants	Bowel sound hypoactive X 4 quadrants
Pulmonary	Breath sounds with scattered rales and rhonchi; diminished on the right and in bases. Diaphoretic, nasal flaring, use of sternocleidomastoids and scaliness accentuated in effort of breathing.	Breath sounds with scattered rales and rhonchi; decreased on the right.

Diagnostic Test	
Chest X-Ray	Diffuse infiltrates bilaterally. The resident says, "it's completely whited out".
Cultures	Cultures (blood, urine) sent to lab.

Laboratory Test Results	0900	1100
SaO_2	88% (venti-mask at 50% O_2)	94% (venti-mask at 50% O_2)
pH	7.25	7.35
PaO_2	70 mm Hg	86 mm Hg
$PaCO_2$	48 mm Hg	40 mm Hg
HCO_3	20 mEq/L (20 mmol/L)	20 mEq/L (20 mmol/L)
BE	2.2	2.4
WBC Count	22,000 mm^3 (22 x 10^9/L)	21,000 mm^3 (21 x 10^9/L)

Question: Will this happen on the Next Generation NCLEX®?

Answer: Yes, remember to pay attention to details as you progress with the questions. This is what happens in clinical practice! Changes occur and plans of care need to be revised ongoing. Now, let's move on to the question evaluating, **Take-action**. Note, I have included two questions for this cognitive skill, so you can experience several approaches to how you may see this on the NGN.

It is important for you not to just memorize a laundry list of nursing actions for specific medical conditions/concepts, but you need to learn to prioritize nursing actions from the list of possible solutions.

Question: What is the fifth cognitive skill?
Answer: The fifth cognitive skill is **Take-action** (First-Do Priority Nursing Interventions).

Question: It looks as if there is some different clinical data in this next case. Is this what is referred to as an unfolding case?
Answer: Yes, this is an unfolding case. In the clinical setting, client's clinical findings change constantly requiring the nurse to be vigilant with the cues (system-specific assessments) and revise the plan of care (generate solutions) based on these changes. Do you observe any trends in the VS changes, laboratory test results, etc.? Based on these findings, you will respond by applying these changes as you answer the question.

5. Case Question for Student: Take-action

5A. Drag and drop or list the top 4 nursing interventions that are priority to implement for the client to the box on the right.

Nursing Intervention	Top 4 Nursing Interventions
Increase oxygen to 50% per venti mask.	
Encourage oral fluids of at least 8 glasses of water per day.	
Promote turning side to side, coughing, and deep breathing every two hours while awake.	
Administer albuterol 2 puffs as an inhalation prn every 4–6 hours as prescribed.	
Elevate the head of the bed 30–45 degrees.	
Instruct client on importance of effective use of incentive spirometer every two hours while awake.	

As you review the list, you most likely recognized the need to elevate the head of the bed, provide supplemental oxygen, increase fluids, and turn client from side to side.

5A. Priority nursing actions should be directed at improving oxygenation and decreasing work of breathing. **Elevation of head of bed** promotes better chest expansion and gas exchange due to change in anatomic position of lungs and diaphragm. The addition of **supplemental oxygen** increases the available oxygen for gas exchange and perfusion which decreases sympathetic "fight or flight" response to poor oxygenation. **Increasing fluid intake** will assist in decreasing the viscosity of secretions making them much easier to mobilize and expectorate. The increased activity of **turning from side to side**, frequent purposeful coughing, and taking slow deep breaths will increase lung expansion, facilitate oxygen exchange, and mobilize secretions to remove from the lungs more easily. Decreased mobility also promotes stasis of secretions which increases the risk of infection. "If it sits, it either clots or cultures". There is no indication to administer albuterol and instruction is not priority over the priority nursing interventions reviewed in rationale. This test-item format requests you to prioritize the top 4 interventions. Note, the next question does NOT limit answers, so the answers will be more inclusive of the nursing interventions (actions). Pay attention to details when reading!

5B. Which of the following actions would the nurse implement for this client with pneumonia who is experiencing respiratory compromise? Select all that apply.

- ☐ 1. Elevate the head of the bed 30-45 degrees.
- ☐ 2. Monitor pulse oximetry every shift.
- ☐ 3. Encourage oral fluids of at least 8 glasses of water per day.
- ☐ 4. Place client in an airborne infection isolation room (negative pressure).
- ☐ 5. Promote turning side to side, coughing, and deep breathing every two hours while awake.
- ☐ 6. Request an order for computer tomography (CT) scan of the chest.
- ☐ 7. Increase oxygen to 50% per venti mask.
- ☐ 8. Instruct client on importance of effective use of incentive spirometer every two hours while awake.

5B. Options #1, #3, #5, #7, and #8 are correct. Note this is another approach to an NGN question. Does this look similar to the "Select all that apply" you currently are evaluated on your nursing exams? Throughout the NGN book,, in-depth rationales will be provided as part of the steps to learning how to become proficient clinical decision makers; however, the rationales for this question have been reviewed in 5A., so these will not be repeated in this rationale. The purpose was to share with you another test format that could be tested on the NGN. Option #8 was not discussed with the previous question, so let's do this now. Incentive spirometry is an important plan of care, since it encourages deep breathing and coughing resulting in increased lung expansion facilitating oxygen exchange. Option #2 is incorrect; the pulse oximetry should be monitored more frequently than once a shift for this client with respiratory compromise. Option #4 is incorrect. There is no current indication the client has an infection that mandates an airborne infection isolation room. Option #6 is not part of the protocol for this client.

> ## I CAN Thinking TIP!
>
> A strategy for answering this fifth cognitive skill, **Take-action**, is to determine the priority order of actions that need to be implemented in a list of possible solutions. Priorities are determined by factors such as urgency, difficulty, or complexity of the client's situation. Ask the question, "What will I do?" "**FIRST**" will assist you in organizing this tip! Ask yourself the following questions:
>
> 1. What are my **first** (priority) nursing actions and medications for this client? (Our current case is a client who is experiencing symptoms of respiratory distress.)
> 2. What nursing actions are priority for an **identified urgency** of the situation?
> 3. What nursing actions are priority for the **complexity** of the situation?
> 4. What nursing actions are priority for the **standards** of care for this case?
> 5. What nursing actions are priority for providing **safe** care?
> 6. What is priority to **teach** client? What **trends** require immediate nursing action?
>
> **F** First (priority)
> **I** Identify urgency
> **R** Review complexity
> **S** Standards of care, Safety
> **T** Teaching, Trends

Question: Will the mnemonic "**BREATHE**" that we referred to with the previous cognitive skill, Generate Solutions, work for this cognitive skill as well?
Answer: Absolutely. In fact, each of the concepts have been organized in the book, *Medical Surgical Nursing Concepts Made Insanely Easy: A New Approach to the Next Generation NCLEX®*, to simplify recall of evidence-based nursing care that can be applied to these NGN questions. The book is written within the framework of the "SAFETY" Model which reflects the NCSBN CJMM. The great news is that "BREATHE" applies to most medical conditions that result in altered oxygenation.

Question: What type of NGN test item format is this question (5A) that we just reviewed for the fifth cognitive skill, Take-action?
Answer: This is referred to as an **Extended Drag-and-Drop** test item. This item format allows you to place response items into spaces for answers. This item is like the current NCLEX® ordered response items but not all the response options may be required to answer the test item. This test item format instructs you on how many findings to include from the response items.

Question: How many response options can I expect with this Extended Drag-and-Drop test item?
Answer: The maximum will be up to nine response options. The format will provide instructions on how many findings to include from the response items.

Question: Question 5B. looks very familiar. This looks like our current "SATA". Have the total number of options been revised for the NGN?
Answer: Yes, the NGN can have a maximum of ten possible options.

Question: Is it safe to say that there will always be more than 1 correct answer?
Answer: That is a very good question! The National Council of State Boards of Nursing have indicated that there could only be one answer, all ten options could be correct, or there could be any number of options between one and ten. The great news is that NGN is all about making safe clinical decisions, and when you understand standards of care based on evidence-based-practice you will recognize the correct options based on the information presented in the case.

Summary for the fifth cognitive skill, Take-action

"**FIRST**" will guide you in organizing **Take-action**. The priority order of actions will be determined from a list of possible solutions.

- **F** First (priority)
- **I** Identify urgency
- **R** Review complexity
- **S** Standards of care, Safety
- **T** Teaching, Trends

There are questions you will consistently ask as you learn to master this fifth skill, **Take-action**. The bottom line for this skill is, "What is important for me to do?"

Question: I believe we are ready to review the last cognitive skill.
Answer: This sixth cognitive skill is **Evaluate Outcomes**. To assist in evaluating outcomes, we reassess the client following the implementation of the nursing actions. This cognitive skill is an essential component for clinical decision making and clinical judgment. Evaluation of Expected Outcomes is the cognitive skill where the nurse makes a judgment regarding the effectiveness of the care. If unmet expected outcomes occur or a decline in assessment findings occur, then the nurse will need to further analyze the findings and decide on a plan for other action revisions that need to be implemented.

6. Case Question for Student: EVALUATE OUTCOMES

For each assessment finding, click or fill in the circle to specify if the finding indicates that the client's condition has improved, not changed, or declined since admission to MICU at 0900.

Assessment Findings	Improved	No Change	Declined
SaO_2: 95% (venti-mask on 40% O_2)	●	○	○
$PaCO_2$: 40 mm Hg	●	○	○
HCO_3: 22 mEq/L (22 mmol/L)	●	○	○
Heart rate (HR): 130 bpm	○	○	●
Breath sounds with coarse rales bilaterally; diminished in bases and in right upper and middle lobe	○	●	○
WBC Count: 22,000 mm^3 (22×10^9/L)	○	●	○

Note: Each column must have at least 1 response option selected.

The desired outcomes in this case are that the client will:

Have adequate oxygenation and present with "No **DYSPNEA**":

D Dyspnea will not be present

Y Yes, vital signs will be within the reference range

S Secretions, sputum, color clear

P Precipitating factors NONE

N No cough

E Evaluation of SaO_2 > 95% on ABGs, O_2 saturation > 92%

A Adventitious breath sounds – NONE

Now remember, we are basing our evaluation on the clinical data from the case since admission to the MICU! In this case, the SaO₂ 95% is an improvement since admission. PaCO₂: 40 mm Hg indicates an improvement in the client's condition. HCO₃: 22 mEq/L (22 mmol/L) – improved. The heart rate (HR) has declined, breath sounds and WBC Count had no change.

> ### I CAN Thinking TIP!
>
> A strategy for answering this sixth cognitive skill, **Evaluate Outcomes**, is following the interventions, the nurse must evaluate effectiveness. The final question is to evaluate any actions implemented based on an updated status of the client. Ask the question, "Did the interventions help?" "**END**" will assist you in organizing this tip! Ask yourself the following questions:
>
> Were the expected outcomes met?
> - ☐ Is the problem likely to recur without nursing interventions?
> - ☐ Does the concept require the same level of intervention or vigilance? If so, continue plan of care.
>
> Were the expected outcomes partially met?
> - ☐ Is more time needed before evaluating?
> - ☐ Are changes needed in interventions to achieve the outcomes?
> - ☐ If no, continue plan of care and ongoing evaluation.
>
> Were the expected outcomes not met?
> - ☐ Did the client's situation change?
> - ☐ Were the interventions not effective?
> - ☐ Is more time needed before evaluating?
>
> **E** Expected outcomes
>
> **N** Not related to care
>
> **D** Determine if ineffective

Question: I notice that the cognitive skill, **Evaluate Outcomes,** is also tested with the Matrix format. I did note that the radio buttons are circular in contrast to the other Matrix format where the radio buttons were square. Does this mean anything to me as a test taker?

Answer: Yes, that is a good observation! The circular radio buttons indicate that you can select one option per row. In contrast, the square radio buttons indicate multiple options can be selected per row.

Question: How can I remember this detail?

Answer: It will not be a challenge because the question will indicate "*each finding may support more than one medical condition or concept*", so there will be more than one response per row. Another hint is the 0=one response! When **Evaluating Outcomes**, the assessment findings per row will only have one response, since the question evaluates "if findings indicate improvement, no change, or a decline in the client's condition".

> ### Summary for the sixth cognitive skill, Evaluate Outcomes
>
> "**END**" will guide you in organizing **Evaluate Outcomes**. Following the interventions, the nurse must evaluate effectiveness. The final questions are to evaluate any actions implemented based on an updated status of the client. It is with this question that you will connect new findings with positive improvement, no change, or decline in clinical presentation. Evaluation of outcomes requires clinical judgment and is crucial in making clinical decisions about the plan of care. This is an ongoing process when caring for your client.
>
> **E** Expected outcomes
>
> **N** Not related to care
>
> **D** Determine if ineffective
>
> There are questions you will consistently ask yourself as you learn to master this sixth skill, **Evaluate Outcomes**. The bottom line for this skill is "Did it help?"

Question: Did you finish the story to help us remember how to organize and recall the details in the questions for strategies including "*Generate Solutions, Take-action, and Evaluate Outcomes*"?

Answer: In review the first mnemonics for the first 3 cognitive skills, "Recognize Cues, Analysis of Cues, Prioritize Hypotheses are (TRIP, CAFE, and RISK). *Before we take a "TRIP", we need to know what matters most in how to get to our destination (Recognize Cues). We are not interested in irrelevant facts! During our "TRIP", we must take a break at the "CAFÉ" to analyze what could this mean (Analysis of Cues).*

Then we need to determine what will present the highest "RISK" (Prioritize Hypotheses) to us on our "TRIP". This "**RISK**" must be "**SOLVED**" by generating solutions and decide to take-action on what to do "**FIRST**". At the "**END**" of our "TRIP" we will evaluate outcomes to determine if the trip was successful! This is a fun and easy way to jog your memory with questions/strategies to assist you in mastering the knowledge for each of the cognitive skills.

Summary Questions

1. What are the six cognitive skills in the Clinical Judgment Measurement Model?
2. What is an example of a question to ask yourself from each of the cognitive skills to assist in becoming a self-directed thinker?
3. Which cognitive skill is used when starting a case to determine what "matters most"?
4. Which cognitive skill is used when determining "what could it mean"?
5. Which cognitive skill is used to decide on "where to start"?

An example of an unfolding case will follow on the next page. For an extensive reference with Next Generation NCLEX® cases, we recommend the book, *A Step-by-Step Approach to Developing Clinical Judgment for the Next Generation NCLEX® and Clinical Success* by Manning, Akins, Brocato.

This can be ordered directly from icanpublishing.com or call 770.495.2488.

Oxygenation: Clotting: Deep Vein Thrombosis (DVT)

1A Clinical Judgment Application

Nurses' Notes: 1200: A 36-year-old female client was admitted to the Medical Unit 2 days ago presenting with severe pain in the right lower abdominal quadrant, nausea, vomiting, and a fever. Diagnosed with appendicitis and was taken to surgery for an appendectomy. The client has a history of smoking cigarettes with an average of a pack every 3-4 days. Client is currently taking oral contraceptives and has not been active since surgery. Most of the past few days have been spent recovering in bed. The initial assessment findings are documented below.

Vital Signs (Admission)	
Temperature	99.9° F (37.7° C)
Heart rate (HR)	88 bpm
Respiratory rate (RR)	24 breaths/min
Blood pressure (BP)	128/88 mm Hg

Clinical Assessment Findings	
Pulmonary	Occasional dry non-productive cough.
Gastrointestinal	Abdominal incision approximated and healing. Hypoactive bowel sounds x 4. Complains of tenderness to incision.
Left calf of leg	Reports pain 5/10. Edema in the left lower extremity. Left lower extremity red and warm to touch.

Laboratory Test Results	
SaO_2	97% on room air
Labs	Pending

1A. 1 Highlight or use an x next to the assessment findings that will require follow up by the nurse.

1200: Vital Signs	
Temperature	99.9° F (37.7° C)
Heart rate (HR)	88 bpm
Respiratory rate (RR)	24 breaths/min

1200: Clinical Assessment Findings	
Pulmonary	Occasional dry non-productive cough.
Gastrointestinal	Abdominal incision approximated and healing. Hypoactive bowel sounds x 4. Complains of tenderness to incision.
Left leg calf	Reports pain 5/10. Edema in the left lower extremity. Left lower extremity red and warm to touch.

1200: Laboratory Test Results	
SaO_2	97% on room air

1A. 2 For each client finding below, click or use an x to specify if the finding is consistent with a DVT, peripheral artery disease, and/or post-op infection. Each finding may support more than 1 disease process.

Client Finding	Deep Vein Thrombosis (DVT)	Peripheral Artery Disease	Post-op Infection
Pain in left calf	☐	☐	☐
Occasional nonproductive cough	☐	☐	☐
Edema in left lower extremity	☐	☐	☐
Left lower extremity red and warm to touch	☐	☐	☐
Tenderness to abdominal incision	☐	☐	☐
Pallor and coolness of lower extremities	☐	☐	☐

Note: Each column must have at least 1 response option selected.

Oxygenation: Clotting: Deep Vein Thrombosis (DVT)

1A   Clinical Judgment Application

Nurses' Notes: 1200: A 36-year-old female client was admitted to the Medical Unit 2 days ago presenting with severe pain in the right lower abdominal quadrant, nausea, vomiting, and a fever. Diagnosed with appendicitis and was taken to surgery for an appendectomy. The client has a history of smoking cigarettes with an average of a pack every 3-4 days. Client is currently taking oral contraceptives and has not been active since surgery. Most of the past few days have been spent recovering in bed. The initial assessment findings are documented below.

Nurses' Notes: 1700: Client had an order for a venous duplex ultrasonography of lower extremities and laboratory studies.

Nurses' Notes: 1900: Heparin sodium bolus ordered 6000 Units IVP followed by continuous infusion at 1350 Units/hour. PTT every 6 hours. Follow up per heparin protocol.

Vital Signs (Admission)	
Temperature	99.9° F (37.7° C)
Heart rate (HR)	88 bpm
Respiratory rate (RR)	24 breaths/min
Blood pressure (BP)	128/88 mm Hg

Clinical Assessment Findings	
Pulmonary	Occasional dry non-productive cough.
Gastrointestinal	Abdominal incision approximated and healing. Hypoactive bowel sounds x 4. Complains of tenderness to incision.
Left calf of leg	Reports pain 5/10. Edema in the left lower extremity. Left lower extremity red and warm to touch.

Laboratory Test Results	1200	1700
SaO$_2$	97% on room air	97% on room air
Hemoglobin	Pending	16 g/dL (9.93 mmol/L)
Hematocrit	Pending	42%
INR	Pending	1.0
aPTT	Pending	28 seconds
PT	Pending	10 seconds
Platelets	Pending	162,000 mm^3 (162 x 10^9/L)
Creatinine	Pending	0.7 mg/dL (61.89 umol/L)
Venous duplex ultrasonography	Pending	Deep vein thrombosis in the left leg calf

1A. 3 Complete the following sentences by choosing from the list of options.

The client is at risk for developing _____

Select (Options 1) ▼
Select...
clotting
hypoxia
infection
gastrointestinal (GI) obstruction

as evidenced by the client's _____ .

Select (Options 2) ▼
Select...
gastrointestinal (GI) assessment
respiratory assessment
neurovascular assessments
vital signs

1A. 4 For each potential nursing intervention, click or fill in the circle to specify whether the intervention is indicted or contraindicated for the client.

Potential Intervention	Indicated	Contraindicated
Monitor and trend heart rate, BP, and for petechiae per protocol.	○	○
Apply sequential compression devices to both legs.	○	○
Apply lotion and massage left lower extremity to decrease pain and edema.	○	○
When sitting in the chair, encourage client to dangle legs.	○	○
Assess for nose bleeds and/or abdominal distention.	○	○
Review the importance of avoiding salicylates.	○	○

Note: Each column must have at least 1 response option selected.

Oxygenation: Clotting: Deep Vein Thrombosis (DVT)

1A   Clinical Judgment Application

Nurses' Notes: 1200: A 36-year-old female client was admitted to the Medical Unit 2 days ago presenting with severe pain in the right lower abdominal quadrant, nausea, vomiting, and a fever. Diagnosed with appendicitis and was taken to surgery for an appendectomy. The client has a history of smoking cigarettes with an average of a pack every 3-4 days. Client is currently taking oral contraceptives and has not been active since surgery. Most of the past few days have been spent recovering in bed. The initial assessment findings are documented below.

Nurses' Notes: 1700: Client had an order for a venous duplex ultrasonography of lower extremities and laboratory studies.

Nurses' Notes: 1900: Heparin sodium bolus ordered 6000 Units IVP followed by continuous infusion at 1350 Units/hour. PTT every 6 hours. Follow up per heparin protocol.

Vital Signs (Admission)	
Temperature	99.9° F (37.7° C)
Heart rate (HR)	88 bpm
Respiratory rate (RR)	24 breaths/min
Blood pressure (BP)	128/88 mm Hg

Clinical Assessment Findings	
Pulmonary	Occasional dry non-productive cough.
Gastrointestinal	Abdominal incision approximated and healing. Hypoactive bowel sounds x 4. Complains of tenderness to incision.
Left calf of leg	Reports pain 5/10. Edema in the left lower extremity. Left lower extremity red and warm to touch.

Laboratory Test Results	1200	1700
SaO$_2$	97% on room air	97% on room air
Hemoglobin	Pending	16 g/dL (9.93 mmol/L)
Hematocrit	Pending	42%
INR	Pending	1.0
aPTT	Pending	28 seconds
PT	Pending	10 seconds
Platelets	Pending	162,000 mm^3 (162 x 10^9/L)
Creatinine	Pending	0.7 mg/dL (61.89 umol/L)
Venous duplex ultrasonography	Pending	Deep vein thrombosis in the left leg calf

1A. 5 Which nursing actions and teaching will the nurse include in the care for this client regarding DVT management and the prevention of a new DVT? Select all that apply.

- ☐ 1. Monitor blood pressure and heart rate per protocol.
- ☐ 2. Begin client education regarding safety concerns with oral anticoagulant therapy.
- ☐ 3. Encourage taking an aspirin daily to prevent further clotting issues.
- ☐ 4. Notify the health care provider for any bruising and/or tarry stools.
- ☐ 5. Discuss importance of keeping legs elevated when up in chair.
- ☐ 6. Explain the importance of wearing sequential compression device while in bed on unaffected leg.
- ☐ 7. Report a sudden onset of chest pain, tachycardia, and tachypnea.
- ☐ 8. Recommend using a soft toothbrush and electric razor.

1A. 6 For each assessment finding, click or fill in the circle to specify if the finding indicates that the client's condition has improved, not changed, or declined.

Assessment Finding	Improved	No Change	Declined
No pain in the left leg calf.	○	○	○
Temperature is the same in bilateral lower extremities.	○	○	○
SaO$_2$: 90%.	○	○	○
Left leg calf is larger in diameter than right calf.	○	○	○
Respiratory rate (RR): 32 breaths/min, Heart rate (HR): 126 bpm.	○	○	○
Edema in left lower extremity.	○	○	○

Note: Each column must have at least 1 response option selected.

Answers and Rationales
Oxygenation: Clotting: Deep Vein Thrombosis (DVT)

1200: Vital Signs	
Temperature	99.9° F (37.7° C)
Heart rate (HR)	88 bpm
Respiratory rate (RR)	24 breaths/min
Blood pressure (BP)	128/88 mm Hg

1200: Clinical Assessment Findings	
Pulmonary	Occasional dry non-productive cough.
Gastrointestinal	Abdominal incision approximated and healing. Hypoactive bowel sounds x 4. Complains of tenderness to incision.
Left leg calf	Reports pain 5/10. Edema in the left lower extremity. Left lower extremity red and warm to touch.

1200: Laboratory Test Results	
SaO_2	97% on room air

1A. 1   Answers

Rationales:

What clinical data presents an immediate concern for the client?

The **temperature** needs to be followed up requiring additional assessments such as breath sounds and abdominal incision to determine if this temperature elevation is becoming a trend, since client has been immobile for several days. **The left leg calf** is a concern for this client with **pain, edema,** and **red/warmth to touch**. As we progress to the next step in clinical decision making and judgment, then we will analyze the potential complication that these system-specific assessments (cues) may indicate. The other assessment findings do not require follow up by the nurse.

Judgment Cognitive Skill
Recognize Cues (System-Specific Assessments)

NGN® Test Item Type
Enhanced Hot Spot (Highlighting)

References
Manning & Zager, 2019, p. 172

1A.2 Answers

Client Finding	Deep Vein Thrombosis (DVT)	Peripheral Artery Disease	Post-op Infection
Pain in left calf	X	X	☐
Occasional nonproductive cough	☐	☐	X
Edema in left lower extremity	X	☐	☐
Left lower extremity red and warm to touch	X	☐	☐
Tenderness to abdominal incision	☐	☐	X
Pallor and coolness of lower extremities	☐	X	☐

Rationales:

What medical conditions are consistent with the clinical data (cues)?

Prior to reviewing the client findings, there is powerful information in the Nurses' Notes indicating the client is currently taking oral contraceptives and has not been active since surgery. The client also has a history of smoking cigarettes with an average of a pack every 3–4 days. This clinical data and client findings of **pain (tenderness), redness, edema, and warmth** to touch in the left lower extremity indicate a potential complication of a deep vein thrombosis (DVT). A deep vein thrombosis (DVT) is an inflammation of the vein where a clot can form. When a clot forms, it can break away as an emboli and travel to different parts of the body, most commonly the lungs. DVTs are common, but they are preventable. Prevention is the key, particularly with clients who have circulatory problems and those who are immobile. An EASY way to remember assessment findings for a DVT is to remember "**DVT**".

Diameter of calf and thighs: compare bilaterally for swelling.

Vein tenderness and redness, note.

Temperature ↑ (also at site of clot, warm to touch).

Peripheral arterial disease (PAD) can also result in pain with activity (i.e., intermittent claudication), but may subside if the activity stops, allowing for an increase in circulation to the lower extremity. The clinical findings did not clarify if this discomfort was secondary to activity. PAD can also result **in skin color changes with pallor and coolness of lower extremities** in contrast to the DVT which presents with rubra and warmth. **Pallor and coolness of lower extremities** are consistent with the diagnosis of peripheral artery disease (PAD) due to a decrease in the arterial circulation to the lower extremities.

The **occasional nonproductive cough** needs further evaluation to determine if there is an alteration in the oxygenation. Assessments such as breath sounds, oxygen saturation, and trending of temperature, etc. need to be further evaluated. The current oxygen saturation is 97% on room air which indicates no current alteration in oxygenation. **Abdominal incision tenderness** is not unusual for the postop client; however, an increase in the tenderness could indicate a post-op infection. It is unlikely though because the incision is approximated and healing, but the temperature is 99.9° F (37.7° C), so this clinical finding will require on-going assessment.

Judgment Cognitive Skill
Analysis of Cues (Analysis)

NGN® Test Item Type
Matrix Multiple Response

References
Manning & Zager, 2019, pp. 170, 172

Chapter 1: ANSWERS & RATIONALES

I CAN Thinking TIP!

REMEMBER the Clinical Judgment Skill: Analyze of Cues (Analysis) for a Deep Vein Thrombosis is to organize these findings within the mnemonic, "DVT"!

D Diameter of calf and thighs; compare bilaterally for swelling

V Vein tenderness and redness, note

T Temperature ↑ (also at site of clot, warm to touch)

© Manning L. & Zager, L. (2019) *Medical Surgical Nursing Concepts Made Insanely Easy. (2nd ed.)* I CAN Publishing®, Inc. Duluth, GA Page 172.

1A.3 Answers

The client is at risk for developing <u>clotting</u> as evidenced by the client's <u>neurovascular assessments</u>.

Rationales:

What is the possible risk that may be occurring with the client and what are the most likely explanations?

The pain in the left calf of the leg, redness, and warmth to touch, and presenting with edema all indicate a complication with a DVT. An occasional nonproductive cough is not enough clinical evidence to indicate hypoxia with the heart rate (HR) and respiratory rate (RR) being in the desired range. The gastrointestinal (GI) assessment does not indicate any complication. Although the abdominal incision is tender, the incision is approximated and healing. If the client had an infection, the temperature would be elevated more with additional clinical findings indicating infection and pain would be more severe and constant. The client is at risk for developing complications with **clotting** (i.e., a deep vein thrombosis) as evidence with the **neurovascular assessment** findings and confirmed with the ultrasound results.

Judgment Cognitive Skill
Prioritize Hypotheses (Analysis)

NGN® Test Item Type
Cloze (Drop-Down)

References
Manning & Zager, 2019, p. 172

1A.4 Answers

Potential Intervention	Indicated	Contraindicated
Monitor and trend heart rate, BP, and for petechiae per protocol.	●	○
Apply sequential compression devices to both legs.	○	●
Apply lotion and massage left lower extremity to decrease pain and edema.	○	●
When sitting in the chair, encourage client to dangle legs.	○	●
Assess for nose bleeds and/or abdominal distention.	●	○
Review the importance of avoiding salicylates.	●	○

Rationales:

What plans based on the hypotheses should be included or contraindicated?

Monitor and trend heart rate, BP, and for petechiae per protocol. The client is at risk for bleeding due to the heparin, so assessments such as a trend with the HR increasing, BP decreasing, and/or symptoms of bleeding such as petechiae need to be monitored ongoing per protocol. Due to the risk of dislodging the thrombus, a client with a DVT should never have sequential compression device (SCD) on the affected extremity nor should massaging ever be done such as applying lotion. It is an important standard of practice to apply the sequential compression device (SCD) to the unaffected leg to prevent a DVT. *An ounce of prevention is worth a pound of cure!* When sitting in the bed or chair, legs should be elevated to improve venous return. If the client had arterial insufficiency, the legs should dangle to assist with increasing arterial blood flow to the extremity. A major complication of heparin is abnormal bleeding which could be indicated by **nose bleeds**, blood in urine and/or stool, and/or **abdominal distention**. Abdominal distention and/or epigastric pain may indicate a complication with gastrointestinal bleeding. The stools should be assessed for bleeding such as tarry and dark stools. Other clinical findings the client may present with indicating bleeding include bleeding gums, ecchymosis, bruising, etc. The nurse should include in the plan of care the importance of avoiding **salicylates** due to the increased risk of bleeding when taking with Heparin.

Judgment Cognitive Skill
Generate Solutions (First-do Plans)

NGN® Test Item Type
Matrix Multiple Choice

References
Manning & Zager, 2019, pp. 170, 172; Manning & Rayfield, 2017, p. 100–101

1A.5 Answers

Options #1, #2, #4, #5, #6, #7, #8, are correct.

Rationales:

What nursing actions are priority for providing safe care?

Options #1 and #4: The client should be monitored per protocol for an **increase in heart rate, decrease in blood pressure,** and evidence of **bruising, and/or tarry stools**. These clinical findings indicate complications of bleeding and the health care provider should be notified.

Option #2: The usual medical treatment for DVT includes follow-up oral anticoagulant therapy. The numerous undesirable effects regarding **anticoagulant therapy** mandate **early education to optimize compliance and safe home medication administration**.

Option #3: Encouraging client to take an aspirin daily is incorrect. Aspirin can contribute to bleeding.

Options #5 and #6: DVT management should include teaching the client to **keep legs elevated** when **in bed and up in the chair**, and the importance of wearing **sequential compression devices on unaffected leg** while in bed for the purpose of preventing additional DVTs.

Option #7: A sudden onset of **chest pain, tachycardia, and tachypnea** may indicate the development of a pulmonary embolism, a potential complication. This must be **reported**.

Option #8: Since anticoagulation therapy has been started, bleeding precautions should be included in the plan of care such as the use of an **electric razor** and **soft toothbrush**. The nurse should also apply prolonged pressure over IV sites, cuts, or scratches to minimize risk of bleeding.

Judgment Cognitive Skill

Take-action (First-Do Interventions)

NGN® Test Item Type

Extended Multiple Response

References

Manning & Zager, 2019, pp.172–173; Manning & Rayfield, 2017, pp. 98–99

1A. 6 Answers

Assessment Finding	Improved	No Change	Declined
No pain in the left leg calf.	●	○	○
Temperature is the same in bilateral lower extremities.	●	○	○
SaO$_2$: 90%	○	○	●
Left leg calf is larger in diameter than right calf.	○	●	○
Respiratory rate (RR): 32 breaths/min, Heart rate (HR): 126 bpm.	○	○	●
Edema in left lower extremity.	○	●	○

Rationales:

Were the expected outcomes met?

Clients with a DVT experience pain in the calf of the leg. This change with no pain indicates an improvement in the condition. Redness and warmth and induration along blood vessels on the affected leg are clinical findings of a DVT. This change in temperature being the same in bilateral extremities indicates an improvement in the condition. This decline in the SaO$_2$ may indicate a complication with a pulmonary embolism. This may result from the DVT dislodging and entering the venous circulation forming a blockage in the pulmonary vasculature. The size of the embolus will have an impact on the severity of this complication. Due to the hypoxia that may occur, the respiratory rate (RR): 32 breaths/min, heart rate (HR): 126 bpm may also be the result of the pulmonary embolism. The nurse must assess further to analyze if client is experiencing chest pain, blood pressure (BP) decrease, changes in the breath sounds, and/or petechiae which support the diagnosis of a pulmonary emboli. Left leg calf is larger in diameter than right calf and edema in the left lower extremity indicate no change in the client's condition. The client is still in need of nursing care with ongoing clinical decision making for safe and effective care. This evaluation requires immediate follow up and communication with the health care provider! A potential blockage in the pulmonary vasculature from a pulmonary embolus can be life threatening.

Judgment Cognitive Skill
Evaluate Outcomes (Evaluation of Expected Outcomes)

NGN® Test Item Type
Matrix Multiple Choice

References
Manning & Zager, 2019, pp. 141, 170, 172

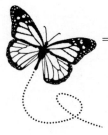

Notes

Section 2

Linking Clinical Judgment to Stand-Alone Cases

Stand-Alone Items

Two types of stand-alone items are included in the NGN-RN and NGN-PN Special Research Sections (SRSs):
- ☐ Bow-tie items
- ☐ Trend items

These items may contain multiple steps from Layer 3 and aspects of Layer 4 of the NCSBN Clinical Judgment Measurement Model (NCJMM) (Spring 2020, Summer 2020). The chart below describes the differences between the stand-alone item and the case study.

Stand-alone	Case Study
Diagnosis: implied or stated	Clinical data
Clinical information for client	Group of six items represents NCJMM
Requires one or more clinical decisions	Requires multiple decisions throughout the NCJMM

All six steps of the NCJMM are addressed in the bow-tie in one item.

The scenario will be on the left for you to review. You will need to:
- ☐ Determine if findings are normal or abnormal (Recognize Cues).
- ☐ Know the possible complications or medical conditions the client may be experiencing (Analyze Cues).
- ☐ Identify possible solutions to address the issues and needs of the client (Generate Solutions).

On the right will be the bow-tie item for you to answer. The item will evaluate your competence with:
- ☐ Determining the most likely cause of the client's clinical presentation (Prioritize Hypotheses).
- ☐ Know the appropriate actions to take (Take-action).
- ☐ Know the parameters to monitor after interventions have been implemented (Evaluate Outcomes).

This is how the item got the name "bow-tie" because the answer area is shaped like a bow-tie. As you can see in the example in this chapter, there are two "Actions to Take" on the left, two "Parameters to Monitor" on the right with a single "Potential Condition" response in the middle.

All targets (placeholders for option responses) must be completed with a token (the option response), that is located below the bow-tie in the labeled columns. Only tokens from the same column are interchangeable. A token from "Actions to Take" cannot fill in a "Parameter to Monitor" target and vice versa. The target boxes and options tokens have similar wording and similar shading of the boxes to facilitate appropriate responses. A token can be removed from the target space by moving it from the target back to the designated token column once the token has been placed on a target. The original token will return to the appropriate column. The following is an examples of the bow-tie item. For the purpose of this book, you can write in the tokens (options) in the designated boxes for the target (answers) in the bow-tie format.

2A Sample NGN Bow-Tie: Post-Op Thyroidectomy

The nurse in the Recovery Room is admitting a 50-year-old female client with a laboratory confirmed hyperthyroidism not responding to medication therapy.

Nurses' Notes	History and Physical
1500	A total thyroidectomy was performed at 1200 yesterday. Peripheral pulses palpable, 1+. **Vital Signs:** Temperature: 98.0°F (36.7° C) Heart rate (HR): 48 bpm with a prolonged QT interval on ECG Respiratory rate (RR): 20 breaths/min Blood pressure (BP): 98/60 mm Hg Pulse oximetry reading 97% on room air Client presenting with Chvostek's sign

> The nurse is reviewing the client's assessment data to prepare the client's plan of care. Complete the diagram by dragging from the choices below to specify what condition the client is most likely experiencing, 2 actions the nurse should take to address that condition, and 2 parameters the nurse should monitor to assess the client's progress.

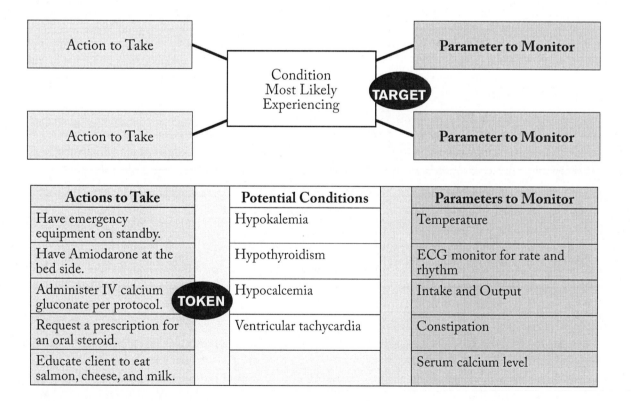

Actions to Take	Potential Conditions	Parameters to Monitor
Have emergency equipment on standby.	Hypokalemia	Temperature
Have Amiodarone at the bed side.	Hypothyroidism	ECG monitor for rate and rhythm
Administer IV calcium gluconate per protocol.	Hypocalcemia	Intake and Output
Request a prescription for an oral steroid.	Ventricular tachycardia	Constipation
Educate client to eat salmon, cheese, and milk.		Serum calcium level

This introduction for the stand-alone test item is to assist you in becoming familiar with the format. The tokens in the left column, "actions to take", will only be used as targets in the answer section in the bow-tie above the row. The token for "potential conditions" will only be used in the middle of the bow-tie for "condition most likely experiencing", and the tokens under "parameters to monitor" can only be used as the targets for the two boxes above the column in the bow-tie section. It may be helpful to remember that tokens are equivalent to options and distractors in traditional questions and target is equivalent to the answer. The answers and rationales can be found below.

2A Hypocalcemia: Post-Op Thyroidectomy

2A   Answers

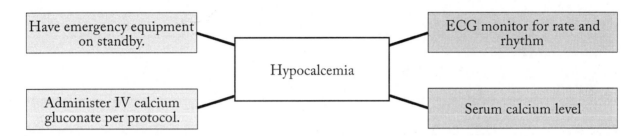

Rationales:

Based on the heart rate (HR)—48 bpm with a prolonged QT interval on ECG, blood pressure (BP)—98/60 mm Hg, presence of the Chvostek's sign, and client had a thyroidectomy, the system-specific assessments (cues) support the complication with the parathyroid gland being injured or accidentally removed during the thyroidectomy. The purpose of the parathyroid gland is to secrete parathyroid hormone (PTH). The PTH increases calcium absorption by the kidneys and therefore increases calcium levels and decreases phosphorus (phosphate) levels through excretion. If the parathyroid gland is removed or injured, the client may develop hypocalcemia. Assessing for decreased calcium (hypocalcemia) is one of the priority assessments following a thyroidectomy. The potential condition is **hypocalcemia**. Due to the risk for a seizure or cardiac complications, it is priority to have **emergency equipment on standby. Administer IV calcium gluconate per protocol** is another priority due to the risk of the parathyroid gland being injured. Amiodarone would be inappropriate for this client due to the risk for a further decline in the heart rate (HR). There is no ventricular or atrial dysrhythmia that would require administering this medication. There is no rationale for this client to receive an oral steroid. Salmon, cheese, and milk are high in iodine and should be avoided, since they can cause a decrease in the stimulation of the thyroid hormones. Priority parameters to monitor include the **electrocardiogram (ECG) for the rate and rhythm** of the heart and the **calcium level**. The low calcium level should not affect the client's temperature. The I & O are not priority to the cardiac assessment and the calcium level. Constipation does not occur from hypocalcemia. Diarrhea may occur from a low calcium level.

Judgment Cognitive Skill

Take-action (First-Do Interventions); Prioritize Hypotheses (Analysis); Evaluate Outcomes (Evaluation of Expected Outcomes)

NGN® Test Item Type

Stand-Alone Item; Extended Drag and Drop (Bow-tie)

References

Manning & Zager, 2019, pp. 381–382

A second type of stand-alone items is the trend items. Trend Items are individual items that will have you review information over a period of time. Trend items can address any item response (Fall 2019). Information may include Nurses' Notes, Admission Notes, Laboratory Values, History and Physical, Vital Signs, Intake and Output, Medications, Diagnostic Results, and Flow Sheet.

2B Sample Trend Item: Intracranial Regulation (Spinal Cord Injury)

The nurse on the spinal cord unit is caring for a 32-year-old male who is post-2 weeks C6 spinal cord injury.

Flow Sheet			
Vital Signs (5/22/21)	**0800**	**0900**	**1000 (current)**
Temperature	98.7° F (37.1°C)	99.0° F (37.2 °C)	99.0° F (37.2 °C)
Heart rate (HR)	78 bpm	68 bpm	48 bpm
Blood pressure (BP)	128/78 mm Hg	130/80 mm Hg	190/100 mm Hg
Nurses' Notes 5/22/21			
0800	Intermittent sequential stockings on client.		
0900	AM care complete. No skin breakdown.		
1000 (current)	Client is experiencing a severe headache, flushed face and neck, diaphoresis, and nasal stuffiness. Intermittent sequential stockings remain on client.		
Intake and Output	**5/20/21**	**5/21/21**	**5/22/21**
Intake Output Bowel movements (BM)	1680 mL 1200 mL 1 firm brown BM	960 mL 1100 mL No BMs	960 mL 1050 mL No BMs

> **Which of the following nursing actions should the nurse implement immediately? Select all that apply.**

☐ 1. Place client in reverse Trendelenburg position.

☐ 2. Administer dopamine as prescribed.

☐ 3. Remove sequential compression device.

☐ 4. Administer sublingual nitroglycerine as prescribed.

☐ 5. Evaluate for impaction and remove.

☐ 6. Teach client about importance of regular fluid intake.

☐ 7. Review with staff importance of not fluctuating room temperature.

2B Perfusion: Autonomic Dysreflexia (Spinal Cord Injury)

2B Answers
Options #1, #3, #4, and #5 are correct.

Rationales:
Options #1, #3, #4, #5 are correct. Based on the trends with the vital signs and bowel movements, the client's potential condition is autonomic dysreflexia. Autonomic dysreflexia can be life-threatening and requires immediate intervention. Clients who have lesions below T6 do not experience dysreflexia since the parasympathetic nervous system is able to neutralize the sympathetic response. This condition only occurs with clients who have a T6 or higher spinal cord injury resulting in an inadequate compensatory response by parasympathetic nervous system. The sympathetic stimulation of the nervous system can result in a sudden severe headache, extreme hypertension, pallor below the level of the spinal lesion, blurred vision, nausea, and diaphoresis. Stimulation of the parasympathetic nervous system can cause bradycardia, flushing above the lesion (flushed face and neck), along with nasal stuffiness. The cause needs to be recognized and treated.

Option #5: Based on the system-specific assessments (cues), the client had limited fluid intake and has not had a **bowel movement** for 48 hours. Stimuli that can result in autonomic dysreflexia may include fecal impaction; a full (distended) bladder from a kinked or blocked urinary catheter, urinary calculi, retention; funny feeling with the skin (i.e., tight clothing or cold draft on lower part of the body). **Option #1:** If autonomic dysreflexia does occur, **elevate the head of the bed without manipulating the neck (reverse Trendelenburg)** to assist with decreasing BP.

Option #3: Any tight clothing such as **sequential compression device** can stimulate this response and should be removed.

Option #4: The current BP is 190/100 mm Hg. **Nitrates** are one classification of medications that are standard practice in decreasing the hypertension. They will relax the vascular smooth system and decrease the left ventricular preload by dilating veins, thus indirectly decreasing afterload.

Option #2 is incorrect; dopamine is prescribed to increase cardiac output. As a result of the vasoconstriction in blood vessels and stimulation of beta 1; the production of an inotropic effect will increase the cardiac output and BP. This is not our goal for this client. We need the BP to decrease!

Options #6 and #7 are incorrect since these do not need to be implemented immediately. They need to be included in the plan of care, but the question is asking for immediate interventions.

Judgment Cognitive Skill
Take-action (First-Do Interventions)

NGN® Test Item Type
Stand-Alone Item; Trend-Item

References
Manning & Zager, 2019, p. 270

Refer below to a comparison of the three different exam item formats for the Next Generation NCLEX®.

	Stand-Alone		Case Study
	Bow-tie	Trend	
Steps from NCJMM	Six steps	One or more of six steps	Six steps
Decisions	Multiple	One or more	Multiple
	One item	One item	Six items

Refer to the next page for an example of an NGN Bow-Tie with answers and rationales. We recommend the book, *A Step-by-Step Approach to Developing Clinical Judgment for the Next Generation NCLEX® and Clinical Success!* by Manning, Akins & Brocato. This book will provide you with a comprehensive review of NGN cases, test items, and excellent rationales with correct and incorrect answers.

2C Perfusion Renal: Chronic Kidney Disease (CKD)

The nurse in the emergency department (ED) is admitting a 48-year-old male client who has a diagnosis of chronic kidney disease (CKD). Client has been on hemodialysis three times a week and missed last dialysis appointment.

Nurses' Notes	History and Physical
0730	The client reports that he is struggling with doing any activity without getting fatigue and having shortness of breath. Client is alert and answering questions. **Vital Signs:** Blood pressure (BP): 192/100 mm Hg Heart rate (HR): 110 bpm Respiratory rate (RR): 30 breaths/min Temperature: 97.6° F (36.4° C) O₂ saturation: 91% on room air **Laboratory Results:** Serum Potassium: 5.4 mEq/L (5.4 mmol/L) Serum Sodium: 144 mEq/L (144 mmol/L) Blood Urea Nitrogen: 51 mg/dL (18.2 mmol/L) Creatinine: 8.2 mg/dL (725.04 umol/L) Hemoglobin: 7.8 g/dL (4.84 mmol/L) Hematocrit: 23.4% Phosphorus: 6 mg/dL (1.94 mmol/L) Calcium: 5 mg/dL (1.25 mmol/L)

> The nurse is reviewing the client's assessment data to prepare the client's plan of care. Complete the diagram by dragging from the choices below to specify what condition the client is most likely experiencing, 2 actions the nurse should take to address that condition, and 2 parameters the nurse should monitor to assess the client's progress.

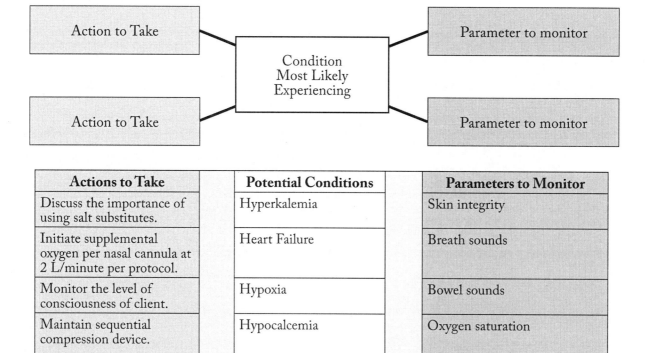

Actions to Take	Potential Conditions	Parameters to Monitor
Discuss the importance of using salt substitutes.	Hyperkalemia	Skin integrity
Initiate supplemental oxygen per nasal cannula at 2 L/minute per protocol.	Heart Failure	Breath sounds
Monitor the level of consciousness of client.	Hypoxia	Bowel sounds
Maintain sequential compression device.	Hypocalcemia	Oxygen saturation
Administer Epoetin alfa subcutaneous injection as prescribed.		Range of motion

2C Perfusion Renal: Chronic Kidney Disease (CKD)

2C Answers

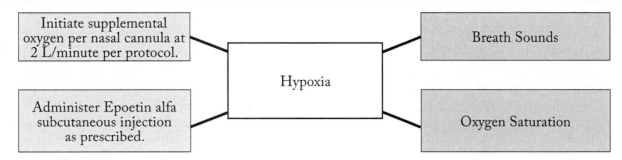

Rationales:

While the client is presenting with a high potassium and decreased calcium levels, the priority clinical assessments support **hypoxia** as being the current potential condition for this client. HR and RR are elevated with a decrease in the oxygen saturation, hemoglobin, and hematocrit. These are indicative of alteration in oxygenation and the need to provide **supplemental oxygen per nasal cannula at 2 L/minute per protocol**. This is based on the low hemoglobin and hematocrit levels, and the fact with chronic kidney disease (CKD), there is a decrease in the renal system's ability to secrete erythropoietin. **Epoetin alfa is DNA recombinant erythropoietin and subcutaneous injections with epoetin will stimulate RBC production and oxygen carrying capacity.** Epoetin alfa is an erythropoietic stimulating agent that stimulates the production of red blood cells. Salt substitutes are high in potassium and should not be administered to this client who is experiencing hyperkalemia from the chronic kidney disease (CKD). While monitoring the level of consciousness (LOC) is important for clients with chronic kidney disease (CKD), this client's priority concern is with oxygenation. Maintaining sequential compression device is an important part of the plan of care, but the immediate concern is the actions to take for supporting the need to optimize oxygenation. The case does not provide any assessment findings to support heart failure such as peripheral edema, ascites, jugular vein distention, adventitious breath sounds, and/or a change in the heart sounds (S3).

The priority parameters to monitor for this client are **breath sounds and oxygen saturation**. The heart rate (HR), respiratory rate (RR), and ability to ambulate or participate in activities of daily living (ADLs) without experiencing fatigue and shortness of breath also need ongoing monitoring to evaluate progress of the client. Skin integrity is important due to the risk of skin breakdown with these clients from fluid retention and from uremic frost, however, it is not priority over oxygenation. Bowel sounds and range of motion are not priorities to monitor for this client. They both should be included in the plan of care, but based on the client's assessment findings, oxygenation is priority. Due to the reduction of calcium from the increase phosphate in clients with chronic kidney disease (CKD), the bone demineralization results in a risk for bone injury. We always begin and end with our client! Safe clinical decision making will provide excellence in nursing care! Did you address the priority system-specific assessments (cues) the client was experiencing? Congratulations if you did! If you did not, did you learn the steps in making the correct clinical decision? Great! This is all about learning!

Judgment Cognitive Skill

Take-action (First-Do Interventions); Prioritize Hypotheses (Analysis); Evaluate Outcomes (Evaluation of Expected Outcomes)

NGN® Test Item Type

Stand-Alone Item; Extended Drag and Drop (Bow-tie)

References

Manning & Zager, 2019, pp. 476–477, 479; Manning & Rayfield, 2017, pp. 242–243

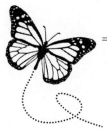

Notes

CHAPTER 2
Prioritization

The Principle of Priority states:
(a) you must know the difference between what is urgent and what is important, and
(b) you must do what's important first.
— STEVEN PRESSFIELD

✔ Clarification of this test ...

This second chapter has been developed to assist you in reviewing strategies on how to PRIORITIZE. The clinical decision-making strategies for this chapter have been adapted from the NCLEX® standards. The NCLEX® requires high-level clinical decision-making and clinical judgment as outlined below in the minimal standards. Prioritize delivery of care, organize time, assess and respond to clinical changes, and recognize complications are a few of these standards requiring the skill in prioritization. These standards will also be organized within each chapter representing the category for the client needs.

- Prioritize the delivery of client care on acuity.
- Organize workload to manage time effectively.
- Assess and respond to changes and/or trends in client vital signs.
- Recognize trends and changes in client condition and intervene as needed.
- Recognize signs and symptoms of client complications and intervene.
- Apply principles of infection prevention (e.g., hand hygiene, aseptic technique, isolation, sterile technique, universal/standard enhanced barrier precautions).
- Prepare and administer medications, using rights of medication administration.
- Provide care within the legal scope of practice.
- Recognize limitations of self and others and utilize resources.
- Delegate and supervise care of client provided by others (e.g., LPN/VN, assistive personnel, other RNs).
- Assess the need for referrals and obtain necessary orders.
- Collaborate with multi-disciplinary team members when providing client care (e.g., physical therapists, nutritionist, social worker).
- Properly identify client when providing care.
- Evaluate client response to medication (e.g., therapeutic effects, side effects, adverse reactions).
- Evaluate appropriateness and accuracy of medication order for client.

Continued ➡

- Educate client about medications.
- Review pertinent data prior to medication administration (e.g., contraindications, lab results, allergies, potential interactions).
- Manage the care of a client with impaired ventilation/oxygenation.
- Manage the care of a client with alteration in hemodynamics, tissue perfusion and hemostasis (e.g., cerebral, cardiac, peripheral).
- Assess client need for pain management.
- Protect client from injury (e.g., falls, electrical hazards).
- Verify appropriateness and/or accuracy of a treatment order.
- Evaluate responses to procedures and treatments.
- Assist with invasive procedures (e.g., central line, thoracentesis, bronchoscopy).
- Use precautions to prevent injury and/or complications associated with a procedure or diagnosis.
- Monitor the results of diagnostic testing and intervene as needed.
- Assess the potential for violence and use safety precautions (e.g., suicide, homicide, self-destructive behavior).
- Use therapeutic communication techniques to provide client support.
- Assess psychosocial, spiritual and occupational factors affecting care, and plan interventions.
- Provide care and education for the newborn, infant, and toddler client from birth through 2 years.
- Provide care and education for the adult client ages 65 and over.
- Provide care for a client experiencing visual, auditory or cognitive distortions.
- Provide post-operative care.

Adapted from: © National Council of State Boards of Nursing, Inc. (NCSBN). (2022). 2021 *RN Practice Analysis: Linking the NCLEX-RN® Examination to Practice*. Chicago: Author.

Adapted from: © National Council of State Boards of Nursing, Inc. (NCSBN). (2023) *Next Generation NCLEX® NCLEX-RN® Test Plan. Chicago*: Author.

2.1 The nurse receives laboratory results for a client and the platelet count is 13,000/mm³ (13 x 10⁹/L). Which action is the priority for the nurse to include in the plan of care?
① Place client on complete bed rest.
② Verify the appropriateness for a new thoracentesis order now.
③ Report to health care provider a HR – 88 bpm and BP - 138/88 mm Hg.
④ Delegate to the UAP to take and report electronic BP readings every 15 minutes for several hours.

2.2 After receiving shift report, which client should the nurse assess first?
① A client newly diagnosed with heart failure and presenting with a moist cough.
② A client who is vomiting and has diarrhea presenting with a heart rate - 88 bpm, BP - 134/80 mm Hg.
③ A client presenting with peripheral edema and a 1 lb. weight gain within 24 hours.
④ A client who has an order for digoxin with a heart rate – 66 bpm at rest that has decreased from 82 bpm in 24 hours.

2.3 Which client should the nurse assess first after receiving report?
① The client diagnosed with deep vein thrombosis (DVT) who is presenting with achy calf pain.
② The client with a T-100.4° F, HR – 90 bpm with a cough.
③ The client with peripheral artery disease refuses to elevate legs.
④ The client with a femoral-popliteal bypass who is presenting with tingling of the foot.

2.4 Which health care provider's orders should the nurse implement first for an elderly client who lives in an assistive living community with a diagnosis of a community-acquired pneumonia and is being admitted to the medical unit?
① Place client in contact precautions.
② Immediately start the new prescription for ceftriaxone 1000 mg IVPB every 12 hours.
③ Administer albuterol 2 puffs as an inhalation as prescribed.
④ Obtain sputum samples for culture and sensitivity.

2.5 What is the priority nursing intervention for a client with chronic lung disease who is presenting with dypspnea, HR – 140 bpm, and labored respirations?
① Administer oxygen at 40% heated mist.
② Assist client to cough and deep breathe.
③ Place client in the orthopneic position.
④ Assess breath sounds.

2.6 Which client is priority for the nurse to assess immediately following shift report?
① A middle-aged client diagnosed with diverticular disease presenting with left lower quadrant abdominal pain accompanied with nausea.
② A middle-aged client diagnosed with pancreatitis presenting with a serum glucose: 160 mg/dL and calcium level: 8 mg/dL (Normal ranges: serum glucose-70-110 mg/dL and calcium level-9-10.5 mg/dL).
③ An older adult client who is 1-day post-operative abdominal surgery presenting with trending in abdominal firmness, HR – 114 bpm, and color pale.
④ An older adult client who is 1-day post-operative for an appendectomy and is reporting abdominal pain of 7 on a pain scale of 1 to 10.

2.7 Which of these clients in the outpatient mental health unit require priority assessment by the nurse?
① An adolescent male client who is mad at his parents and is threatening to run away from home.
② A middle-aged female client diagnosed with schizophrenia who is hearing voices telling her to kill herself.
③ An older-adult male client who refuses to eat and is not sleeping since his wife was diagnosed with cancer.
④ An elderly female client who is depressed after the death of her husband.

2.8 The nurse is providing care for children on the pediatric unit. Which client will be priority for the nurse to assess following shift report?
① A 2-year-old with Kawasaki's disease and is presenting with a red rash on trunk and a strawberry red tongue.
② A 4-year-old with asthma who has expiratory wheezing and a pulse oximeter reading of 91%.
③ A 5-year-old with a T-100.8° F and diagnosed with otitis media.
④ A 7-year-old with Hemophilus influenza meningitis and is irritable.

2.9 The 7-year-old child is admitted to the Pediatric Unit with a positive Brudzinski's sign, a positive Kernig's sign, nuchal rigidity, and a T – 102.2° F. Which nursing action is priority for the nurse to implement?
① Place the client in droplet infection prevention precautions.
② Administer morphine for complaints of headache.
③ Position client in the supine position.
④ Immediately start antibiotics as prescribed.

2.10 What would be the priority of care for the nurse to include in the preoperative teaching plan for a client scheduled for a cholecystectomy?
① Assess client's concerns regarding the surgery.
② Instruct client regarding the importance of coughing and deep breathing exercises.
③ Teach client passive range of motion exercises.
④ Review the importance of resuming a regular low-fat diet.

2.11 Which client requires immediate intervention after shift report?
① The client diagnosed with atherosclerosis and is presenting with slurred speech and drooling.
② The client diagnosed with endocarditis and is staying in bed.
③ The client diagnosed with heart failure and is presenting with peripheral edema and weight gain of 1.7 lbs (0.77 kg) in 24 hours.
④ The client diagnosed with pericarditis who is with inspiration complaining of chest pain.

2.12 Which client would be the priority to evaluate immediately after admission?
① The client admitted with heart failure who has +1 edema in feet and ankles.
② The client admitted with atrial fibrillation and is complaining of chest pain.
③ The client admitted with hypertension who has a BP of 149/90.
④ The client admitted with angina and a depressed ST wave on ECG.

2.13 Which medication is priority to administer after morning report?
① Nifedipine for a client with a blood pressure of 108/66.
② Furosemide to a client with a serum potassium level of 3.3 mEq/L (3.3 mmol/L).
③ Digoxin to an elderly client who is presenting with a new symptom of confusion.
④ Amiodarone to a client in ventricular fibrillation.

2.14 Which of these clinical findings is priority to report for a client in the acute phase of Guillain-Barré syndrome?
① Weakness in the lower extremities.
② Alteration in coordination.
③ pH—7.32, pCO$_2$—48 mm Hg, HCO$_3$—23 mEq/L (23 μmol/L).
④ Tingling and numbness in the lower extremities.

2.15 What is the priority of care for a client who is presenting with a peaked T-wave on the ECG monitor?
① Report a potassium level of 2.2 mEq/L (2.2 mmol/L).
② Administer lisinopril for hypertension.
③ Provide a salt substitute with client's diet.
④ Notify the health care provider regarding a new order for spironolactone.

2.16 What is the priority information to include in the teaching plan for a young female client who suffered a head injury, began having seizures, and is now being sent home on phenytoin?
① "If you stop taking the medication suddenly, an unpleasant, acute withdrawal syndrome is likely along with renal failure."
② "You may stop taking this drug when you have had no seizures for six months."
③ "Let's talk about what kind of contraception you plan to use while you are taking this medication."
④ "I know it's depressing to face this, but you absolutely must take this drug the rest of your life."

2.17 What is the priority of care for a client who becomes unresponsive and the blood pressure is 82/52 with pulse oximetry reading 88% on 50% face mask?
① Ask family to go to the waiting room.
② Initiate CPR.
③ Notify the Rapid Response Team.
④ Prepare to administer code drugs.

2.18 What is the priority intervention when admitting a client with a diagnosis of posttraumatic stress disorder (PTSD) to the mental health unit who becomes confused and disoriented during the process?
① Accept the client and help to make client feel safe.
② Orient the client to the unit and introduce to the staff.
③ Review the unit rules and provide a booklet outlining them.
④ Stabilize the client's physical needs.

2.19 Which client should the nurse assess initially after receiving reports on these pediatric clients?
① An 8-week-old client admitted 4 hours ago with substernal retractions and an oxygen saturation of 90%.
② An 11-month-old client admitted 8 hours ago with dehydration whose vital signs are as follows: T—99.7° F (37.6° C), HR—126, R—28.
③ A school-age child who had closed reduction of a fractured left tibia 2 hours earlier and has swelling of the left toes.
④ An adolescent client who had an appendectomy 10 hours ago and has a 2.0 cm (1-inch) circular area of serous drainage on the dressing.

2.20 Which of these clients would be assessed first following shift report?
① A client with COPD presenting with diminished breath sounds in bilateral lung fields with a pH—7.34, pCO_2—47 mm Hg.
② A client with burns on head, neck, chest, has an O_2 saturation of 90%, and is presenting with wheezes in bilateral lung fields.
③ A client with asthma presenting with a HR—90 bpm after receiving a treatment with albuterol.
④ A client with pneumonia who has a temperature of 102° F (38.9° C) and just received first-dose of IV antibiotics 2 hours ago.

2.21 Which client would the nurse assess initially after receiving shift report on these obstetric clients?
① A primigravida client who is presenting in the last trimester with a small amount of painless, bright red blood and FHR—130 bpm with good variability.
② A primipara client, with an oxytocin infusion, who delivered an 8 lb. 4 oz. (3.74 kg) daughter 45 minutes ago.
③ A postpartum client who delivered 20 hours ago, is presenting with a temperature of 100° F (37.8° C) and in last 20 hours diuresed 2000 mL.
④ A multipara client, one hour after a precipitate delivery, presenting with a BP—98/62, HR—102 bpm, with pale and clammy skin.

2.22 Which of these maternity clients would be assessed initially?
① A client who is 36 weeks gestation with a BP 150/88, periorbital edema, +3 protein in urinalysis.
② A client who is 36 weeks gestation with a BP 160/90, headache, blurred vision, and epigastric pain.
③ A client who is 36 weeks gestation presenting with painless bright red blood, FHR—140 bpm, and good variability.
④ A client who is 36 weeks gestation presenting with rectal pressure, loss of mucous plug, and 2 cm dilated.

2.23 Which of these infants in the newborn nursery would be assessed first following shift report?
① A 14-hour-old neonate with RR—45 breaths per minute and irregular.
② A 24-hour-old neonate who has a bulging anterior fontanel when crying.
③ A 48-hour-old neonate with a HR—180 beats per minute when quiet.
④ A 2-week-old neonate with seedy yellow stools after breastfeeding.

2.24 Which of these older adult clients would be assessed initially during AM rounds?
① An older client who is presenting with anorexia.
② An older client who presents with incontinence following the AM cup of coffee.
③ An older client who presents with confusion and a new symptom of incontinence.
④ An older client who complains of dizziness when getting up quickly after taking oxybutynin and dicyclomine, so remains sitting on bedside until nurse arrives.

2.25 Which client would the nurse assess immediately?
① The middle-aged client who was admitted 2 days ago with heart failure, BP of 126/76, and has a respiratory rate of 21 breaths per minute.
② The middle-aged client who was admitted one day ago with thrombophlebitis and is receiving IV heparin.
③ The older client who was admitted 1 hour ago with new-onset atrial fibrillation and is receiving IV diltiazem.
④ The elderly client with end-stage right-sided heart failure, BP of 78/50, and a DNR order.

2.26 Which of these clients is a priority to assess?
① A client with chronic renal failure who is preparing for hemodialysis in one hour and is presenting with HR—100 bpm and BP—160/92 with weight increase of 2 kg/48 hours.
② A newly diagnosed client with chronic renal failure who has begun hemodialysis and is presenting with nausea/vomiting, change in LOC, and agitation.
③ A client who is receiving an initial round of peritoneal dialysis is draining straw-colored dialysis return.
④ A client who is receiving peritoneal dialysis with an order to infuse in 500 mL of dialysate and only drains out 450 mL.

2.27 Which of these clients is a priority to assess?
① A client who is taking, dexamethasone and has a HR—118 bpm, presenting with an increase in abdominal distention, pain, and vomiting.
② A client presenting with some blood tinged sputum and a depressed gag reflex following a bronchoscopy.
③ A client presenting with rebound tenderness in the right lower abdominal quadrant, associated with decrease in the bowel sounds and vomiting.
④ A client who is third day post-op after a gastric resection and the nasogastric tube is draining bile-colored liquid containing coffee-ground material.

2.28 Which of these lab values is a priority to report to the provider of care prior to inserting a chest tube in a client with a spinal cord injury?
① Platelets—90,000/mm^3 (90 x 10^9/L)
② Hgb—11 g/dL (110 g/L)
③ Hgb A1C—7%
④ Hct—37%

2.29 What is the priority of care for a client with a pH—7.55, pCO$_2$—25 mm Hg, HCO$_3$—24 mEq/L (24 mmol/L)?
① Encourage turning, coughing, and deep breathing.
② Increase the frequency for using the incentive spirometer.
③ Monitor the client's weight daily as prescribed.
④ Encourage client to slow down the breathing and relax.

Chapter 2: PRIORITIZATION

2.30 Which clinical assessment findings for a client with a decrease in cardiac output require priority intervention?
① Expiratory wheezing, substernal retracting, and SpO$_2$ 89% on 4 liters nasal cannula.
② BP—140/90, weight gain of 1.5 kg in 2 days, mild shortness of breath and dyspnea with activity.
③ Urine output 50 mL for last 2 hours, restless, and orthopnea.
④ BP—110/72, atrial flutter with HR—90, bibasilar crackles.

2.31 What is the priority psychosocial plan of care for a client who is dying?
① Administer pain medication, so the client will be comfortable.
② Encourage family to sit with client at bedside and touch and talk.
③ Recommend that only one family member should be in the room at a time.
④ Allow family members to only talk with client while nurse assists with food, hygiene, and physical comfort.

2.32 What is the priority plan of care for a client with severe Alzheimer's Disease who has a new prescription for memantine?
① Identify wrist bracelet for correct client identity prior to administering.
② Hold the medication and report a blood urea nitrogen (BUN): 38 mg/dL and creatinine level: 3.5 mg/dL.
③ Educate family that medication can cure the Alzheimer's Disease.
④ Initiate fall and safety precautions.

2.33 Forty-five minutes after a client with a C 4-5 vertical compression injury is admitted to the ED, the oxygen saturation drops to 86% and presents with rapid and shallow respirations. During the auscultation, the breath sounds are decreased in bilateral lung fields. What would the nurse implement next?
① Notify the provider of care immediately.
② Call the respiratory therapist for a non-rebreather mask.
③ Increase the oxygen flow to 6 L/minute.
④ Suction the client for oral and nasal secretions.

2.34 What is the priority plan of care for an elderly client on a medical unit who has minimal vision?
① Softly touch client to let client know the nurse is present.
② When guiding client while walking, walk behind client and place client's hand in the nurse's hand.
③ Assist with meal enjoyment by placing the meal in terms of the face of a clock (e.g., "meat at 6 o'clock").
④ When administering medications, provide client with a full glass of water and explain the number of medications.

2.35 What is the priority of care for a middle-aged client with severe epigastric pain due to acute pancreatitis?
① Assess client for tremors and diaphoresis.
② Discuss foods that are low in carbohydrates and high in protein.
③ Monitor client for CNS depression, decreasing muscle tone.
④ Position client with the head of the bed in semi-Fowler's position with knees flexed toward the chest.

2.36 Which of these interventions by the rehabilitation nurse is priority for a client who is a quadriplegic with a diagnosis of a C3-C4 fracture 4 months ago, has a tracheostomy, and is being maintained on a ventilator following a motor vehicle accident?
① Assist family in locating a support group and community resources following discharge.
② Maintain a regular bowel program to prevent impaction.
③ Offer fluids that promote alkaline urine.
④ Suction client when the low-pressure ventilator alarm sounds.

2.37 Which of these orders would the nurse initiate first for a post-operative client who has been in the recovery room for one hour and presents with the following vital signs: BP—100/70, HR—90 bpm, RR—22/min, and urine output is 45 mL/hour?
① Administer intravenous fluids to maintain a CVP of 5-8 mm Hg.
② Position client in the Trendelenburg position.
③ Place several blankets on the client to increase the temperature.
④ Administer nifedipine as ordered.

2.38 What is the priority of care for a client who is scheduled for a thoracentesis?
① Place the client in a sitting position with arms raised and resting on an over bed table.
② Encourage the client to cough during the needle insertion.
③ Ensure that no more than 100 mL of fluid is removed from the pleural cavity within the first 30 minutes.
④ Ensure that clean technique is used during needle insertion.

2.39 What is the priority outcome for a client with renal failure who is receiving epoetin?
① Calcium—8 mg/dL (2.0 mmol/L)
② Magnesium—3.2 mEq/L (1.6 mmol/L)
③ Hematocrit 48%
④ RBC—2.2×10^{12}/L

2.40 What is the priority outcome for a client with cirrhosis of the liver that has progressed to portal-systemic encephalopathy and has a new order for lactulose?
① Decrease in the normal flora in the intestine
② Increase in the number of stools
③ Serum blood ammonia level—60 mcg/dL (35.2 µmol/L)
④ Serum pH—7.33

2.41 Which of these clinical findings indicate the priority outcome for the treatment of syndrome of inappropriate antidiuretic hormone (SIADH)?
① Specific gravity—1.029
② Serum sodium—149 mg/dL (149 mmol/L)
③ Serum osmolality—310 mOsm/kg of water
④ Hemoglobin (Hgb) 13 g/dL (130 g/L), Hematocrit (Hct)—39%

2.42 Which of these laboratory reports is the highest priority to evaluate and report to the health care provider for a client with Addison's disease?
① Serum calcium—7 mg/dL (1.75 mmol/L)
② Serum potassium—3.1 Eq/L (3.1 mmol/L)
③ Serum glucose—50 mg/dL (2.78 mmol/L)
④ Serum sodium—148 mEq/L (148 mmol/L)

2.43 Which of these clinical findings indicate a desired outcome from terbutaline?
① Contractions absent with a fetal heart rate—130 bpm
② Contractions occurring occasionally and lasting for 30 seconds
③ Fetal heart rate—140 bpm with late decelerations
④ Fetal heart rate—170 bpm with decrease in variability

2.44 The client with a C-7 spinal cord injury (SCI) is admitted to the Neurological Unit with a BP of 210/115 mm Hg and a throbbing headache. What would be the priority nursing action?
① Complete a neurological assessment.
② Place the client in the semi-Fowler's position.
③ Request an MRI.
④ Place in an indwelling urinary catheter.

2.45 Which of these nursing actions by the unlicensed assistive personnel (UAP) for a client admitted to the cardiac unit with suspected heart failure require intervention by the charge nurse due to the standard of care not being followed?
① Reports to the RN the client who is taking digoxin is complaining of nausea.
② Positions client in the low-Fowler's position with legs elevated.
③ Assists client to the bathroom due to frequent urination after receiving furosemide.
④ Coordinates care with the RN to provide uninterrupted sleep.

2.46 Which of these nursing actions by the licensed practical nurse (LPN) would the charge nurse intervene with for a client who has an internal arteriovenous fistula on the right arm for hemodialysis?
① Palpates for a thrill over the site.
② Auscultates for a bruit over the site.
③ Takes blood pressure on the right arm.
④ Assesses the pulses distal to the access site.

2.47 Which of these clinical situations should the charge nurse intervene with due to not following the appropriate standard of practice?
① The licensed practical nurse (LPN) reinforces the instruction to a client that Hepatitis A can be transmitted through infected food handlers.
② The licensed practical nurse (LPN) puts on gloves to administer an injection with a client who has Hepatitis B.
③ The registered nurse (RN) discusses the need to avoid sexual activity for a client with Hepatitis A.
④ The unlicensed assistive personnel (UAP) puts on a gown and mask prior to giving a bath to a client with Hepatitis B.

2.48 Which of these nursing actions by the nurse require immediate intervention by the charge nurse due to lack of understanding regarding the standard of care?
① The RN accesses the vein in the antecubital area when initially starting the IV.
② The RN uses an 18-gauge needle when accessing the vein for a blood administration.
③ The RN flushes a heparin lock with heparin solution 100 units per 1 mL as prescribed based on the hospital policy.
④ The RN documents the time and date of insertion, the type of catheter and size and the status of fluid infusing.

2.49 Which nursing action by the licensed practical nurse (LPN) requires immediate intervention by the RN for a client who had a cardiac catheterization two hours ago?
① Compares the quality of the pulses on the right and left legs.
② Evaluates the vital signs every 2 hours.
③ Encourages early ambulation to the bathroom to prevent a deep vein thrombosis.
④ Encourages oral intake of fluids following the procedure.

2.50 What is the priority of care for a client with the diagnosis of tuberculosis and has an order to receive Isoniazid and Rifampin twice daily orally?
① Administer with lunch and dinner.
② Verify identity of client prior to giving meds.
③ Check and verify accuracy of order with provider of care.
④ Teach client that the urine and tears will turn orange.

2.51 Which of these orders need to be questioned?
① Increase the pyridoxine (B_6) as prescribed for a client who takes Levodopa for Parkinson's Disease.
② Administer spironolactone for a client with a potassium level of 3.2 mEq/L (3.2 mmol/L).
③ Administer Lithium for a client who is manic.
④ Administer atenolol for a client with a BP—150/90; HR—90 bpm.

2.52 The health care provider's orders are: continue all previous medications which include digoxin 0.25 mg po each AM, and Propranolol 20 mg po tid; oxygen at 2L/minute via nasal cannula, establish an IV, and give furosemide 40 mg IV now, bathroom privileges, full liquid diet. Which part of the order is priority for the nurse to discuss with the health care provider for a client with a history of cardiac disease who is admitted to the hospital with a diagnosis of heart failure (HF) and COPD?
① Digoxin 0.25 ng/mL (0.3 nmol/L) PO in AM
② Level of oxygen concentration
③ Propranolol 20 mg tid
④ The rate the IV should infuse

2.53 An older adult-client with diabetes mellitus has an order for an intravenous pyelogram (IVP). What is the priority of care for this client?
① Assess for allergies to dyes.
② Educate client regarding the procedure.
③ Obtain a consent from the client.
④ Verify appropriateness for procedure with health care provider.

2.54 Which of these clinical findings is priority to report for a client who is experiencing cardiogenic shock?
① Cardiac output has gone from 4 L/min to 6 L/min in 2 hours.
② 8 AM: Breath sounds—clear in bilateral lung fields; 10 AM: Crackles in bilateral lung fields
③ 8 AM: central venous pressure (CVP)—3 mm Hg; 10 AM: CVP—6 mm Hg
④ 8 AM: pulmonary artery wedge pressure (PAWP)—6 mm Hg; 10 AM: PAWP—8 mm Hg

2.55 Which of these post-op clients would the nurse assess immediately after shift report?
① A client with a 8 AM: HR—84 bpm; urine output 60 mL/hr; 10 AM: HR 92 bpm; urine output 50 mL/hr and anxious.
② A client who at 8 AM: has a CVP of 8 mm Hg, BP—150/86; 10 AM: CVP 6 mm Hg, BP—142/78.
③ A client at 8 AM with a BP—120/78, restless and HR—92 bpm; 10 AM: BP—132/80, HR—88 bpm.
④ A client 8 AM with a HR—92 bpm, BP—120/82; 10 AM: HR 120 bpm; decrease in LOC, and BP—92/58.

2.56 When the nurse is educating a new graduate regarding the appropriate infection prevention measures for a client with tuberculosis, which of these statements are most important to include during the teaching?
① "The nurse should wear gown, gloves, and a surgical mask when in client's room."
② "The nurse should restrict visitors to immediate family only."
③ "The isolation precautions should be discontinued after one of the sputum smears is negative."
④ "The nurse should wear an N95 respirator when in client's room with monitored negative airflow."

2.57 What is priority for the nurse to include in a teaching plan for a mother who has a child diagnosed with varicella?
① Instruct to keep fingernails short.
② Isolate child until all the vesicles have crusted.
③ Provide quiet activities to keep child occupied.
④ Recommend bathing the child in warm baths with a mild soap.

2.58 When making shift assignments, which of these clients is highest risk for suicidal precaution?
① An elderly Caucasian client who lives alone following the death of his wife and has been giving away his favorite items.
② An older African-American client who has been diagnosed with diabetes mellitus.
③ A middle-aged Asian client who has been diagnosed with cancer.
④ A young adult, single Hispanic client who has recently had a mastectomy.

2.59 What is the priority nursing action for a client who has an order for clopidogrel and warfarin?
① Advise to take meds on an empty stomach.
② Continue to monitor AST / ALT.
③ Notify health care provider and verify appropriateness of this new drug order.
④ Review with client that a sore throat and chills are expected with these drugs.

2.60 Which information is priority for the nurse to include in the discharge teaching for a client being discharged on amphojel and amlodipine?
① Discuss the importance of taking on an empty stomach.
② Review the possible side effect of a rapid heart rate and importance of reporting.
③ Discuss the importance of increasing dietary intake of fiber and fluid.
④ Review the possible side effect of diarrhea and the importance of drinking Gatorade.

2.61 What is most important to monitor for a client with a spinal cord injury who is taking naproxen and dexamethasone?
① Decrease in daily weights
② Hemoglobin and Hematocrit
③ Muscle cramps in legs
④ Presenting with cool and clammy skin

2.62 Which of these plans indicates the priority additional information needed regarding how to safely provide home care for a client with Multiple Sclerosis?

① Advise client to conserve energy by using a cane to assist with ambulation.
② Encourage client to wear non-slip, flat, tie shoes.
③ Discuss the importance of only having a few throw rugs in the living and dining room.
④ Recommend client schedule major activities in the AM and rest in the afternoon.

2.63 What is priority of care for a client with a C4 spinal cord injury who begins complaining of a throbbing headache that suddenly started a short time ago? Assessment findings include: blood pressure—188/100, heart rate—48 bpm, diaphoresis, and flushing of the face and neck.

① Adjust room temperature.
② Administer the ordered acetaminophen.
③ Evaluate the Foley catheter for kinks or obstruction.
④ Initiate a complete neurological exam.

2.64 Which client would be priority to delegate to the LPN on the mental health unit?

① A client who has anorexia nervosa and presenting with dizziness.
② A client who has panic attacks and is starting to ramble and hyperventilate.
③ A client who has dementia and is wandering in the hallway.
④ A client who has anxiety and has a new order for a blood transfusion.

2.65 What nursing task would be priority to delegate to the licensed practical nurse (LPN/VN) for a client on the medical surgical unit?

① Assist client in getting out of bed the first time in the post-op period.
② Measure and record intake and urine output.
③ Prior to surgery insert an indwelling catheter.
④ Assist client in turning and repositioning every 2 hours.

Answers & Rationales

2.1 ② Option #2 is correct. This is the priority due to the risk of bleeding with the procedure. The normal platelet count is between 150,000 and 400,000/mm³ (150 to 400 x 10⁹ /L). 13,000/mm³ (13 x 10⁹ /L) is very low and will increase risk of bleeding. Option #1 is not priority over #2. It is more of a priority to minimize any needle insertions such as a "centesis", biopsy, and/or epidural. Option #3 is incorrect since the vital signs are not consistent with bleeding which may be a result of a low platelet count. Option #4 is incorrect because maintaining electronic BP readings ongoing may result in bleeding due to the low platelet count.
I CAN HINT: Prioritizing Strategy: Organize the plan of care based on the laboratory value provided in the stem of the question. Link labs to think plans! Which of these options provide the SAFEST care?
NCLEX® Standards: Prioritize delivery of care. Monitor the results of laboratory results and intervene as needed

2.2 ① Option #1 is correct. After comparing the options, the priority is the heart failure presenting with a moist cough. The moist cough may be indicative of left sided heart failure which can result in alteration in oxygenation. Option #2 does not need to be assessed first because the vital signs are not consistent with fluid deficit which could result from vomiting and diarrhea. Option #3 is incorrect since the weight increase is not significant enough to be concerned with the edema. The weight increase would be > 2 lbs. for the increase to be significant. Option #4 is incorrect since the decrease remains within the desired range and there is no indication of alteration in perfusion.
I CAN HINT: Prioritizing Strategy: Organize the plan of care with the client presenting with a potential pump issue that could result in alteration in oxygenation.
NCLEX® Standard: Prioritize delivery of care. Recognize changes in client condition and intervene as needed.

2.3 ④ Option #4 is correct. The client may be experiencing a complication with arterial perfusion from the surgical procedure and is priority to assess. Option #1 is an expected assessment finding for a client with a DVT. Option #2 is not a priority over #4. Option #3 is incorrect. The client should not be elevating legs, but dangling legs to assist with circulation. Peripheral artery disease is a complication with blood being delivered to the extremity.
I CAN HINT: Prioritizing Strategy: Organize the plan of care with the client presenting with a potential alteration in perfusion following a surgery.
NCLEX® Standard: Prioritize the delivery of care. Recognize changes in client condition and intervene as needed

2.4 ④ Option #4 is correct. Based on the diagnosis, antibiotics are important to administer. The sputum samples for culture and sensitivity should be obtained first to provide valid data for administering the correct antibiotic. The antibiotic can be discontinued after the sputum samples are reviewed if it is not sensitive to the organism the client has. This is an important test taking strategy to always get samples for culture and sensitivity prior to starting the antibiotics to provide a reliable plan of care. Option #1 is incorrect. The infection prevention precautions would include droplet and standard precautions (based on the component of care the client requires). Option #2 should not be implemented prior to option #4. Option #3 has no indication to receive a beta₂ adrenergic agonist which decreases airway resistance.
I CAN HINT: Prioritizing Strategy: Organize the plan of care with the client presenting with an infection. Recognize the importance of obtaining specimens other than blood for diagnostic testing (e.g., sputum, etc.) prior to starting antibiotics.

NCLEX® Standard: Prioritize delivery of care.

2.5 ③ Option #3, orthopneic position, will help optimize lung expansion resulting with easier breathing for the client. This position is when the client is using several pillows being used to prop client up in bed. Option #1 is incorrect. Clients with chronic lung disease must not be prescribed oxygen levels greater than 3 L/min. With elevated oxygen levels, these clients can lose their drive to breathe. Option #2 is incorrect. The priority is to position client correctly to optimize pulmonary expansion. Option #4 is not priority. The stem of the question indicates client is in distress, so the nurse needs to intervene prior to further assessment.
I CAN HINT: Prioritizing Strategy: Organize the plan of care with the client presenting with alteration in oxygenation secondary to a chronic lung disease.
NCLEX® Standards: Prioritize delivery of care.

2.6 ③ Option #3 is correct. These assessments indicate a possible complication of GI bleeding. Options #1 and #2 are expected based on the pathophysiology that occurs with these conditions. Option #1 does not indicate any assessments supporting fluid volume deficit. Option #2 does need to be addressed but is not priority over option #3 that is a complication of bleeding. This could result in complications with alteration in perfusion if the issue is not resolved. Option #4 is important to address, but is not priority over option #3.
I CAN HINT: Prioritizing Strategy: When you compare the four options, the most acute client is #3 who is presenting with bleeding. The other options are expected assessment findings with the medical conditions. Each of the assessments are a concern and need a plan of care but are not priority to the client who is bleeding.
NCLEX® Standards: Prioritize the delivery of care. Recognize changes in client condition and intervene as needed.

2.7 ② Option #2 is correct. This is a safety issue and without assessment and intervention there is a risk for suicide. Option #1 is not priority over #2. Options #3 and #4 are a concern, but not priority over #2. These two clients do not have energy to hurt themselves.
I CAN HINT: Prioritizing Strategy: Assess the potential for violence and use safety precautions.
NCLEX® Standards: Prioritize delivery of care.

2.8 ② Option #2 is correct. The normal reference range for the pulse oximeter is (93% - 100%). This value of 91% is low in addition to the clinical assessment finding of expiratory wheezing. Option #1 is not priority. These clinical assessment findings do occur with Kawasaki's disease, but do not support a complication such as option #2 who is presenting with hypoxia. Options #3 and #4 are not correct. They do need further assessment and plans of care, but these are not priority to option #2 who is experiencing hypoxia.
I CAN HINT: Prioritizing Strategy: ABC strategy (airway, breathing, and circulation).
NCLEX® Standards: Prioritize delivery of care.

2.9 ① Option #1 is correct. The nurse would anticipate the diagnosis of bacterial meningitis based on the clinical assessment findings and place the child in the appropriate infection prevention precautions. Option #2 is incorrect. Nonopioid analgesics are administered for headache to avoid masking an alteration in the level of consciousness. Option #3 is incorrect. The bed should be maintained at 30 degrees. Option #4 is incorrect. CSF from the lumbar puncture will need to be performed for a definitive diagnosis of bacterial meningitis. This is not priority over protecting others from the disease through effective infection prevention.
I CAN HINT: Prioritizing Strategy: Infection prevention.
NCLEX® Standards: Prioritize delivery of care.

2.10 ② Option #2 is correct. Following a cholecystectomy, client's breaths may be shallow due to the pain that deep breathing may present due to the location of the surgical procedure. Option #1 is important to include in the plan of care but is not a priority over option #2 based on the strategy of ABC's (airway, breathing, and circulation). Option #3 is incorrect because the exercises would be active range of motion with special attention to the leg exercises to prevent deep vein thrombosis. Option #4 is not the priority teaching plan for this client.
I CAN HINT: Prioritizing Strategy: ABC's strategy (airway, breathing, and circulation).
NCLEX® Standards: Prioritize delivery of care.

2.11 ① Option #1 is correct. Clients with atherosclerosis do not present with slurred speech and drooling unless they are experiencing a cerebrovascular accident (stroke). This client mandates immediate assessment and intervention. Option #2 is not priority, since the standard of care for a client with endocarditis is rest. Strict bed rest is encouraged during the active disease process to decrease the cardiac workload. Option #3 is incorrect. The weight gain is not significant and can occur with heart failure. While this does require attention, it is not an emergency like option #1. Option #4 is incorrect. The client with pericarditis is expected to have chest pain with inspiration, so there is not a need for immediate intervention.
I CAN HINT: Time pressure is a clinical judgment skill and is the key to answering this question appropriately. Early intervention is imperative for a client who is presenting with symptoms of a cerebrovascular accident.
NCLEX® Standard: Prioritize the delivery of care.

2.12 ② Option #2 is correct. This client is high risk to have a pulmonary emboli which is a potentially life-threatening complication. Option #1 is incorrect. A client with heart failure would be expected to have edematous feet. This is not priority over option #2. Option #3 is incorrect. This BP is elevated, but is not a priority over a potentially life-threatening complication such as option #2. Option #4 is not a priority. This ECG pattern is consistent with angina. While this client does need attention, it is not as urgent as option #2.

I CAN HINT: Time pressure is a clinical judgment skill and is the key to answering this question appropriately. Early intervention is imperative for a client who is presenting with chest pain and has a diagnosis of atrial fibrillation.
NCLEX® Standard: Prioritize the delivery of care.

2.13 ④ Option #4 is correct. Ventricular fibrillation can be life-threatening. The antidysrhythmic, amiodarone, should be administered first. Another option for an antidysrhythmic may be lidocaine. Option #1 is incorrect. The BP is above 90/60, so it can be administered; however, it is not priority over a client presenting in a life-threatening situation. Option #2 is incorrect. With a low potassium, the furosemide should be questioned prior to administering. The loop diuretic can result in a further decrease in the potassium and cause cardiac dysrhythmias. Option #3 is incorrect. This new symptom of confusion is a sign of digoxin toxicity for the elderly.
I CAN HINT: Consequences and risks require clinical judgment skills and are the keys to answering this question appropriately. The consequences of administering options #1, #2, and #3 have risks due to the current clinical findings.
NCLEX® Standard: Prioritize the delivery of care.

2.14 ③ Option #3 is correct. Guillain-Barré is an acute, rapidly progressing motor neuropathy involving the nerve roots in the spinal cord and medulla. This inflammatory, demyelinating disorder can result in edema, and compression of the nerve roots leading to a rapidly ascending paralysis. Motor and sensory impairment may occur. The client is experiencing respiratory acidosis which means the lungs are not expanding well and may be leading to pulmonary compromise. Options #1 and #4 would be a concern for Myasthenia Gravis and could result in alteration in coordination. While option #2 is a concern, it is not priority over option #3.
I CAN HINT: Cue recognition is a skill in clinical judgment. The key to answering this question correctly is to remember one priority is to monitor the respiratory status closely.
NCLEX® Standard: Manage the care of a client with impaired ventilation/oxygenation.

2.15 ④ Option #4 is the correct answer. Spironolactone is a potassium-sparing diuretic and will contribute to the hyperkalemia if administered. Peaked T waves occur from hyperkalemia. Option #1 is incorrect. The T wave would be depressed if client was experiencing hypokalemia. Option #2 is incorrect. Lisinopril suppresses the renin-angiotensin-aldosterone system. The excretion of sodium and water may occur, but retention of K+ by actions in kidneys. This will also result in hyperkalemia which is already occurring with this client. Option #3 is incorrect. Salt substitute is high in potassium.
NCLEX® Standards: Evaluate appropriateness and accuracy of medication order for client. Manage client with fluid and electrolyte imbalance.

2.16 ③ Option #3 is the priority. Due to the drug interactions, birth control pills will not be as effective and may result in pregnancy. It is important for the client to be educated regarding the importance of using a barrier contraceptive when taking phenytoin and oral contraceptives together. Options #1 is not a true statement. Option #2 is not correct since this is not the standard of care for this medication. Option #4 is not the priority over option #3.
I CAN HINT: Prioritizing Strategy: Assess, the first step in the Nursing Process. If you did not know the information, you could get this correct by understanding that option #3 is the only option that is focused on the client and is further assessing additional information regarding birth control. Note that when the developmental stage and the gender are in the stem and/or an option and the question evaluates a drug that goes through the first by-pass, there is a great possibility it is addressing a need for further information about contraceptives due to the risk for an interaction.
NCLEX® Standards: Review pertinent data prior to medication administration (e.g., potential interactions). Educate client about medications.

2.17 ③ Option #3 is correct. The Rapid Response Team should be notified immediately. The client needs evaluation and immediate treatment. Option #1 is incorrect. As long as the team can get to the client at the bedside, there is no reason to ask family to leave. In reality, it can be very comforting to the family to know all of the care that is possible is being provided for their loved one. Option #2 is incorrect. There is no indication that CPR should be implemented. Option #4 is incorrect. Additional assessment and evaluation need to be done prior to preparing meds for a code.
I CAN HINT: Prioritizing Strategy: Notify the Rapid Response Team. The client is presenting with trends of rapid deterioration in clinical status. There is a blood pressure even though it is low and the client has become unresponsive both of which indicate ominous findings. The Rapid Response Team is crucial at this time. You can group option #2 and option #4 together, since these address a code which hasn't occurred yet, but is right around the corner. Option #1 is a psychosocial action and typically will be secondary to an intervention that is addressing the grave clinical findings.
NCLEX® Standards: Assess and respond to changes in client vital signs. Collaborate with inter-professional team members when providing client care (e.g., health care professionals, Rapid Response Team).

2.18 ① Option #1 is correct. The priority of care is all about making the client with posttraumatic stress disorder to feel safe. Options #2 and #3 are very similar in that they both address a general orientation to the unit versus focusing on the priority of care for the client. Option #4 is incorrect. Due to the diagnosis and the current clinical assessments the client is presenting with, safety is a priority over the physical needs.
I CAN HINT: Prioritizing Strategy: Maslow's Hierarchy of Needs. The goal for client care is all about safety! If you knew nothing about this diagnosis, you could still get this correct by using the strategy of Maslow's Hierarchy of Needs.
NCLEX® Standards: Prioritize the delivery of client care. Protect client from injury (e.g., self-harm).

2.19 ① Option #1 is correct due to the ABC's. Option #2 is not correct. The vital signs do not indicate a major complication with dehydration for the developmental stage. Option #3 is incorrect. This clinical finding would be an expected assessment 2 hours following a closed reduction of a fractured femur. Option #4 may be an expected finding following this surgical procedure. There are no additional assessments indicating a complication with hemorrhaging.
I CAN HINT: Prioritizing Strategy: ABC's. As you compare and contrast each of these options, you begin to observe that there is only one option focusing on airway.
Refer to the book, *Nursing Made Insanely Easy* for review of clinical findings indicating hypoxia for an infant. The bottom line is that if the infant presents with "GRUNTS," there is a complication with hypoxia. This will be the priority client.

    Grunting, grimacing

    Retracting, restless

    Uninterested in feeding

    Nasal flaring

    Tachycardia, tachypnea

    Stridor

You may have selected option #3 due to risk of compartmental syndrome. The swelling of the toes is a result of the procedure. Notice the time frame when this is included in the question or option. There is typically a reason. If there was a complication with compartmental syndrome, the time would not be as close to the procedure and there would have been several assessments such as change in pulse, pain, pallor, paresthesia, and/or paralysis.
NCLEX® Standards: Prioritize the delivery of client care. Recognize signs and symptoms of complications and intervene appropriately when providing client care.

2.20 ② Option #2 is the priority due to the location of the burns may result in smoke inhalation. With the O_2 saturation and bilateral wheezing, this client is in acute distress mandating immediate intervention. Option #1 is not a priority due to the client experiencing a chronic medical condition with expected clinical findings. Option #3 is not a priority over #2 since the only assessment provided was an elevation in the HR and this can be an expected finding after albuterol. Option #4 is a concern, but is not the priority since the client just received IV antibiotics. The client will remain febrile until the medication becomes effective.
I CAN HINT: Prioritizing Strategy: ABC's. The key to answering this question successfully is to recognize that COPD is a chronic condition. Option #3 is an expected outcome from the medication, and the HR is not high enough to cause problems with perfusion. Option #4 is not presenting with any acute respiratory assessments. While the ABC's are your strategy, another strategy is to recognize ACUTE will typically be a priority over CHRONIC!
NCLEX® Standard: Prioritize the delivery of client care.

2.21 ④ Option #4 is correct. This client is presenting with alterations in perfusion as indicated by the BP, HR, and skin color and temperature. Although the fundus is firm and midline, there are two other causes of hemorrhaging after a precipitate delivery. These include a retained placental fragment or cervical lacerations. Option #1 is a concern with placenta previa, but the bleeding is only small and the FHR is WDL and the variability indicates adequate oxygenation of the fetus. Option #2 is incorrect, since oxytocin can assist in minimizing bleeding by stimulating the uterus to contract. Option #3 is incorrect, since these are normal findings during the first 24 hours in the postpartum period.
I CAN HINT: Prioritizing Strategy: Identify the client who is unstable or highest risk for developing complications. Even if you did not know anything about maternity, you could get this question correct due to your understanding of the concept of perfusion. Bleeding is bleeding! No matter the location of the hemorrhaging, the hemodynamics will be the same. The difference that you will need to know for the NCLEX® is the system-specific assessment findings. For example, if the maternity client is hemorrhaging due to an abruptio placenta the abdomen will be firm, blood will be dark if it is visible, and client will experience pain. If the hemorrhaging is from a placenta previa, bleeding will be bright red and client will not experience any pain. If the pediatric client is bleeding from a tonsillectomy, the clinical findings will be frequent swallowing. If the client is bleeding post op, bleeding will most likely be at the area

of the surgery. Whenever the client bleeds from any complication, the earliest signs include an increase in the HR and RR. Later signs of bleeding include a decrease in CVP, BP and urine output.
NCLEX® Standards: Prioritize the delivery of client care. Recognize trends and changes in client condition and intervene as needed.

2.22 ② Option #2 is correct since these symptoms represent late signs of preeclampsia. Mild preeclampsia is gestational hypertension with the addition of proteinuria of 1 to 2+ and a weight gain of more than 2 kg (4.4 lb.) per week in the second and third trimesters. Mild edema will also begin to appear in the upper extremities or face. Severe preeclampsia consists of blood pressure that is 160/100 mm Hg or greater, proteinuria 3 to 4+, oliguria, elevated serum creatinine greater than 1.2 mg/dL (106 μmol/L), cerebral or visual disturbances (headache and blurred vision), hyperreflexia with possible ankle clonus, pulmonary or cardiac involvement, extensive peripheral edema, hepatic dysfunction, epigastric and right upper-quadrant pain, and thrombocytopenia. Eclampsia is severe preeclampsia symptoms along with the onset of seizure activity or coma. Eclampsia is usually preceded by headache, severe epigastric pain, hyperreflexia, and hemoconcentrations, which are warning signs of probable convulsions. Option #1 is incorrect since these would indicate moderate signs of preeclampsia, and is not a priority over option #2. Option #3 indicates the client may be presenting with placenta previa, but the FHR is WDL, and there is good oxygenation as indicated by the good variability which would not make this a priority over option #2. Option #4 is not a priority. This is a normal sign that the body is preparing for labor, but there are no complications pending that would mandate immediate assessment following report.
I CAN HINT: Prioritizing Strategy: Identify the client who is unstable or highest risk for developing complications. The key in answering this question appropriately is to organize the signs and symptoms for preeclampsia between what occurs early versus late. When taking the NCLEX®, recognize the expected findings for clients. These will NOT be the priority. This is an effective strategy for any question evaluating prioritizing. As you study, remember "*early assessments versus late assessments*" for perfusion, hypoxia, increased intracranial pressure, etc.
NCLEX® Standards: Prioritize the delivery of client care. Recognize signs and symptoms of complications and intervene appropriately when providing client care.

2.23 ③ Option #3 is correct. The normal neonatal heart rate is 120 to 160 beats per minute. A heart rate of 180 beats per minute at rest mandates assessment first, since other clinical findings need to be evaluated such as RR, neonate's color, O₂ saturation, any grunting, flaring, or retracting, etc. Option #1 is not a priority. The rate is WDL and the RR will still be irregular at 14 hours. Option #2 is an expected finding when crying. Option #4 is an expected finding for a breast fed neonate. The formula-fed newborn's stool is typically tan, brown, or green and about the consistency of peanut butter. The breast-fed newborn's stool is typically seedy yellow. The formula-fed newborn's stool is a bit firmer than the breast-fed newborn's stool.
I CAN HINT: Prioritizing Strategy: Identify the client who is unstable or highest risk for developing complications. *Remember "the 4's for the neonate":* HR—120 to 160 with 140 in the middle; RR—30 to 50 with 40 in the middle. The key word in the option is when "quiet." Key words can be your best friend as you answer these questions! They will be there! Use them!
NCLEX® Standards: Prioritize the delivery of client care. Provide care for the newborn less than 1 month.

2.24 ③ Option #3 is a priority since these clinical findings indicate a complication from a urinary tract infection. Older clients do not respond to infections as younger clients. They do not present with dysuria, a fever, an elevation in the WBCs, etc. The first clinical finding is acute confusion with a new symptom of incontinence. Many professionals believe that this incontinence is a normal part of the aging process, so this may be ignored. Notice that for your clinical decision making strategy, the key word was "new" symptom. Option #1 is a concern, but the anorexia is not connected to any medication which would change the focus for this question, and would require option #3 to be revised. The way it is currently written, however, the answer remains option #3 due to

the symptoms of infection. Option #2 is not a priority, since this may be an expected outcome from drinking the coffee. Option #4 may occur if client rises quickly. Anticholinergic side effects may occur with these medications. This still would not be a priority over option #3, since client is not attempting to get out of bed without the nurse.
I CAN HINT: Prioritizing Strategy: Identify the client who is unstable or highest risk for developing complications. In addition to the prioritizing strategy, using the strategy of expected outcomes versus new symptom will assist you in answering the question correctly.
NCLEX® Standards: Prioritize the delivery of client care. Provide care and education for the adult client ages 65 through 85 years and over.

2.25 ③ Option #3 is correct. This client is presenting with a new onset of atrial fibrillation, and is receiving a calcium channel blocker that is not being effective in preventing the new onset of atrial fibrillation. The client must be evaluated prior to the other clients due to the new onset. Option #1 is in no acute distress in comparison to option #3. Option #2 has no indication of any undesirable effects from the treatment, so this is not a priority over the client with a new dysrhythmia. Option #4 is a DNR, so is not the priority in comparison to option #3.
I CAN HINT: Prioritizing Strategy: Identify the client who is unstable or highest risk for developing complications.
NCLEX® Standards: Prioritize the delivery of client care. Recognize changes in client condition and intervene as needed.

2.26 ② Option #2 is correct. This client is presenting with disequilibrium syndrome which may be caused by too rapid a decrease of BUN and circulating fluid volume. It may result in cerebral edema and increased intracranial pressure (ICP). Early recognition of disequilibrium syndrome is essential. Signs include nausea, vomiting, change in level of consciousness, seizures and agitation. Option #1 is incorrect. This is the reason the client is preparing for hemodialysis in one hour due to the renal failure and with an increase in fluid there would be an increase in the HR, BP and weight. Option #3 is an expected outcome. Option #4 does require some repositioning of the client in order to facilitate the drainage, but it is not a priority to option #2 which is a complication.
I CAN HINT: Prioritizing Strategy: Identify the client who is unstable or highest risk for developing complications. In addition to disequilibrium syndrome, other complications that may occur from dialysis and require prioritization may include sepsis and hepatitis B and C.
NCLEX® Standards: Prioritize the delivery of client care. Recognize trends and changes in client condition and intervene as needed.

2.27 ① Option #1 is correct. This client is taking corticosteroids which can lead to a bleeding ulcer. The HR is elevated and the other assessments in this option indicate an intestinal perforation requiring immediate nursing action. Option #2 is an expected outcome following this procedure, so this would not be a priority client to assess. Option #3 is incorrect; this client is presenting with appendicitis. Rebound pain is elicited by pressing firmly over the area known as the McBurney's point; pain occurs when pressure is released. The rebound pain, decreased bowel sounds, fever, and tender abdomen are all characteristic of the clinical findings of appendicitis. This is important to assess, but not a priority over the clinical findings of a perforated intestine. Option #4 is not a priority. Coffee-ground material is old blood. This is normal on the third post-operative day and should be assessed and correlated with the vital signs. The tube must be in the correct position since it is draining gastric secretions. There is no indication that the tube is obstructed or needs to be irrigated.
I CAN HINT: Prioritizing Strategy: Identify the client who is unstable or highest risk for developing complications.
NCLEX® Standards: Prioritize the delivery of client care. Recognize trends and changes in client condition and intervene as needed.

2.28 ① Option #1 is the priority due to the risk for bleeding. The normal platelet count is between 150,000 and 400,000/mm³ (150 to 400 x 10⁹/L). This count in option #1 is very low which increases the risk for bleeding. Option #2 is only slightly low. Range is from 12.0 to 16.0 g/dL (120 to 160 g/L). The Hct is within the normal range: 37% to 47% (0.370 to 0.470). Option #3 should be 6% or less, but it is evaluating the management of diabetes mellitus and is not a priority for evaluating

prior to chest tube insertion. The priority concern with this procedure is the risk for bleeding.
I CAN HINT: Prioritizing Strategy: Organize priority nursing plan/interventions based on the key concepts. If you were uncertain of the answer, focus on the fact that the procedure will require a tube being inserted which could result in bleeding. This can apply to biopsies, any centesis, or any procedure that may result in bleeding. Note that the other options have a focus on anemia or diabetes mellitus. Option #1 is the only option that has a focus on the concept of risk of alteration in perfusion due to hemorrhage. See you CAN do this by incorporating your nursing knowledge. Refer to *Nursing Made Insanely Easy* for a review of all of the procedures that involve a "centesis".
NCLEX® Standards: Use precautions to prevent injury and/or complications associated with a procedure. Prioritize delivery of care.

2.29 ④ Option #4 is correct. The labs in the stem of the question indicate a complication with respiratory alkalosis. Options #1 and #2 would require implementation for a client presenting with respiratory acidosis. Option #3 is incorrect. This would be appropriate for a client who was either vomiting or had diarrhea which would be reflective of a client with a metabolic problem versus a respiratory complication.
I CAN HINT: Prioritizing Strategy: Organize priority nursing plan/interventions based on the key concepts. In this question, the pH is high and the $PaCO_2$ is low; which means the client is breathing off too much CO_2. Remember the strategy "ROME." Refer to the book *Nursing Made Insanely Easy*, for more review of this strategy. The goal is to "SLOW" down the breathing and assist with rebreathing in order to hold on to more CO_2.
NCLEX® Standards: Prioritize delivery of care. Manage the care of a client with impaired ventilation/oxygenation. Monitor the results of the diagnostic test (labs) and intervene as needed.

2.30 ③ Option #3 is correct. A low urine output (*UO of 50 mL for 2 hours is < 30 mL/hr*), restless, and orthopnea are signs of decreased cardiac output. These would be the priority since these clinical findings are linked to the problem with decreased cardiac output, and with the oliguria there is a need for immediate intervention. Keep in mind the importance of linking the pathophysiology with the clinical findings and nursing assessment. Option #1 is incorrect. These assessments would be for a client who had asthma. Option #2 is incorrect. While these do need to be monitored, the key is the client in the stem of the question has a decreased cardiac output, and these do not represent a decrease in cardiac output. These exemplify fluid overload. Option #4 is incorrect. Atrial flutter can result in a decrease in the atrial output, but the blood pressure and heart rate are stable and not irregular. No additional signs of decreased cardiac output.
I CAN HINT: Priority Strategy: Organize priority nursing plan/interventions based on the key concepts. The key here is to connect the clinical assessment findings with the complication of decreased cardiac output. Remember, the entire option must be correct for the option to be the correct answer.
NCLEX® Standards: Prioritize the delivery of client care. Manage the care of a client with alteration in hemodynamics, tissue perfusion and hemostasis (e.g., cerebral, cardiac, peripheral).

2.31 ② Option #2 is the best answer. It is important for the family to be with client and support during the end-of-life care. Option #1 is incorrect. There is no indication that client is in pain. Option #3 is incorrect, since family should be there to support. Option #4 is incorrect, since family should be allowed to assist and participate in care.
I CAN HINT: Priority Strategy: Organize priority nursing plan/interventions based on the key concepts. "SPIRIT" will assist you in organizing your facts regarding "end of life."

Support for clients who are dying "Hospice or palliative care."

Promote spiritual comfort—encourage/assist client to contact spiritual advisors.

Isolation feelings by client—prevent by responding quickly to call lights, check on client often.

Recommend client's family to be at bedside to talk, sit and touch client and help with basic care.

Incorporate cultural needs by providing personal preferences and cultural implications regarding death.

Treatment decisions—assist client and family to make decisions such as in preparing advance directives.

NCLEX® Standards: Prioritize the delivery of client care. Assess psychosocial, spiritual and occupational factors affecting care, and plan interventions. Providing end-of-life care to clients and families. Assisting client and family to cope with end-of-life interventions.

2.32 ② Option #2 is correct. Clients with renal impairment as evidenced by an elevated BUN and creatinine should not receive memantine. Option #1 is important prior to administering the medication; however, if the BUN and creatinine are elevated the medication should not be administered due to renal insufficiency. Option #3 is incorrect. Clients taking this medication will experience an improvement in cognitive function (memory, attention, language, ability to perform activities of daily living); however, the medication does not provide a cure. Option #4 is important to include in the plan of care but is not a priority over option #2 due to the renal insufficiency.
I CAN HINT: Prioritizing Strategy: Link laboratory values to medication.
NCLEX® Standard: Prioritize delivery of care. Review pertinent data prior to medication administration (e.g., lab results, allergies, potential interactions, etc.).

2.33 ① Option #1 is the correct answer. The greatest risk to the client with a spinal cord injury (SCI) at the level of C 4–5 is respiratory compromise secondary to involvement of the phrenic nerve. Maintenance of an airway and provision of ventilator support would be the priority interventions both of which would need medical intervention. Option #2 is incorrect since the mask will have no effect on the phrenic nerve. Option #3 is incorrect due to the same rationale as option #2. Option #4 is incorrect since this level of the spinal cord injury is about the phrenic nerve and is not about secretions.
I CAN HINT: Priority Strategy: Organize priority nursing plan/interventions based on the key concepts. Notice that options #2 and #3 are both about oxygen devices and option #4 is about suctioning. The key words in the stem of the question include the type of spinal cord injury, the clinical presentation of the oxygen saturation dropping to 86%, and client presenting with rapid and shallow respirations.
NCLEX® Standard: Recognize signs and symptoms of complications and intervene appropriately when providing client care.

2.34 ③ Option #3 is correct. Organizing the meal in a consistent placement will facilitate the client enjoying the foods by knowing where each type of food is located on the plate. A few additional plans that may be helpful for this client with minimal vision may include: identifying self upon entering the room, always raising side rails for newly sightless persons (e.g., clients wearing post-operative eye patches), walking client around the room and acquainting client with all objects: bed, TV, telephone, etc. Option #1 is incorrect. The nurse should never touch a client unless client knows nurse is present. Option #2 is incorrect. When guiding client while walking, walk ahead of client and place client's hand in the bend of the nurse's elbow. Option #4 is incorrect. When administering medications, inform client of number of pills; however, what makes this option incorrect is that only a half glass of water should be given in order to avoid spills.
I CAN HINT: Priority Strategy: Organize priority nursing plan/interventions based on the key concepts. Remember for the option to be correct, the entire information must be correct. If part of the option is wrong, the entire option cannot be used as an answer. SAFETY is a big key to success!
NCLEX® Standards: Prioritize delivery of care. Provide care for a client experiencing visual, auditory or cognitive distortions.

2.35 ④ Option #4 is correct. The client is more comfortable sitting up with knees flexed toward the chest or in side lying position with knees drawn up to the chest. Option #1 is incorrect since the potential complication with acute pancreatitis may be hyperglycemia versus hypoglycemia. These assessments represent hypoglycemia.
Option #2 is incorrect since the client should be NPO during an acute episode. Typically the client will not take in any food until they are pain free. Diet should be bland, low fat, high carbohydrate, protein recommendations vary when not in an acute exacerbation. Option #3 is incorrect. These

are signs of hypercalcemia and the client with acute pancreatitis may experience signs and symptoms of hypocalcemia. Including the following: tetany, Chvostek's sign, Trousseau's sign, neuromuscular irritability, numbness and tingling in extremities or around mouth, seizures.
I CAN HINT: Priority Strategy: Organize priority nursing plan/interventions based on the key concepts.
NCLEX® Standards: Prioritize delivery of client care. Implement measures to promote circulation (e.g., active or passive range of motion, positioning and mobilization).

2.36 ② Option #2 is correct. A priority for this client is to prevent autonomic dysreflexia which can result from bladder distention and/or bowel impaction. Out of these options, maintaining a regular bowel program to prevent impaction is a priority of care to prevent complications with bowel impaction. Other plans that may decrease additional complications for this client include the following: administer chest physiotherapy; provide kinetic bed to promote blood flow to extremities; apply antiembolic stockings or SCDs; facilitate ROM exercises; turn frequently; keep skin clean and dry; observe for impending skin breakdown; bowel and bladder retraining, etc. Option #1 is an important part of the care, but is not the priority over option #2 which can result in an emergency situation with a significant increase in the blood pressure, a decrease in the HR and RR, and a pounding headache. Option #3 is incorrect. Bacteria grow best in alkaline media, so keeping urine dilute and acidic is prophylactic against infection. A common cause of death after spinal cord injury is a urinary tract infection. Fluids the client should drink in order to promote acidic urine include: cranberry juice, prune juice, bouillon, tomato juice, and water. Option #4 is incorrect. When the low-pressure ventilator alarms this is indicative of an air leak. The high-pressure alarm indicates the need for suctioning.
I CAN HINT: Priority Strategy: Organize priority nursing plan/interventions based on the key concepts. Following a spinal cord injury of T6 or higher, it is important to monitor the "3 F's": **F**unny feeling with the skin, **F**ecal impaction, and/or **F**ull bladder to prevent complications with autonomic dysreflexia.

NCLEX® Standards: Prioritize delivery of care. Assess and manage client with an alteration in elimination (e.g., bowel, urinary).

2.37 ① Option #1 is correct. The key to answering this is to review the time frame and the vital signs. The time out of the operating room is one hour. There are no other vital signs to compare, so you have to make a clinical decision based on the information you are given. BP may be normal or may be low (no comparison); HR may be elevated but no comparison, RR is ok; however, urine output is only 45 mL/hr. Is this a trend? No, this is one hour post-op. Is this a complication? No. The client needs to maintain hydration with IV fluids to maintain a CVP of 5 to 10 mm Hg to help with renal perfusion. (This is normal range for CVP reading.) Option #2 is incorrect. There can be complications involved with this intervention, but in reality there is no need to place this client in this position. The client is not in shock. Option #3 is incorrect. There is no indication the client is hypothermic. Options #4 is incorrect. This is a calcium channel blocker and would result in the BP being decreased. This is not our goal! We want to keep the client perfused. BP needs to be maintained or increased, but definitely not decreased!
I CAN HINT: Priority Strategy: Organize priority nursing plan/interventions based on the key concepts.
NCLEX® Standards: Prioritize delivery of care. Provide post-op care.

2.38 ① Option #1 is correct. This is the position that aids in spreading out the spaces between the ribs for needle insertion. Option #2 is incorrect as the client should not cough while the needle is inserted in order to avoid puncturing the lung. Option #3 is incorrect as no more than 1,000 to 1,500 mL should be removed in the first 30 minutes. Approximately 100 mL of pleural fluid is used for diagnostic studies. Option #4 is incorrect as a thoracentesis requires a sterile technique.
I CAN HINT: Priority Strategy: Organize priority nursing plan/interventions based on the key concepts. Refer to the book *Nursing Made Insanely Easy* for a review of the priority care for diagnostic procedures such as thoracentesis, bronchoscopy, any test ending in "gram," etc.
NCLEX® Standards: Use precautions to

prevent injury and/or complications as associated with a procedure or diagnosis. Prioritize delivery of care. Assist with invasive procedures (e.g., central line, thoracentesis, bronchoscopy).

2.39 ③ Option #3 is correct. Epoetin (Epogen) stimulates the production of red blood cells. The desired outcome would be the hematocrit is within the defined range. Options #1 and #2 are incorrect for this medication. Option #4 is still too low and does not indicate a desired outcome from this medication.
I CAN HINT: Priority strategy: Remember to think about the desired outcome. It is important to also know the normal ranges for the values in each of the options:
Calcium—9.0 to 10.5 mg/dL (2.25 to 2.62 mmol/L); Magnesium—1.3 to 2.1 mEq/L (0.7 to 1.1 mmol/L); Hematocrit—37 to 47%; RBC—4.2 to 5.4 x 10^{12}/L.
NCLEX® Standard: Evaluate response to medications.

2.40 ③ Option #3 is the correct answer. Lactulose is used to reduce the amount of ammonia in the blood of clients with liver disease by drawing out the ammonia from the flood that is in the colon where it is removed from the body. Lactulose may also be used to treat constipation since it pulls water into the colon to facilitate movement of waste through the GI system. Option #1 is incorrect. Neomycin decreases the normal flora in the intestines to reduce bacterial activity on protein. This is the action of the drug versus the outcome. Option #2 does occur as a result of the action of the drug, but the question is asking about the desired outcome from the medication. Option #4 is not correct. A potential complication from this medication may be metabolic acidosis if too much bicarbonate is lost in the stools. If anything, this pH would indicate an undesirable effect versus a desired outcome.
I CAN HINT: Priority Strategy: Remember to think about the desired outcome. "POO," from the book *Pharmacology Made Insanely Easy*, will help you remember the major concepts for lactulose.

- **P**SE (portal system {hepatic} encephalopathy) and constipation are indications
- **O**rientation (LOC) should be monitored
- **O**utput (stools) and electrolytes should be monitored; outcome: Serum ammonia WDL (or at least decreasing)

NCLEX® Standard: Evaluate response to medications.

2.41 ④ Option 4 is correct. The desired outcome is that the client is no longer demonstrating symptoms of fluid overload due to the inappropriate antidiuretic hormone. The hematocrit should be 3x the hemoblobin and it is. The value would be dilutional if SIADH treatment was not effective. Option #1 is incorrect since the specific gravity remains elevated. Remember the range is from approximately 1.003 to 1.030. The low values indicate the urine is dilute and the high values indicate concentrated urine. The range in the middle, 1.012 to 1.017 indicates appropriate hydration. Option #2 is incorrect. It would be low due to being diluted. Option #3 is incorrect; this value is elevated. If this occurred following treatment, then the client lost too much fluid.
I CAN HINT: Priority Strategy: Remember to think about the desired outcome. Refer to the book *Nursing Made Insanely Easy* for a review. The key to answering this correctly is to link the labs with fluid volume overload and cluster the labs together. Note that with fluid overload, the BUN, serum sodium, serum osmolality, and Hct values will be decreased. The urine specific gravity will be elevated since the client has an inappropriate amount of inappropriate antidiuretic hormone.
NCLEX® Standard: Evaluate response to medications/treatment.

2.42 ③ Option #3 is correct. Decreased hepatic gluconeogenesis and increased tissue glucose uptake may result in hypoglycemia in clients with Addison's disease. Option #1 is incorrect. There may actually be an elevation in the calcium. The normal calcium level is 9 to 10.5 mg/dL (2.25 to 2.62 mmol/L). Option #2 is incorrect. Serum potassium actually may be increased with Addison's disease, and option #4 is incorrect, since the sodium is typically decreased. The normal serum potassium is 3.5 to 5.0 mEq/L (3.5 to 5.0 mmol/L); normal serum sodium is 135 to 145 mEq/L (135 to 145 mmol/L); and the serum glucose is 70 to 110 mg/dL (3.9 to 6.1 mmol/L).
I CAN HINT: Priority Strategy: Remember to think about the desired outcome. Addison's

disease is caused by a decrease in secretion of the adrenal cortex hormones. There is a decrease physiologic response to stress, vascular insufficiency, and hypoglycemia. There is a decrease in the aldosterone secretions (mineral corticoids), which normally promote concentration of sodium and water and excretion of potassium. As a result of this, the sodium may be low and potassium elevated.
NCLEX® Standard: Evaluate response to medications/treatment.

2.43 ① Option #1 is correct. Terbutaline is a tocolytic agent which decreases contractions from occurring in preterm labor. It activates beta 2 receptors resulting in smooth muscle relaxation in the uterus. The objective is to prevent labor until fetus is ready for extra-uterine life. Option #2 is incorrect. Oxytocin would stimulate contractions, but not terbutaline. Options #3 and #4 are incorrect. Option #3 would not be a desired outcome since late decelerations indicate utero-placenta insufficiency. Option #4 is incorrect since a decrease in variability indicates a decrease in oxygenation.
I CAN HINT: Priority Strategy: Remember to think about the desired outcome. Refer to the book *Pharmacology Made Insanely Easy* to further review terbutaline and the priority information necessary to remember. If you were unable to remember this, just think about the other reason a client may be prescribed terbutaline. Does asthma ring a bell? If not, let's ring it for you! Now, think about this for a minute ... if this drug is used for clients with asthma to relax the alveoli, then it would make sense that it would relax the uterus since they both have beta 2 receptors. See you can do this! Focus on what you know!
NCLEX® Standard: Evaluate response to medications.

2.44 ④ Option #4 is correct. This clinical presentation could be a problem with autonomic dysreflexia. A major cause of this is a full bladder. Option #1 is incorrect. The assessment has been provided; it is time for a nursing action. Option #2 is incorrect. The position needs to be the reverse Trendelenburg position to assist in lowering the blood pressure. The head of the bed needs minimal manipulation since the spinal cord and head need to remain in alignment. Option #3 is not priority with this client.
NCLEX® Standard: intervene in an emergency.

2.45 ② Option #2 is correct. This nursing action is incorrect for this client. The client should be almost upright in bed with the feet and legs on the mattress in order to decrease venous return to the heart, which will result in a decrease cardiac workload. The elevation of the legs will increase the venous return causing an increase in the preload. This could be unsafe for this client due to the suspicion of heart failure. Options #1, #3, and #4 are all within the standards of care for a client with heart failure.
I CAN HINT: Prioritizing Strategy: Organize the priority nursing interventions based on the key concepts. *(Recognize limitations of staff members.)*
NCLEX® Standards: Recognize limitations of self and others and seek assistance. Implement measures to promote circulation (e.g., active or passive range of motion, positioning and mobilization).

2.46 ③ Option #3 is correct. There is a need for further intervention and teaching about the standard of care for this client with an AV fistula. Blood pressure, blood samples, or infusing fluids or medications in the access site of the extremity that has a vascular access site should NOT be performed. Options #1, #2, and #4 are appropriate standards of care for this client.
I CAN HINT: Prioritizing Strategy: Organize the priority nursing interventions based on the key concepts. *(Recognize limitations of staff members.)*
"PATENT" will help you remember the care of the AV fistula:

Patency is evaluated by "hearing a bruit or feeling a thrill."

Assess the pulses distal to the access site.

The blood pressure or blood samples should NOT be taken on this extremity.

Evaluate weight, blood pressure, peripheral edema, lung and heart sounds, and vascular access site before and after dialysis.

Note: Most common side effects from dialysis include hypotension, headache, muscle cramps, and bleeding from site.

The COMPLICATIONS that may occur include: dialysis disequilibrium

syndrome (cerebral edema and neurologic complications, including headache, nausea, vomiting, seizures). Others include: sepsis, Hepatitis B and C.
NCLEX® Standards: Provide care for a client with a vascular access site before and after hemodialysis. Recognize limitations of self and others and seek assistance.

2.47 ④ Option #4 is the answer. Standard precautions are the appropriate type of infection prevention for all clients with hepatitis. Droplet precautions are not necessary for these clients. There is no need for a mask due to how Hepatitis B is transmitted which is by blood and blood products. The nurse would need to put on gloves while giving a bath as outlined in the infection prevention protocol for Standard precautions from the CDC. The UAP needs to put on gloves and review the appropriate infection prevention standards for this infection. Options #1, #2, and #3 do not require further intervention, since they are following the appropriate standards of care.
I CAN HINT: Prioritizing Strategy: Organize the priority nursing interventions based on the key concepts. *(Recognize limitations of staff members.)* The key to answering this question correctly is to understand that hepatitis requires the infection prevention guidelines of standard precautions that include blood and body fluids. Refer to *Nursing Made Insanely Easy* for an overview of the different kinds of infection prevention procedures.
NCLEX® Standards: Apply principles of infection prevention. Recognize limitations of self and others and seek assistance.

2.48 ① Option #1 is correct. Areas of flexion, especially the antecubital area should be avoided on the initial attempt. Other IV sites to avoid would include the veins that were previously injured by infiltration or phlebitis; veins of an affected extremity: mastectomy, dialysis access; veins of an extremity affected by a stroke or neurologic trauma; veins in the lower extremities and sclerosed or irritated veins; and/or areas of previous venipuncture sites, areas of inflammation or bruising. This nurse needs additional information regarding the standard of care for IV access with a focus on IV sites to avoid. Option #2 is acceptable practice and does not require additional intervention. 18- or 20-gauge needle or catheters are recommended for blood or rapid administration of fluids. Remember the larger the gauge of needle or cannula, the smaller the needle or cannula. A 22-gauge needle or catheter is the most common size for typical IV fluids. Option #3 is correct practice. There is no need for further teaching with the RN. A note to remember, however, is that it can be easy to mistake the heparin 1–10,000 units as a flush solution. Be alert and CAREFUL! Option #4 is correct practice. This information should all be documented clearly in the nursing notes.
I CAN HINT: Prioritizing Strategy: Organize the priority nursing interventions based on the key concepts. *(Recognize limitations of staff members.)* Note that ANTecubital is NOT the first place to start an IV because the client CAN'T bend arm or be as mobile with this location.
ANT = CAN'T
NCLEX® Standards: Insert, maintain or remove a peripheral intravenous line. Recognize limitations of self and others and seek assistance.

2.49 ③ Option #3 is correct. The client should maintain bed rest; avoid flexion; keep extremity straight for 3 to 6 hours following the procedure. The LPN needs direction from the RN regarding the standard of care for the client. This is dangerous to have the client up to the bathroom. Options #1, #2, and #4 are within the standard of care for this procedure. There is no need to immediately intervene with these nursing actions.
I CAN HINT: Prioritizing Strategy: Organize the priority nursing interventions based on the key concepts. *(Recognize limitations of staff members.)*
NCLEX® Standards: Use precautions to prevent injury and/or complications associated with a procedure or diagnosis. Recognize limitations of self and others and seek assistance.

2.50 ③ Option #3 is the correct answer. These medications should only be administered one time a day. The current order reads twice daily, so the order needs to be verified with the provider of care. Option #1 is incorrect since these should be administered on an empty stomach. Option #2 is incorrect since the medication order is incorrect, and needs to be rewritten prior to even getting to the bedside to administer the medication. Option #4 is incorrect. Once again, the priority is the incorrect order that is written in the stem of the question. While the client does need to know that orange colored tears and urine are expected outcomes, the question is inquiring about the "priority of care".

I CAN HINT: Priority Strategy: Verify if order is appropriate and accurate. The book *Pharmacology Made Insanely Easy*, by Manning, Loretta and Rayfield, Sylvia outlines an easy way to remember both of these drugs. *Nursing Made Insanely Easy* has a quick approach to the "Rights to Medication Administration." The key to answering the question is to know the frequency the medication is being administered in the stem of the question is incorrect.

NCLEX® Standards: Evaluate appropriateness and accuracy of medication order for client. Prepare and administer medications, using rights of medication administration.

2.51 ① Option #1 is correct. It does need to be questioned. The order for pyridoxine (B_6) should be decreased instead of increased. Pyridoxine (B_6) decreases the effect of Levodopa and can result in toxic effects. This also means that foods high in pyridoxine (B_6) should also be decreased. These foods include avocado, bananas, bran, eggs, hazelnuts, legumes, organ meats, shrimp, tuna, and wheat germ. Option #2 does not need to be questioned. Spironolactone is a potassium sparing diuretic and will assist in holding on to potassium that will assist with this low level. (Potassium-Normal—3.5 to 5.0 mEq/L or 3.5 to 5.0 mmol/L) Options #3 and #4 are correct for these clients.

I CAN HINT: Priority Strategy: Verify if order is appropriate and accurate. An easy way to remember when to increase or decrease pyridoxine can be found in the book *Pharmacology Made Insanely Easy*, by Manning and Rayfield. Just remember there is an "L" in Levodopa to assist you in remembering the need to Lower the pyridoxine and an "I" in Isoniazid to assist you in remembering the need to increase the pyridoxine. See how EASY that is! You CAN do it!

NCLEX® Standards: Evaluate appropriateness and accuracy of medication order for client. Review pertinent data prior to medication administration (e.g., contraindications, lab results, allergies, potential interactions).

2.52 ③ Option #3 is the correct answer. Propranolol (Inderal) is contraindicated in clients with HF and COPD. It is possible the health care provider overlooked this in reordering all of the client's previous medications. The oxygen, and digoxin are appropriate. There is no specific order regarding the rate of infusion or any fluids to be infused. Since the client is on po fluids, this is probably a heparin/saline lock. This order should be clarified. However, option #3 is a priority due to the risk involved with a nonselective beta blocker for a client with COPD and with HF. The nonselective beta part is a risk for the COPD. Any type of beta blocker can slow the heart rate down, and should not be administered if a client has HF. Option #2 does not need to be discussed, since the client has COPD. These clients typically do not receive large amounts of oxygen.

I CAN HINT: Priority Strategy: Verify if order is appropriate and accurate. The key to successfully answering this question is to focus on the diseases and the medications. Beta blockers decrease the contractility, renin release, and sympathetic output. Beta 1 affects one heart. Beta 2 affects 2 lungs. The book *Pharmacology Made Insanely Easy* will assist you with the names of these. For now, however, keep in mind that propranolol (Inderal) is a nonselective beta blocker, which means it affects both beta 1 and beta 2. If a client has COPD, do we want the drug to block the beta receptors in the lungs? Of course not, you are so correct! The client would get into further respiratory problems. Remember the "*Road Block to Beta Blockers.*" If the client has a slow heart rate, we would not administer the med. Low blood pressure may need to hold. Asthma —not if nonselective. Diabetics—masks low blood sugar. Safety is the issue!

NCLEX® Standards: Evaluate appropriateness and accuracy of medication order for client. Review pertinent data prior to medication administration (e.g., contraindications, lab results, allergies, potential interactions).

2.53 ④ Option #4 is correct. Due to the age of the client, the medical diagnosis, and the procedure, there may be a risk for this test. There is a risk for a decrease in renal perfusion and the IVP requires a dye which requires the client to have effective renal function to excrete the dye. Since the renal function is unknown, the order needs to be verified due to the possible risk to the client. Option #1 is incorrect since the order may not even be appropriate for this client.

Options #2 and #3 are incorrect since the order may not be implemented due to the risks involved. Remember, as clients age the renal function decreases, diabetes mellitus may also result in alteration in renal perfusion, and the dyes used in the procedure require renal excretion of the dye.

I CAN HINT: Priority Strategy: Verify if order is appropriate and accurate .Refer to the book *Nursing Made Insanely Easy* for a review of the priority of care for the diagnostic procedures requiring dyes, such as grams, CAT Scan with contrast, and cardiac catheterizations.

NCLEX® Standards: Verify appropriateness and/or accuracy of a treatment order. Use precautions to prevent injury and/or complications associated with a procedure or diagnosis. Provide care and education for the adult client ages 65 through 85 years and over.

2.54 ② Option #2 is correct. Cardiogenic shock occurs secondary from heart/pump failure. This may be the result of heart failure, cardiomyopathy, valvular rupture, valvular stenosis, or dysrhythmias. The hemodynamic changes include crackles in the lungs, elevation in the central venous pressure reading (CVP) and the pulmonary artery wedge pressure (PAWP). Crackles must be reported due to the need for further intervention. This is indicative of fluid overload. Options #1, #3, and #4 are incorrect since the readings are still within the desired limits. The range for the cardiac output is 4 to 6 L/min and the range for the CVP is 1 to 8 mm Hg. The PAWP range is from 4 to 12 mm Hg.

I CAN HINT: Priority Strategy: Identify trends and changes. *Nursing Made Insanely Easy*, by Manning and Rayfield, will assist you in remembering these values.

NCLEX® Standards: Recognize trends and changes in client condition and intervene as needed. Manage the care of a client with alteration in hemodynamics, tissue perfusion and hemostasis (e.g., cardiac, peripheral).

2.55 ④ Option #4 is correct due to the trending of the vital signs. The HR increased and the BP dropped in addition to a decrease in the LOC. Option #1 is incorrect because the HR and urine output do not present with a significant change. Option #2 is incorrect because the CVP remains in the normal range and the BP has decreased. Option #3 is incorrect since the HR decreased; BP not increased significantly.

I CAN HINT: Priority Strategy: Identify trends and changes.

NCLEX® Standards: Recognize trends and changes in client condition and intervene as needed. Prioritize the delivery of client care.

2.56 ④ Option #4 is correct. Due to the infectious agents being smaller than 5 mcg, this client will be placed in Standard/Airborne precautions. The private room will have monitored negative airflow (air exchange and air discharge through HEPA filter). If the client is transported outside of negative-airflow room, then the client will wear a surgical mask. Option #1 is incorrect. The gown is not necessary, and the mask is not the appropriate mask. The mask should be the N95 respirator. Option #2 is not necessary. The visitors will just need to be educated about the appropriate infection prevention precautions in order to adhere to the standards. Option #3 is incorrect. The Standard of Care is three negative sputum smears.

I CAN HINT: Priority Strategy: Infection Prevention.

NCLEX® Standard: Apply principles of infection prevention (e.g., hand hygiene, surgical asepsis).

2.57 ② Option #2 is the correct answer. The key to answering this question is to understand the diagnosis of varicella (chickenpox) and the communicability. These are transmitted via contact and airborne. The incubation period is 14 to 16 days. Varicella is highly contagious, usually occurring in children under 15 years of age and presenting with maculopapular rash with vesicular scabs in multiple stages of healing. The communicability is 1 day prior to the lesions appearing to the time when all

lesions have formed crusts. The child should be isolated, and family members, health care providers, etc. need to follow the appropriate infection prevention precautions in order to prevent others from being exposed to the infection. Option #1, while it is important to keep the fingernails short to prevent scratching, is not a priority over option #2 due to the risk for others being exposed and possibly resulting in an infection. Option #3 is also important, but not a priority over option #2. Option #4 is incorrect; the water would be cool-tepid and no soap would be used.
I CAN HINT: Priority Strategy: Infection prevention.
NCLEX® Standard: Apply principles of infection prevention (e.g., hand hygiene, surgical asepsis).

2.58 ① Option #1 is correct. The high-risk factors for suicide include Caucasian males, advanced age, hopeless, living alone, family history of suicide, psychosis, substance abuse. Males 65 and older are high risk, especially males 85 and older. Diagnoses (psychiatric) are some of the most reliable factors for suicide such as substance disorders, schizophrenia, and depression. This client who is alone following the death of his wife is a high risk for suicide. Options #2, #3, and #4 are not within this category. They will be concerned, but typically do not consider suicide.
I CAN HINT: Priority Strategy: Environmental Safety. (Keep client/environment safe (suicide, falls, equipment, etc.). It would be important for you to be able to compare and contrast who is highest risk for suicide. "SUICIDE" will assist you in organizing who these clients may be. Refer to *Nursing Made Insanely Easy*.
NCLEX® Standard: Assessing the potential for violence and use safety precautions (e.g., suicide, homicide, self-destructive behavior).

2.59 ③ Option #3 is correct. Clopidogrel (Plavix) is a platelet aggregation inhibitor and works by inhibiting the first and second phases of ADP-induced effects in platelet aggregation. Warfarin (Coumadin) interferes with the hepatic synthesis of vitamin K-clotting factors (II, VII, IX, and X). When these drugs are taken together, the risk is bleeding. Consequently, these drugs should not be administered together due to the drug-drug interaction resulting in bleeding. Option #1 is incorrect because they should be taken with food to minimize GI discomfort, but please note that even if this was stated appropriately for the client to take with food this still would not the PRIORITY. The drugs should NOT be administered together due to risk for bleeding. Remember, this is all about CLINICAL DECISION MAKING. Option #2 is important to monitor if the client is taking clopidogrel (Plavix), but in this situation the PRIORITY still remains that the health care provider should be notified due to the risk involved with taking these drugs together. Option #4 would be a concern for clopidogrel (Plavix), but once again this is not the PRIORITY, since it would be unsafe to administer these drugs together.
I CAN HINT: Prioritizing Strategy: Safe Medication Administration.
While you are in school, you learn to focus on facts and connect these facts to nursing concepts or drugs. Now that you are preparing for the NCLEX® and clinical practice that is all about clinical decision making, it is important to wire your brain for the importance of "comparing and contrasting" the options. Several of the options will actually be close to being correct; however, the stem of the question will drive you to the right answer! Now that you reflect back on the question, you may be able to see that the key is there are two drugs that should NEVER be administered together. This is where we begin!
NCLEX® Standards: Medication Administration. Review pertinent data prior to medication administration (e.g., contraindications, lab results, allergies, potential interactions). Evaluate appropriateness and accuracy of medication order for client.

2.60 ③ Option #3 is correct. Amphojel is an aluminum based antacid and can cause a complication with constipation. Amlodipine (Norvasc) is a calcium channel blocker with the action of inhibiting calcium ion influx across the cardiac and smooth-muscle cells. It can reduce myocardial contractility and oxygen demand. This drug can also result in an undesirable effect with constipation. The last effect we want for a client taking amlodipine (Norvasc) for the heart is a problem with constipation. This would result in stress to the heart. Option #1

is incorrect since amlodipine (Norvasc) can be taken with meals. Yes, you are correct that Amphojel can be and should be taken on an empty stomach, but the question reads that they are being discharged on both drugs. As a result of this statement, the option must be correct for both drugs. Option #2 is incorrect. Due to the action of this drug (as outlined in the correct rationale), the possible side effect would be bradycardia versus tachycardia. Option #4 is incorrect since the possible side effect is constipation versus diarrhea. The extra sodium in Gatorade would also not be great for a client with cardiac involvement requiring the amlodipine (Norvasc).
I CAN HINT: Prioritizing Strategy: Safe Medication Administration. When two drugs are referred to in the stem of the question, pay attention to these since the options must address both drugs. If part of the option is incorrect, the entire option is wrong. This is a great clinical decision making strategy.
NCLEX® Standards: Medication Administration. Educate client about medications.

2.61 ② Option #2 is correct. Both of these drugs can cause GI irritation which can result in peptic ulcers that can cause bleeding. Monitoring the hemoglobin and hematocrit will assist the nurse in determining if the client is developing any complications from bleeding. Option #1 is incorrect; although the dexamethasone (Decadron) may result in fluid retention, naproxen (Aleve) would not contribute to this clinical finding. The focus of the question is for both of these drugs. Option #3 could be an issue with dexamethasone (Decadron) alone, but not with naproxen (Aleve). Option #4 is incorrect since the concern would be more with hyperglycemia, but still not an issue for naproxen (Aleve).
I CAN HINT: Prioritizing Strategy: Safe Medication Administration. The key to answering this question appropriately is to remember the common undesirable effects both medications have in common. The book, *Pharmacology Made Insanely Easy*, by Manning, L. and Rayfield, S. has great images to help this information stick in the long-term memory. One look at "Cushy Carl" and you will remember forever the major undesirable effects from dexamethasone (Decadron).
NCLEX® Standards: Medication Administration. Evaluate client response to medication (e.g., therapeutic effects, side effects, adverse reactions).

2.62 ③ Option #3 is correct. Multiple sclerosis (MS) is an autoimmune disorder characterized by development of plaque in the white matter of the central nervous system (CNS). This plaque damages the myelin sheath and blocks impulse transmission between the CNS system and the body. As a result of this medical condition, there is an impairment of the physical mobility. The nurse's responsibility is to promote and maintain a safe home and hospital environment to reduce the risk of injury. Even a few throw rugs in the living room can be a safety hazard to this client. Option #3 should read "have no rugs due to the risk for falling" for this option to be correct. Options #1, #2, and #4 are correct plans for this client.
I CAN HINT: Prioritizing Strategy: Environmental Safety. (Keep client/environment safe (falls, equipment, etc.)
There is no "CURE" for the disease. The goals are to prevent complications and provide support for client/family.

- **C**ommunication is effective due to complication with (dysarthria) i.e., use a communication board or a speech language therapist; Cognitive changes – maintain function (reorient, place routine objects in routine places).
- **U**rinary tract infections—decrease risk of UTI by encouraging fluid intake, assist with bladder elimination (intermittent self-catheterization, bladder pacemaker, Crede).
- **R**esources and respite services for the client and family as the disease progresses.
- **E**ye patches should be alternated to treat diplopia. Teach scanning techniques. Environment—safety precautions.

NCLEX® Standard: Protect client from injury (e.g., falls, electrical hazards).

2.63 ③ Option #3 is correct. This client is experiencing autonomic dysreflexia which can occur in clients with spinal cord injuries at T6 or higher. A noxious stimulus below the level of injury triggers the sympathetic nervous system, which causes a release of catecholamines (epinephrine, norepinephrine). Most common stimuli causing the response are a full bladder or bowel, UTI, pressure ulcers, and/or skin stimulation. Severe hypertension, nausea, pounding headache, bradycardia, restlessness, flushing piloerection, and blurred vision are the most common body responses. Option #3 needs evaluated since a catheter kink or obstruction could result in this complication. Options #1, #2, and #4 are incorrect for this clinical presentation of autonomic dysreflexia. The key to answering this question is to understand the complication that can occur from the spinal cord injury. Option #4 is incorrect. Due to the clinical assessment findings, there is not time to complete a neurological exam. The exam needs to be a focused or a system specific assessment.
I CAN HINT: Prioritizing Strategy: Environmental Safety. Keep client/environment safe (falls, equipment, etc.) The key to answering this question correctly is to link the assessment findings in the stem of the question with the cause which is most likely the obstructed Foley. The key assessments were bradycardia, hypertension, diaphoresis, and flushing. *Nursing Made Insanely Easy*, by Manning and Rayfield, will further assist you in organizing the priority care for autonomic dysreflexia.
NCLEX® Standard: Protect client from injury (e.g., falls, electrical hazards).

2.64 ③ Option #3 is correct. This is an expected finding and is appropriate for the LPN/VN. The client is not experiencing any changes or complications that would contraindicate this assignment. Option #1 requires further assessment to analyze the cause of the dizziness. This is not an expected finding for this condition. Option #2 should be assigned to the RN due to the acute clinical presentation. Option #4 requires the RN due to the blood transfusion. This may cause complications with an allergic, hemolytic, or febrile reaction.
NCLEX® Standard: Delegate and supervise care of client provided by others (e.g., LPN/VN, assistive personnel, other RNs).

2.65 ③ Option #3 is correct. The LPN's scope of practice includes performing sterile procedures. This is an appropriate assignment. Option #1 should be the RN due to risks involved following surgery. Options #2 and #4 are appropriate for the UAP and within their scope of practice.
NCLEX® Standards: Delegate and supervise care of client provided by others (e.g., LPN/VN, assistive personnel, other RNs).

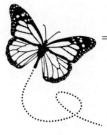
Notes

CHAPTER 3
Alternate-Item Format Questions

Acceptance doesn't mean resignation; it means understanding that something is what it is and that there has got to be a way through it.
— MICHAEL J. FOX

✔ Clarification of this test ...

The minimal standards evaluated with these alternate-item format questions are included below. Examples include: infection prevention, system-specific assessment, medication administration, management and prevention of complications with diagnostic procedures, safe use of equipment, education, and health promotion. Alternate-item format questions will also be integrated throughout the book. The minimal standards outlined below will also be organized within the specific client need category throughout the book.

☛ Apply principles of infection prevention (e.g., hand hygiene, aseptic technique, isolation, sterile technique, universal/standard enhanced barrier precautions).

☛ Properly identify client when providing care.

☛ Prepare and administer medications, using rights of medication administration.

☛ Educate client about medications.

☛ Recognize signs and symptoms of complications; intervene appropriately when providing care.

☛ Prioritize the delivery of client care based on acuity.

☛ Perform focused assessment/system-specific assessment.

☛ Use precautions to prevent injury and/or complications associated with a procedure or diagnosis.

☛ Obtain/Monitor/Intervene/Evaluate response to diagnostic tests (i.e., O_2 sat, glucose monitoring, etc.).

☛ Delegate and supervise care of client provided by others (e.g., LPN/VN, assistive personnel, other RNs).

☛ Use ergonomic principles when providing care (e.g., safe patient handling, proper lifting).

☛ Provide client nutrition through continuous or intermittent tube feedings.

☛ Assess client's need for sleep/rest and intervene as needed.

☛ Assess and manage client with an alteration in elimination (e.g., bowel, urinary).

☛ Assess client for abuse or neglect and intervene as appropriate.

Continued

- Collaborate with multi-disciplinary team members when providing care (e.g., physical therapist, nutritionist, social worker).
- Evaluate client response to medication (e.g., therapeutic effects, side effects, adverse reactions).
- Administer blood products and evaluate client response.
- Monitor IV infusion and maintain site (central, PICC, epidural, and venous access).
- Perform calculations needed for medication administration.
- Insert, maintain, and remove a peripheral IV line.
- Facilitate appropriate and safe use of equipment.
- Educate client about treatment.
- Assess need for pain management/intervene with nonpharmacological care.
- Provide post-operative care.
- Assist client to compensate for a physical or sensory impairment (e.g., assistive devices, positioning, compensatory techniques).
- Perform skin assessment and/or implement measures to maintain skin integrity (e.g., turning, respositioning).
- Provide pulmonary hygiene (e.g., chest physiotherapy, incentive spirometry).
- Manage the care of the client with a fluid and electrolyte imbalance.
- Provide care and education for the newborn, infant, and toddler client from birth through 2 years.
- Provide care and education for the adult client ages 65 and over.
- Manage the care of a client receiving hemodialysis or continuous renal replacement therapy.
- Follow security plan and procedures (e.g., newborn nursery security, violence, controlled access).

Adapted from: © National Council of State Boards of Nursing, Inc. (NCSBN). (2022). 2021 *RN Practice Analysis: Linking the NCLEX-RN® Examination to Practice*. Chicago: Author.

Adapted from: © National Council of State Boards of Nursing, Inc. (NCSBN). (2023) *Next Generation NCLEX® NCLEX-RN® Test Plan. Chicago*: Author.

Chapter 3: ALTERNATE-ITEM FORMAT QUESTIONS

3.1 What nursing interventions would be included in the plan of care for a client who is receiving chemotherapy with a WBC—3,000 mm³ (3 x 10⁹/L), Hgb—5.8 g/dL (58 g/L), Hct 21.2%, and platelets 72,000 mm³ (72 x10⁹/L)? **Select all that apply.**
① Verify appropriateness for invasive procedures with provider of care.
② Initiate fall precautions.
③ Assess temperature q shift.
④ Screen visitors and staff prior to entering room.
⑤ Initiate airborne precautions.

3.2 Which of these clinical findings would be the highest priority to report for an obstetrical client who is presenting with hyperemesis gravidarum? **Select all that apply.**
① Blood pressure increase from 110/70 to 130/84
② BUN—15 mg/dL (5.36 mmol/L)
③ Pulse increase from 68 bpm to 98 bpm
④ Urine output decrease from 95 mL /hour to 45 mL/hour
⑤ Serum sodium 146 mEq/L (146 mmol/L)

3.3 What personal protective equipment (PPE) is needed to suction a client with a tracheostomy tube that is coughing forcibly thick yellow secretions from the tube? **Select all that apply.**
① Gloves
② Face shield
③ Sterile gloves
④ Gown
⑤ Goggles

3.4 What are the appropriate plans of care for a client admitted with the diagnosis of Hepatitis C (HCV)? **Select all that apply.**
① Admit client to a private room with monitored negative-airflow.
② Apply gown, mask, and gloves whenever nurse is in contact with the client.
③ Apply a mask when in direct contact with client.
④ Place in a semi-private room with a client with HIV; wear gloves when in contact with blood/body secretions.
⑤ Discard all needles and sharps in the appropriate containers; do not recap.

3.5 Place in chronological order of priority regarding the process the triage nurse working in the outpatient clinic will return calls. **All of the options must be used.**

① The call from a client who had an electroencephalogram (EEG) 3 days ago and is requesting the results from the diagnostic test.
② The call from a daughter who states her elderly mother who is taking lithium is vomiting and lethargic.
③ The call from a new client who recently lost his job and is sharing with the nurse that he has no money to get his antihypertensive medication that was just prescribed.
④ The call from a client with Cushing's Disease who is presenting with muscle cramps and hot and dry skin.
⑤ The call from the daughter of an elderly client who is requesting her mother's medication be changed from a pill to a liquid to decrease risk of choking.

3.6 What actions would be appropriate for the client with meningitis who has just been admitted to the unit? **Select all that apply.**
① Institute droplet precautions.
② Prepare for a lumbar puncture.
③ Place the client near the nurses' station.
④ Encourage visitors.
⑤ Monitor neuro signs every 8 hours.

3.7 Which of these clinical assessment findings are most important to monitor and report for a client admitted to the medical surgical unit one-hour post abdominal surgery? **Select all that apply.**
① BP—150/90
② CVP—7 mm Hg
③ HR—120 bpm (weak)
④ Pulses bounding
⑤ RR—40/min

3.8 Put in chronological order the steps for transferring an older client from the bed to chair. **Use all of the options.**

| ① Lower the bed to the lowest setting. |
| ② Instruct client how to assist when possible. |
| ③ Assist the client to stand, and then pivot. |
| ④ Position the bed or chair, so that the client is moving toward the strong side. |
| ⑤ Assess if client understands the steps of getting up from bed to chair. |

3.9 What are the most important nursing actions to prevent back injury to the nurse when assisting a client out of bed to the standing position with no weight bearing to the left leg? **Select all that apply.**
① Apply an immobilizer to the left leg as prescribed and position client on side of bed.
② Position nurse's feet close together to assist with stability.
③ Instruct client to position arms around the waist of the nurse.
④ Instruct client to lean slightly forward and bear weight on the right foot as the left foot and leg are held forward.
⑤ Apply a transfer belt around the waist of the client.

3.10 An older client who is being seen on the medical unit by the health care provider complains of having difficulty sleeping at night. Which interventions are appropriate to include in the plan of care for this client? **Select all that apply.**
① Advise client to have a cup of warm tea 1 hour prior to going to bed.
② Avoid all caffeinated beverages.
③ Advise to drink a glass of water 20 minutes prior to going to bed.
④ Limit naps throughout the day.
⑤ Recommend the routine bath that is taken at home in the evening.

3.11 Point and click on the image where the nurse would initiate a gastrostomy feeding for an elderly client in the long-term facility.

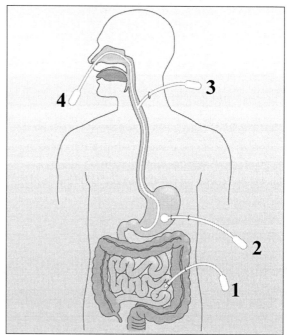

3.12 Following report, the nurse needs to assess each of these clients. Place in chronological order of care delivery how the nurse would assess this group of clients. (1 = highest priority)

| ① Client with a Theophylline level of 22 micrograms/mL. |
| ② Client with Pheochromocytoma and heart rate = 155 beats per minute. |
| ③ Client with carbamazepine level of 10 micrograms/mL. |
| ④ Client with Addison's disease and peaked T-waves on the ECG. |

3.13 What clinical observation findings indicate safety standards have been met for an elderly client one-day after experiencing a cerebrovascular accident (CVA) presenting with complete right-sided hemiplegia? **Select all that apply.**
① Bed exit alarm set for client.
② Restraint mitts in place after client attempted to pull out nasogastric tube.
③ Client left on bedside commode for privacy.
④ Client instructed to ambulate often, including toileting to assist with independence.
⑤ Nurses apply gloves prior to having any contact with the client.

3.14 What nursing plans are most appropriate for a client with chronic renal failure receiving dialysis and is presenting with constipation? **Select all that apply.**
① Discuss the importance of eating fruits such as oranges and bananas.
② Encourage the use of the laxative magnesium citrate.
③ Encourage a diet high in fiber.
④ Encourage exercise in plan of care working within the dialysis management protocol.
⑤ Discuss the importance of increasing fluids in the diet such as orange juice.

3.15 Following a comprehensive assessment of an older adult, what documentations indicate the nurse understands the normal physiological sensory function changes that occur in the older client? **Select all that apply.**
① Increased sensitivity to glare
② Decreased number of taste buds
③ Decreased ability in discriminating consonants
④ Decreased sensitivity to pain
⑤ Increased temperature sensation
⑥ Increased sensitivity to high pitched sounds

3.16 During the admission process for a toddler, what clinical findings will cause the nurse to suspect the parents are abusing the child? **Select all that apply.**
① The child cries when the parents leave.
② The child has a bruise on the right knee.
③ The parents blame the child for being so active and not sitting down when told.
④ The parents demand the child give the parents the stuffed animal the child is clinging to or child will get a whipping.
⑤ The child has some scars on abdomen that are small circular; parents had no idea they were present.

3.17 Which of the laboratory reports require the nurse to notify the provider of care for a client in labor who is now 6 centimeters dilated and is requesting an epidural for relief of pain?

Serum Laboratory Test	Client's Value
RBC	4,800 mm³ (48 x 10⁹/L)
WBC	9,000 cells mm³ (9 x 10⁹/L)
PLATELETS (PLT)	49,000/mm³ (49 x 10⁹/L)
Hemoglobin (Hgb)	11.5 g/dL (115 g/L)
Hematocrit (Hct)	34.5%

① Red blood cells (RBC)
② White blood cells (WBC)
③ Platelets (PLT)
④ Hemoglobin (HGB)

3.18 Which of these clinical findings for a client following a thoracentesis needs to be reported to the provider of care? **Select all that apply.**
   ① A small amount of drainage on the dressing
   ② Discomfort around the incision site
   ③ BP change from 130/80 to 100/68
   ④ SaO_2 86%
   ⑤ Hemoglobin 8 g/dL

3.19 Which of the clinical findings indicate the client is experiencing a therapeutic effect from a Dopamine hydrochloride drip? **Select all that apply.**
   ① Peripheral pulses difficult to palpate
   ② Urine output from 38 mL/hr to 62 mL/hr
   ③ 8 AM: BP—148/98, 10 AM: BP—96/66
   ④ 8 AM: BP—96/66, 10 AM: BP—130/88
   ⑤ Glasgow Coma Scale at 8 AM: 8, 10 AM: 14

3.20 What dose is the client receiving of lidocaine hydrochloride if it is infusing at 20 mL/hr and the dilution is 1,000 mg/250 mL?

   _____ mg/min.

3.21 Which of these recommendations would be included in a health promotion session for women experiencing stress incontinence? **Select all that apply.**
   ① Reduce fluid intake to 400–600 mL/day.
   ② Carry and wear incontinence pads when at home and away from home.
   ③ Discuss that incontinence is always secondary to an infection.
   ④ Review how to perform Kegel exercises.
   ⑤ Reduce the intake of tea, coke, and alcoholic beverages.

3.22 There is an order to administer 1000 mL of D5.45NS over 12 hours. The tubing calibration factor is 15 gtt/mL. The infusion would be set to_____ drops/min.

3.23 Place in chronological order the sequence of events for the nurse to implement in a Code Red (fire alarm). **Use all the options.**

| ① Contain the fire. |
| ② Aim the extinguisher to the base of the fire. |
| ③ Activate the alarm. |
| ④ Pull the pin on the extinguisher. |
| ⑤ Extinguish the fire from side to side. |
| ⑥ Remove any clients from the fire. |

3.24 Which of the clinical findings would a nurse document in the chart, report to health care provider, and include in the plan of care for client with Addison's disease? **Select all that apply.**
   ① Melanosis of skin
   ② Temperature: 97.8°F (36.6°C)
   ③ Spiked T waves on ECG monitor
   ④ BP—98/64
   ⑤ Weight gain of 2 lbs. (0.9 kg) over last two days

3.25 Which nursing actions would a nurse implement for a client with tuberculosis? **Select all that apply.**
   ① Restrict visitors to immediate family only.
   ② Apply on a gown.
   ③ Wear N95 respirator mask.
   ④ Place in a negative airflow room.
   ⑤ Wear gloves when in contact with the client's secretions.

3.26 Point and click to the clinical findings that would require the RN to seek physician consultation for an older adult client. **Select all that apply.**

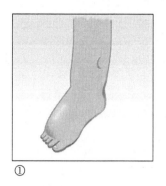
①

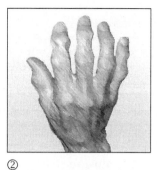
②

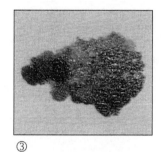
③

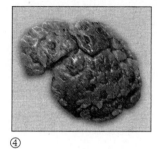
④

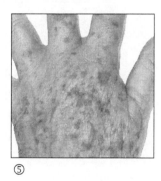
⑤

3.27 Which nursing actions are important to include in the plan of care for an older adult client who is on bed rest and the goal is to decrease the risk of developing pressure ulcers? **Select all that apply.**
① Reposition client every 3 to 4 hours to prevent pressure.
② When the client is lying on side, use the 30-degree lateral inclined position.
③ Massage bony prominences.
④ Use donut-type devices to minimize pressure.
⑤ Maintain the head of the bed at or below 30 degrees.

3.28 The client with a diagnosis of ulcerative colitis is scheduled for an ileostomy. Which area of the stomach would the nurse assess the stoma?

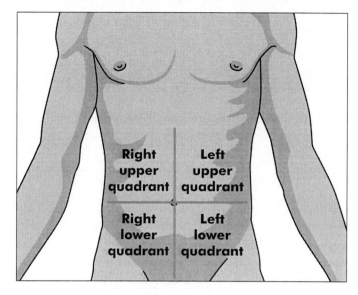

① Right lower quadrant
② Left lower quadrant
③ Transverse colon
④ Right upper quadrant

3.29 Which of these actions indicate the client understands the appropriate and safe use of the cane? **Select all that apply.**
① The cane and the unaffected leg move together.
② The cane is used on the side opposite of the affected leg.
③ The cane is placed approximately 3 feet in front.
④ The cane and the affected leg move together.
⑤ The cane is placed on the affected side and moved with the affected leg.

3.30 Which assessment findings for a client post-abdominal surgery indicate a positive outcome from the hourly use of an incentive spirometer? **Select all that apply.**
① The absence of fever.
② The absence of atelectasis on x-ray.
③ A decrease in pain on inspiration.
④ The absence of crackles upon auscultation.
⑤ A decrease in forced vital capacity.
⑥ A decrease in respiratory rate.

3.31 What actions are appropriate for the client with meningitis who has just been admitted to the unit? **Select all that apply.**
① Institute droplet precautions.
② Maintain head of bed at 30 degrees.
③ Place the client near the nurses' station.
④ Encourage visitors.
⑤ Monitor neurological signs every 8 hours.

3.32 In what order would the nurse prioritize the client assessments following the evening shift report. **Use all options.**

① A client with a decubitus on the sacral area with a temperature of 101°F (38.3°C).
② A client with type 1 diabetes mellitus and Bells Palsy scheduled for discharge in AM.
③ A client with a tracheostomy tube and was just admitted to the Med Surg unit from ICU.
④ A client receiving D5.2 NS at 80 mL/hour with 90 mL remaining in the bag.

3.33 What plans would be included for a client diagnosed with AIDS and has developed Pneumocystis jirovecii pneumonia (PCP)? **Select all that apply.**
① Apply an N95 mask when entering the client's room.
② Wear a gown when assisting the client with personal hygiene.
③ Wear a mask when assisting the client with personal hygiene.
④ Explain to client the reason he cannot have any visitors.
⑤ Wear gloves when assisting with personal hygiene.

3.34 Using the options below, place the steps in the order the nurse should follow to administer the unit of packed red blood cells (PRBCs) for a client who is diagnosed with anemia. **Use all the options.**

① Flush the intravenous tubing and line with normal saline solution.
② Verify the identifiers on the blood bag, ABO group, and compatibility against the client identifiers with another RN.
③ Remain with the client and watch for signs of a transfusion reaction during the start of transfusion.
④ Record the client's vital signs.
⑤ Check the PRBC's for abnormal color, clumping, gas bubbles and expiration date.

3.35 Which of these nursing actions would be implemented by the nurse to prevent an air embolus from occurring during the removal of the central venous catheter (CVC)? **Select all that apply.**
① Instruct client to bear down while removing the catheter.
② Position client in the recumbent position.
③ Position client in the semi-Fowler's position with head turned away from the insertion site.
④ Advise client to breathe in when CVC tube is being removed.
⑤ Encourage frequent coughing during the procedure.

3.36 Prior to administering the prescribed exenatide subcutaneous, which observations are most important? **Select all that apply.**
① Bed number
② Medical record number
③ Name band
④ Name of health care provider
⑤ Room number

3.37 Which nursing actions are appropriate for an obstetric client in labor and delivery who is receiving an I.V. infusion of oxytocin by an infusion pump? **Select all that apply.**
① Check the pump prior to starting the infusion to make certain it is working appropriately.
② Check the alarm settings when the client is repositioned in the bed.
③ Check the alarm settings after the client receives an epidural.
④ Check the alarm settings when infusion is started.
⑤ Check the alarm settings at the beginning of each shift.

3.38 Left heart cardiac catheterization indicated 40% ejection fraction with a cardiac output of 3.5 L/min, cardiac index – 2.2 L/min/m2, pulmonary artery diastolic-18 mm Hg. A stent was placed in client's proximal left anterior descending artery. During the post-procedure recovery, which actions would the nurse implement? **Select all that apply.**
① Encourage ambulation after procedure.
② Assess the neurovascular status of the left lower extremity distal to the catheter site per protocol and comparing to the right lower extremity.
③ Assess insertion site for bleedinge.
④ Evaluate BUN and creatinine post-procedure.
⑤ Measure intake and output every shift.
⑥ Place client on continuous cardiac monitor.
⑦ Start clopidogrel as ordered.
⑧ Encourage oral fluids.

3.39 During a teaching session, which of these foods would the nurse include when discussing foods that are good sources of iron? **Select all that apply.**
① Beans
② Dried fruit
③ Spinach
④ Tuna fish
⑤ Yogurt

3.40 Which interventions are appropriate for an older client to decrease complications with incontinence and also has a diagnosis of glaucoma? **Select all that apply.**
① Teach client how to perform Kegel exercises daily.
② Review the importance of taking the newly prescribed dicyclomine as ordered.
③ Review the importance of avoiding or decreasing the intake of caffeine.
④ Discuss the importance of increasing the use of a daily vitamin.
⑤ Review the rationale for avoiding alcohol consumption.

3.41 Which of these clinical observations would the unlicensed assistive personnel (UAP) report to the nurse for a client with a brain tumor who is taking dexamethasone? **Select all that apply.**
① Weight gain of 3 lbs (1.4 kg) since yesterday
② Tremors and diaphoretic skin
③ Blood pressure change from 150/90 to 120/78
④ Complains of a sore throat
⑤ Moist cough

3.42 The health care provider (HCP) prescribes phenytoin IV. The child weights 120 lbs. (55 kg). The order is to administer 20 mg/kg in three divided doses in 2-hour intervals. How many milligrams (mg) would the nurse administer per dose?
_____ mg (Record as a whole number.)

3.43 Which additional clinical findings would the nurse assess and document in the chart for a client presenting with a S_3 during the cardiac assessment? **Select all that apply.**
① Weight gain
② Enlarged abdominal girth
③ Photosensitivity
④ Headache
⑤ Swollen ankles

3.44 What are the appropriate nursing actions for a client with undiagnosed abdominal pain? **Select all that apply.**
① Give client sips of water.
② Apply heat on the abdomen.
③ Maintain client on bed rest.
④ Administer morphine for acute pain.
⑤ Assess intake and output.

3.45 Which nursing actions would the nurse delegate to the unlicensed assistive personnel (UAP) for a client with renal failure who has Fluid Volume Excess related to compromised regulatory mechanisms? **Select all that apply.**
① Monitor and record vital signs every 4 hours.
② Weigh client every morning using standing scale.
③ Listen to breath sounds every 4 hours.
④ Teach client the importance of eating oranges and bananas.
⑤ Remind client to save all urine for intake and output record.

3.46 The client with a spinal cord injury has been diagnosed with Clostridium Difficile. Which of these nursing actions indicate the nurse understands how to safely provide care for this client? **Select all that apply.**
① Place a client in a room with another client who has MRSA.
② Wash hands with hand sanitizer outside the client's room.
③ Put on a gown when in contact with the client.
④ Put on gloves when in contact with the client.
⑤ Refuses to share blood pressure cuff with the licensed practical nurse (LPN) who needs one for another client.

3.47 The staff nurse is leading an in-service orientation program regarding informed consents. Which of these statements indicates the nurse understands the manner for obtaining these consents? **Select all that apply.**
① "The nurse will assess knowledge level of surgical procedure and answer any questions client may have."
② "The client indicates a voluntary consent with this signature."
③ "The client's spouse must be present during the process of signing the informed consent."
④ "The information discussed with client prior to the signature will be adequately disclosed."
⑤ "The client was informed clearly of the risks involved with the procedure, surgery, etc., and verbalized this understanding prior to signing the consent."

3.48 Put in chronological order the nursing actions for a female client in labor and after membranes ruptured the umbilical cord prolapsed and was visible from the vagina. **Use all options.** (1 is the first step and 4 the last step.)

| ① Notify the health care provider. |
| ② Put sterile saline soaks loosely around the exposed cord. |
| ③ Assist client in the knee-chest position and administer oxygen. |
| ④ Increase the current IV flow rate. |

| |
| |
| |
| |

3.49 Based on the nurse's documentation, what is the priority of care for a client who is 6 hours postpartum?
Progress Notes: 9/16/23
Client's VS: HR—88 bpm
RR—22/min
BP—10 AM 128/80

Fundus palpated left of the umbilicus. Small amount of serosanguinous drainage on the perineal pad. ---------L.Shera, RN

① Notify the health care provider.
② Elevate the head of the bed.
③ Encourage client to empty bladder.
④ Prepare to insert a catheter to assist with voiding.

3.50 Which of these clinical assessment findings require immediate intervention by the nurse for a maternity client who is receiving oxytocin? **Select all that apply.**
① A maternal heart rate of 72 bpm.
② A maternal blood pressure of 168/90.
③ Fetal heart monitor displaying late decelerations.
④ Fetal heart monitor displaying a decrease in variability.
⑤ Crackles in client's bilateral lung fields.

3.51 Which of these clinical findings require further evaluation for the maternity client in labor? **Select all that apply.**
① FHR—140 bpm and increase in variability.
② Early decelerations noted on the external fetal monitor.
③ Complaints of pain throughout the contraction.
④ Amniotic fluid is meconium stained.
⑤ Variable decelerations noted on the external fetal monitor following the rupture of the membranes.

3.52 Which information would be included in the discharge teaching for the parents of a newborn? **Select all that apply.**
① The newborn can be bathed in a tub while the circumcision heals.
② Notify the health care provider for apnea lasting 5-10 seconds.
③ The diaper should be placed under the cord.
④ Antibiotic ointment should be applied to the cord three times a day.
⑤ Use alcohol to clean the length of the cord several times a day.

3.53 Which of these positive clinical symptoms for schizophrenia should be reported to the health care provider? **Select all that apply.**
① Alogia
② Anergia
③ Anhedonia
④ Delusions
⑤ Hallucinations

3.54 A client in diabetic ketoacidosis has an order to start an insulin drip with 40 units of insulin in 100 mL of Normal Saline, and the infusion pump is set at 10 mL/hr. How many units of insulin per hour is the client receiving?

_____ units/hour

3.55 Place in chronological order the steps for starting an IV. **All options must be used.**

| ① Release tourniquet. |
| ② Cleanse site thoroughly; re-cleanse if area is palpated prior to insertion. |
| ③ Insert needle with bevel up at 15-degree to 30-degree angle. |
| ④ Apply gloves. |
| ⑤ Apply the tourniquet 4 to 6 inches above the site. |
| ⑥ Cover the insertion site with a transparent dressing. |

| |
| |
| |
| |
| |
| |

3.56 Place in chronological order the steps the nurse would take when caring for a client and assisting a physician who is going to perform a liver biopsy for a client. **Use all of the options.**

| ① Review blood coagulation study results and make certain on the chart. |
| ② Position client on bed rest for 12 to 14 hours and on right side for 2 hours. |
| ③ Assess for right upper abdominal pain or referred shoulder pain; observe for tachycardia, hypotension. |
| ④ Verify the client has signed the informed consent. |
| ⑤ Instruct client to take a deep breath, exhale completely, and hold breath. |

| |
| |
| |
| |
| |

3.57 Which order would the nurse teach the client to use when taking albuterol with a metered-dose inhaler (MDI)? Place in chronological order. Use **all of the options.**

| ① Breathe out through the nose. |
| ② Activate the MDI when inhaling. |
| ③ Wash hands. |
| ④ Hold breath for 5 to 10 seconds and then exhale. |
| ⑤ Shake the inhaler. |

3.58 The nurse has an assignment of four clients. Prioritize in order from highest to lowest priority how the nurse would assess the clients following report. Use **all of the options.**

| ① A middle-aged client who is presenting with COPD and is sleeping up in a chair at night. |
| ② A young adult client with asthma who has a scheduled dose of a steroid inhaler to be administered. |
| ③ A middle-aged client with pneumonia who has been on antibiotics for 24 hours and needs pain medicine to assist with coughing and deep breathing. |
| ④ An older adult client who is presenting with a new onset of incontinence and does not seem to be as oriented as yesterday. |

3.59 Which clinical findings are most important to report to the health care provider during the immediate post-operative period for a client who is the recipient of a kidney transplant? **Select all that apply.**

① Pink and bloody urine
② BP—122/78 at 8 AM; BP—118/68 at 10 AM
③ T—99.1°F (37.3°C) at 8 AM; T—101°F (38.3°C) at 12 Noon
④ Day 1: Weight—120 lbs (54.4 kg) at 8 AM; Day 2: Weight—123 lbs (55.8 kg) at 8 AM
⑤ Serum postassium—4.8 mEq/L (4.8 mmol/L)

3.60 Which clinical findings would be documented in the progress notes for an older adult admitted with delirium? **Select all that apply.**

① The client is experiencing a progressive loss of judgment.
② The client has a recent history of a respiratory infection.
③ The change in behavior has been acute.
④ The client's family report a progressive loss of memory.
⑤ The client is becoming more disoriented over the last year.

3.61 Which of these dietary selections would the client limit indicating an understanding of the discharge teaching from the nurse with a new prescription for spironolactone.

① Rice
② Oranges
③ Bananas
④ Potatoes
⑤ Tomatoes

3.62 What information would be included in the discharge teaching for a client with a new prescription for levothyroxine? **Select all that apply.**

① Instruct to take a single dose before breakfast.
② Review the importance of not changing brands.
③ Advise to expect the normal change of a rapid weight loss.
④ Review how to take heart rate and to hold med if above 88 bpm.
⑤ Review the importance of notifying HCP if experiences tremors.

3.63 Which of these clinical findings for a client diagnosed with schizophrenia and is taking risperidone would require further evaluation by the health care provider? **Select all that apply.**

① Dry mouth
② Sore throat
③ Temperature—101°F (38.3°C)
④ Reddish brown urine
⑤ Complaints of dizziness when rising quickly

3.64 What information would be included in the discharge teaching plan for a client who is taking prednisone? **Select all that apply.**

① Monitor the BP three times a week and keep a log to share with HCP.
② Avoid potatoes, bananas, and cantaloupe.
③ Use salt instead of salt substitutes.
④ Report to health care provider any feelings of being hot, dry, and flushed.
⑤ Identify potential hazards for falls, after completing a home assessment.

3.65 Which information would be included in the teaching for a client who is prescribed alendronate tablets? **Select all that apply.**

① Instruct client regarding the importance of taking with 6-8 oz of water in AM.
② Review importance of taking med at least 30 min. prior to first beverage, food, or med of the day.
③ Review that client should expect some pain with swallowing when taking this medication.
④ Discuss importance of not lying down for at least 30 minutes after taking medication.
⑤ Remind client that if a dose is skipped to take two tablets on the same day.

Answers & Rationales

3.1 ①, ②, ④ — Options #1, #2, and #4 are correct. The strategy for answering this is to connect the laboratory values with the nursing interventions. Option #1 needs to be implemented due to the low platelet value. The client could hemorrhage from an invasive procedure if the platelets are this low. Option #2 is important to implement due to the low Hgb and platelets. With the low Hgb, the client may experience some weakness and the low platelet count may result in bleeding if the client was to fall. Option #4 is important due to the low WBC count that could result in infection. Option #3 is not correct, due to the frequency. This should be assessed more than q shift. Option #5 is not correct. The precautions should be protective.

NCLEX® Standards: Review pertinent data prior to medication administration (e.g., contraindications, lab results, allergies, potential interactions) and develop plan of care. Apply principles of infection prevention.

3.2 ③, ④, ⑤ — Options #3, #4, and #5 are correct. The strategy for answering this question correctly is to recognize obstetrical clients who present with hyperemesis gravidarum may present with fluid and electrolyte imbalance. The clinical findings will be the same as for any client who experiences vomiting for a significant period of time. Option #3 is correct. The heart rate is having to work harder and faster due to less volume in the client. Option #4 is correct. The fluid deficit is resulting in a trending down of the urine output. Option #5 is correct. The serum sodium is high which can occur with fluid deficit because it is more concentrated. Option #1 is not correct. The BP would not increase if a client is presenting with vomiting from hyperemesis gravidarum. Option #2 is not correct. The BUN would be elevated if client had been presenting with hyperemesis gravidarum.

NCLEX® Standard: Manage the care of the client with fluid and electrolyte imbalance.

3.3 ②, ③, ⑤ — Options #2, #3, and #5 are correct. Based on the Standard Precaution Guidelines from the Center for Disease Control, a face shield, sterile gloves, and goggles are necessary PPE to wear when suctioning a tracheostomy tube. Option #1 is not correct, since they are not sterile. Option #4 is not part of the PPE that is required for this procedure.

NCLEX® Standard: Apply principles of infection prevention (e.g., hand hygiene, surgical asepsis, isolation, sterile technique, universal/standard precautions).

3.4 ④, ⑤ — Options #4 and #5 are correct. Standard precautions in addition to appropriate needle disposal are required precautions. Option #4 has a client that would require the same infection prevention standards. Hepatitis C is transmitted through blood and body fluids. Twenty percent of HCV cases result from high-risk sexual behavior. Option #1 is incorrect based on CDC standards. There is not a need for a private room based on the type of organism/infection prevention guidelines necessary for the care of HCV. The negative airflow room would be a part of care for a client in airborne precautions. Option #2 is incorrect due to how Hepatitis C is transmitted. These PPE in this option are not included in standard of care when just "in contact" with client. If blood and / or body secretions are going to be splashed, then this will need to be stated in the option to assist you in making the correct decision. Option #3 is not necessary for this client.

I CAN HINT: Refer to *Nursing Made Insanely Easy* for an easy approach to remembering Infection Prevention Precautions.

3.5

② The call from a daughter who states her elderly mother who is taking lithium is vomiting and lethargic. *This is the priority client to return the call to since the symptoms indicate lithium toxicity.*
④ The call from a client with Cushing's Disease who is presenting with muscle cramps and hot and dry skin. *This client is most likely experiencing low potassium as evidenced by the muscle cramps and increase in the blood sugar as evidenced by the hot and dry skin, both of which can occur with this medical condition.*
⑤ The call from the daughter of an elderly client who is requesting her mother's medication be changed from a pill to a liquid to decrease risk of choking. *The order needs to be revised to prevent any possible risk for aspiration.*
③ The call from a new client who recently lost his job and is sharing with the nurse that he has no money to get his antihypertensive medication that was just prescribed. *The nurse needs to discuss the client's current situation and explore if there are any alternative medication support programs available.*
① The call from a client who had an electroencephalogram (EEG) 3 days ago and is requesting the results from the diagnostic test. *There is no immediate danger to the client, and the nurse needs to do some problem solving to determine what was the cause of the lack of communication.*

I CAN HINT: Apply the clinical judgment/cognitive skill, (generate solutions), to the triage nurse who will be returning calls based on priority of need.
NCLEX® Standard: Prioritize delivery of care.

3.6 ① ② Options #1 and #2 are correct. Clients with meningitis need to be in a quiet environment with limited stimulation. The nurses' station would be a lot of stimulation. Checks of neuro status should be done more frequently than 8 hours or per hospital protocol for this diagnosis.
NCLEX® Standard: Apply principles of infection prevention (e.g., hand hygiene, surgical asepsis, isolation, sterile technique, universal/standard precautions).

3.7 ③ ⑤ Options #3 and #5 are correct. The key words in the stem of the question are *"clinical assessment findings"* and *"one hour post abdominal surgery."* Option #3, HR—120 bpm (weak) is correct, since it is compensating from loss of blood. Option #5, RR—40/min is correct, since tachypnea indicates shock is progressing.

I CAN HINT: The strategy is to organize the system specific assessment findings around the types of shock. Note, BP and CVP are not low as would be the case if there was a decrease in volume. The CVP is within the defined limits. There is no need to report. The CVP would be decreased in a complication with bleeding or hypovolemia. Refer to the book *Nursing Made Insanely Easy* by Manning & Rayfield, for an easy way to remember the values. The pulse may be bounding in distributive shock. After you have an understanding of the concept, then when answering questions evaluating *"Select all that apply,"* each of the options can be treated like a *"true or false"* question. Remember, one step at a time. Stay focused on what you do know!

3.8

⑤	Option #5 is the initial step. Assess if client understands the steps of getting up from bed to chair. *Assessment is a great place to begin! Helps the nurse know what information to include when teaching.*
②	Option #2 is the second step. Instruct client how to assist when possible. *Remember, nurses must educate prior to interventions.*
①	Option #1 is the third step. Lower the bed to the lowest setting. *Remember client safety is always important prior to moving ahead with intervention!*
④	Option #4 is the fourth step. Position the bed or chair, so that the client is moving toward the strong side. *Now focus on the equipment or chair, and the side it must be on (strong side leads).*
③	Option #3 is the last step. Assist the client to stand and then pivot. *This is the last step to the goal!*

3.9 ① ④ ⑤ Options #1, #4, and #5 are correct. Option #1: The nurse should make certain the immobilizer is applied as prescribed and the client is positioned to the side of the bed to assist with the transfer. If the client has been in the supine position for an extended period of time, this will also facilitate decreasing the risk of orthostatic hypotension. Option #4 is correct. To assist with the client's center of gravity, have the client lean slightly forward from the hips. This will assist in positioning the trunk and head in the same direction as the transfer. The nurse should remain in front of the client positioning one foot forward and one back while flexing the hips, knees, and ankles. The nurse should use the leg muscles to assist the client to the standing position. Option #5: To assist with holding onto the client, the transfer belt will provide this security by providing a way for the nurse to control the movements. Option #2 is incorrect since the nurse should be positioned in a broad stance. The narrow stance will only provide the nurse with a narrow base of support. Option #3 may result in the nurse losing balance.

3.10 ④ ⑤ Options #4 and #5 are correct. Clients may be instructed in developing a bedtime routine. In addition to limiting naps throughout the day and continuing with routines from home, such as an evening bath, older clients can be encouraged to exercise regularly at least 2 hours prior to bedtime. Organize the sleep environment for comfort. Caffeine, alcohol, and nicotine should be limited at least 4 hours prior to bedtime. Fluids should be limited to 2 to 4 hours prior to bedtime. If client is anxious or stressed, engage in muscle relaxation. If someone is available for a back rub 15 min. prior to going to bed, this can also be very therapeutic. Warm milk and crackers can be soothing prior to going to bed. Options #1, #2, and #3 are incorrect for assisting with sleep.

I CAN HINT: Refer to *Nursing Made Insanely Easy* for an easy approach to remembering priority nursing care for geriatrics.

3.11 Line 2 is the correct option. The gastrostomy tube (Line 2) is surgically placed through an abdominal incision into the stomach. The distal end of the gastrostomy tube is secured to the anterior gastric wall, a tunnel is created, and a permanent stoma is formed by the proximal end of the tube being brought through the abdomen. Line 1 is a jejunostomy tube that is similarly placed as the gastrostomy tube; however, the distal end of the jejunostomy tube extends pass the pylorus into the jejunum. Line 3 is an esophagostomy tube. Line 4 is a nasogastric tube. This tube ends in the stomach.

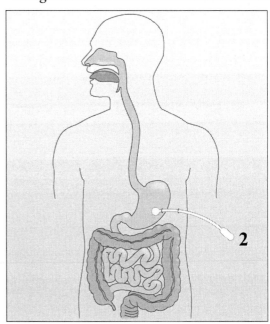

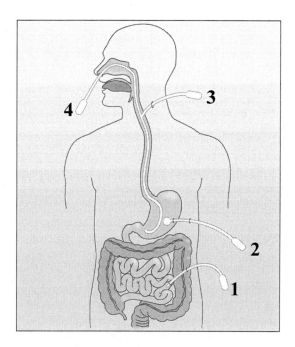

3.12

④ Client with Addison's and peaked T-waves on the ECG. *(Risk for dysrhythmias)*
② Client with Pheochromocytoma with heart rate of 155 beats per minute. *(tachycardia)*
① Client with Theophylline level of 22 micrograms/mL. *(slightly elevated; normal 10–20 micrograms/mL.)*
③ Client with Carbamazepine (Tegretol) level of 10 micrograms/mL. *(normal range)*

3.13 ① Options #1 and #2 are correct. Option #1:
② Bed exit alarm for client following a CVA is a safety need. Option #2: Restraint mitts are less restrictive and may be very effective to alleviate client pulling tubes and decreasing safety risks related to treatments and care. Option #3 is incorrect: Leaving client on bedside commode alone following a CVA can pose a safety risk due to the new paralysis from the CVA. Option #4 is incorrect. Client ambulation and toileting unassisted following a CVA can pose a safety risk as #3 above. Option #5 is incorrect. Applying gloves prior to any contact with the client is not necessary and is not included in the guidelines for infection prevention. If the nurse is going to handle blood or come in contact with body secretions, then yes, gloves would be imperative.

I CAN HINT: Note that the two correct options include doing something for the client to assist with safety. Options #3 and #4 both focus on client performing an aspect of care alone. Option #5 requires an understanding of Standard/Universal precautions.

3.14 ③ Options #3 and #4 are correct. Increasing fiber
④ will increase bulk and result in a decrease in constipation. Exercise will facilitate motility. Option #1 is incorrect. These two fruits are high in potassium and should not be given to clients in chronic renal failure due to risk with hyperkalemia which may lead to cardiac dysrhythmias. Option #2 is incorrect. Magnesium laxatives should not be given to clients in renal failure because this can lead to hypermagnesemia. Option #5 is incorrect since the client is in renal failure. If the option would have read "Take fluids within the client's fluid restriction", then this could have been an answer if orange juice was not included. It is unsafe to increase fluids without a limit due to the renal failure as well as including fluids high in potassium, such as orange juice.

I CAN HINT: Refer to *Nursing Made Insanely Easy* for an easy approach to remembering priority nursing care for chronic renal failure and dialysis.

3.15 ① Options #1, #2, #3, and #4 are correct. These
② are all sensory function changes that occur in
③ the older adult. Options #5 and #6 are both
④ decreased. They are cooler even when it is warm outside. The older client has a challenge hearing high-pitched sounds. The voices of women and children are difficult for older client to hear.

I CAN HINT: A quick and easy way to remember the physiological changes that occur in the older adult is that everything is decreased with the exception of "fat and sensitivity to glare". This is not fair, but this is just how the aging process goes!

3.16 ③ Options #3, #4, and #5 are correct. Option #3
④ indicates parents do not have an appropriate
⑤ understanding of growth and development for the 3 year old, and may have unrealistic expectations for this developmental stage. Option #4 also indicates a lack of understanding of how the child is feeling and not understanding that a decrease in the

child's sense of security is the reason the child is clinging to the familiar object. Option #5 is correct. Parents should have an idea the reason for the scars that are on their young child; at least the parents should have known these scars were present. Option #1 does not cause any suspicion of abuse since this is normal behavior for a toddler experiencing separation anxiety. Option #2 can occur with any active child.

I CAN HINT: Refer to *Nursing Made Insanely Easy* for an easy approach to remembering the clinical findings for a child who is suspected of being abused.

3.17 ③ Option #3 is correct. Platelets less than 100,000/mm³ are considered abnormal. Due to the risk for hemorrhaging, regional anesthesia would be contraindicated with a platelet count below 50,000/mm³. Options #1, #2, and #4 may be slightly abnormal in pregnancy and labor, but these would not be a contraindication for the provider administering the regional anesthesia.

I CAN HINT: "Plate" in platelet has 5 letters and if these are < 50,000/mm³, then the epidural should not be administered due to risk for bleeding. Refer to *Nursing Made Insanely Easy* for an easy approach to remembering these lab values.

3.18 ③ Options #3, #4, and #5 are correct. Options #3
④ and #5 should be reported due to the
⑤ significant drop which could be a result from a complication with bleeding. Option #4 should be reported due to the low value. This could indicate a complication from a pneumothroax due to the injury to the lung during the procedure. In addition to the SaO_2—86%, the nurse should monitor the vital signs, respiratory rate and rhythm, breath sounds hourly for the first several hours after the thoracentesis. Options #1 and #2 are expected findings following the thoracentesis, and should not be reported.

I CAN HINT: Refer to *Nursing Made Insanely Easy* for an easy approach to remembering the priority care for a client who had a "CENTESIS."

3.19 ② Options #2, #4, and #5 are correct. The
④ therapeutic effects of dopamine hydrochloride
⑤ are due to its positive inotropic effect on the myocardium, increasing cardiac output and improving circulation to the renal vascular bed. Therefore, the nurse would observe for an increase in hourly urine output, increased blood pressure and an increased state of alertness from the client. Options #1 and #3 indicate that the effect has not proven therapeutic or that the client is experiencing an adverse effect of the medication. These clinical findings indicate hypovolemia.

3.20 <u>1.3</u> mg/min.

STEP ONE: Calculate the concentration of mg/mL:

$$\frac{\cancel{1{,}000} \text{ mg}}{\cancel{250} \text{ mL}} = \frac{4 \text{ mg/mL}}{1}$$

STEP TWO: Multiply the number of milligrams per milliliter by the pump setting in milliliters per hour:

$$\frac{4 \text{ mg}}{1 \text{ mL}} \times \frac{20 \text{ mL}}{1 \text{ hr}} = 80 \text{ mg/hour}$$

STEP THREE: Divide the milligrams per hour by 60 to obtain milligrams per minute: 80 mg/hour divided 60 minutes = <u>1.3</u> mg/minute.

3.21 ④ Options #4 and #5 are correct. Option #4
⑤ will assist in strengthening the sphincter and structural supports of the bladder. Option #5 should be included because dietary irritants and natural diuretics, such as caffeine and alcoholic beverages, may increase stress incontinence. Option #1 is incorrect. If clients are non-restricted to the fluid intake, they should have a fluid intake of at least 2 to 3 L/day. Clients with stress incontinence may reduce their fluid intake to avoid incontinence at the risk of developing dehydration and urinary tract infection. This needs to be discouraged! Option #2 is incorrect. It would be more effective for a client to establish a voiding schedule that is regular than to carry incontinent pads. Option #3 is an incorrect statement. While a NEW symptom of incontinence may definitely occur in older clients if they have a UTI, the option reads "always" which does not take into account the numerous reasons for incontinence.

3.22　The answer is **21** drops/min.

STEP ONE: What is the volume to be infused? 1000 mL

STEP TWO: What is the duration of time for the infusion? 12 hours

STEP THREE: What is the drop factor? 15 gtt/mL

STEP FOUR:
Equation

$$\frac{\text{Volume (mL)} \times \text{Drop factor (gtt/mL)} \times 1 \text{ hour}}{\text{Time (hr)} \quad\quad\quad\quad\quad\quad 60 \text{ min}}$$

IV flow rate (gtt/min) =

$$\frac{1000 \text{ mL}}{12 \text{ hr}} \times \frac{15 \text{ gtt}}{\text{mL}} \times \frac{1 \text{ hr}}{60 \text{ min}}$$

Cancel out identical units. Multiply the numerator. Multiply the denominator. Divide the numerator by the denominator.

Answer = 20.8333 = **21** gtt/min

I CAN HINT: Always reevaluate to determine if the calculated number makes sense!!! You do NOT want to provide unsafe care. Always THINK and make great decisions.

3.23

⑥ Remove any clients from the fire.
③ Activate the alarm.
① Contain the fire.
④ Pull the pin on the extinguisher.
② Aim the extinguisher to the base of the fire.
⑤ Extinguish the fire from side to side.

I CAN HINT: The strategies for answering this question is to use the acronym "RACE" to assist you in remembering the emergency fire response. Fire extinguisher safety can be recalled by another acronym: "PASS"

RACE: Rescue, Activate, Contain, Extinguish

PASS: Pull the pin, Aim at the base of the fire, Squeeze the trigger, and Sweep from side to side

3.24　① Options #1, #3, and #4 are correct. Addison's
　　　③ disease is caused by a decrease in secretion
　　　④ of the adrenal cortex hormones. There is a decrease physiologic response to stress, vascular insufficiency, and hypoglycemia. The decrease in the aldosterone secretions (mineral corticoids) normally promotes concentration of sodium and water and excretion of potassium. As a result of this, the sodium may be low and potassium elevated. The clinical outcome is the client development of Addison's disease. The clinical findings have a very slow onset, and skin hyperpigmentation (melanosis) is a classic sign. This bronze coloring of the skin is seen primarily in those areas exposed to the sun, pressure points, joints, and in skin creases (especially on the palms). Option #3 is correct due to the elevated potassium level. Option #4 is correct due to the decrease in aldosterone. Option #2 is not a true statement. Option #5 should read "weight loss versus gain" in order for this option to be correct.

I CAN HINT: The key to answering this question successfully is to understand the pathophysiology for Addison's disease, and connect the clinical assessment findings and interventions to the medical condition. Refer to *Nursing Made Insanely Easy* for an easy approach to remember this concept with the image *"Anemic Adam"*!

3.25　③ Options #3, #4, and #5 are correct. Airborne
　　　④ precautions are used in addition to standard
　　　⑤ precautions for clients who are known or suspected to be infected or colonized with infectious organisms. Diseases known to be transmitted by air for infectious agents smaller than 5 micrometers (measles, varicella, pulmonary or laryngeal tuberculosis) must follow these precautions as outlined by CDC. Personal protective equipment (PPE) should include gloves due to being in contact with secretions, mask (N95 respirator) for known or suspected TB. In addition to standard precautions, the client should be in a monitored negative airflow (air exchange and air discharge through HEP filter). Doors of the room should be kept closed. If client leaves the room for a medical necessity, a small particulate mask should be applied to the client. Options #1 and #2 are not essential in airborne precautions.

3.26 ① Options #1 and #3 are correct. These would
③ definitely need physician consultation.

I CAN HINT: It is useful to understand the normal changes that occur with the aging process to assist in answering questions requiring further consultation.

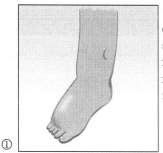

Option #1 is pitting edema, which can be a sign of fluid overload from medications, cardiac, renal, endocrine, or other medical conditions.

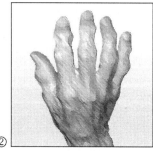

Option #2 may occur with clients who have osteoarthritis, but does not require a consultation. Heberden's nodes are palpable protuberances that are often associated with flexion and lateral deviation of the distal phalanx. These nodes may become tender, red, and swollen, often beginning in one finger and spreading to others. Usually, there is no significant loss of function, but clients are often distressed by the resulting disfigurement.

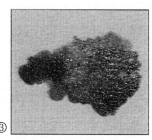

Option #3 is a melanoma which is malignant.

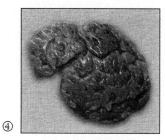

Option #4 is a seborrheic keratosis which is a commonly occurring normal skin lesion in older people. This lesion can be macular-papular lesion seen on neck, chest, back, and at hair line; can be warty, scaly or greasy in appearance. There is no need for consultation for this finding.

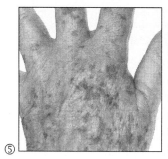

Option #5 is a senile lentigine. It is an irregular gray-brown macular lesion found on sun-exposed areas of the face, arms, and hands. This is also a commonly occurring normal skin lesion in the older adult which does not require further consultation.

3.27 ② Options #2 and #5 are correct for preventing
⑤ pressure ulcers. Both of these positions will assist in decreasing pressure ulcers. Option #1 is incorrect. It should have read "every 1 to 2 hours" for this to be correct. Option #3 is incorrect; Bony prominences should not be massaged. Option #4 is incorrect; these donut-type devices should not be used due to the risk for ulcers.

I CAN HINT: The key to answering this question accurately is to understand and remember the care necessary for preventing or relieving pressure. "PRESSURE" will assist you in organizing this care.

  Position change every 1–2 hours.

  Remember, nutrition is important; increase carbohydrates, protein, vitamin C, and zinc.

  Eggcrate—style or other foam mattress to allow circulation under the body and keep area dry.

  Special bed with mattresses that provides for a continuous change in pressure across the mattress.

  Silicone gel pads placed under the buttocks of clients in wheelchairs; sheepskin pads to protect skin.

  Use active and passive exercises to promote circulation.

  Remoisturize after bathing with lotion or protective moisturizer; remember to maintain head of the bed at/or below 30° or at the lowest degree of elevation.

  Eliminate rubbing excessively and hot water with skin care.

"AVOID" will assist you in reviewing what nursing care should NOT be done when preventing pressure.

  Avoid massaging bony prominences.

  Very important to teach chair-bound clients, who are able, to shift weight every 15 minutes.

  Omit using donut-type devices.

  If lying on side is used in bed, avoid positioning client directly on the trochanter; use 30° lateral inclined position.

  Do not rub excessively, and do not use hot water with skin.

3.28 ① Option #1 is correct. Ulcerative colitis usually affects only the innermost lining of your large intestine (colon) and rectum. To perform surgery for ulcerative colitis usually means removing your entire colon and rectum (proctocolectomy) which would result in the stoma being created in the right lower quadrant.

I CAN HINT: Refer to quadrants to assist you in organizing your physical assessment.

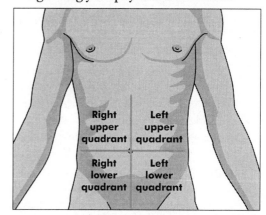

Right upper quadrant includes these anatomic structures: liver and gallbladder, pylorus, duodenum, head of pancreas, right adrenal gland, portion of right kidney, hepatic flexure of colon, portions of ascending and transverse colon.

Left upper quadrant includes these anatomic structures: left lobe of liver, spleen, stomach, body of pancreas, left adrenal gland, portion of left kidney, splenic flexure of colon, portions of transverse and descending colon.

Right lower quadrant includes these anatomic structures: lower pole of right kidney, cecum and appendix, portion of ascending colon, bladder (if distended), ovary and salpinx, uterus (if enlarged), right spermatic cord, right ureter.

Left lower quadrant includes these anatomic structures: lower pole of left kidney, sigmoid colon, portion of descending colon, bladder (if distended), ovary and salpinx, uterus (if enlarged), left spermatic cord, left ureter.

3.29 ② Options #2 and #4 are correct. The cane is
④ used on the side opposite of the affected leg for safety reasons. It provides more balance. Option #4 is correct; the cane and affected leg should be moved together. This will provide the necessary support for the balance due to one leg being weaker or not able to provide much support and will assist in the prevention

of falls. Option #1 is incorrect based on the rationale above. Option #3 is too far in front. This distance may result in a fall. Option #5 is incorrect; correct rationale in previous options.
I CAN HINT: Cane is used on the side opposite the affected leg. The affected leg and cane move together. Note, that the cane should be advanced simultaneously with the opposite affected lower limb. Evaluating for correct size ... Measure from the wrist to the floor. *Nursing Made Insanely Easy* will provide you with an EASY approach to remember the use of "CANES."

3.30 ① Options #1, #2, #4, and #6 are correct. A goal of incentive spirometer use is to reverse lung atelectasis, as noted by a decrease or absence of crackles upon lung auscultation, and to decrease the body temperature of a post-operative client with a fever. When atelectasis improves, so does gas exchange. As such, the client's respiratory rate decreases. Option #3 is incorrect as deep breathing may increase pain in the post-op client. Therefore, pre-medication of the client using an incentive spirometer should be considered. Option #5 is incorrect as forced vital capacity reflects the maximum amount of air that can be inhaled or exhaled from the lung, and should increase with the continued use of an incentive spirometer.
②
④
⑥

I CAN HINT: "BREATHE" will assist you in organizing the desired outcomes from the incentive spirometer.

Breath sounds improve

Respiratory rate decreased

Evaluate absence of atelectasis on x-ray

Absence of crackles upon auscultation

Temperature decreased

Heart rate within normal range

Evaluation of the oxygen saturation needs to be ongoing

3.31 ① Options #1 and #2 are correct. Clients with meningitis need to be in droplet precautions until antibiotics have been administered. The head of the bed should be elevated 30 degrees to assist with the cerebral brain flow. Option #3 is incorrect. A quiet environment is important for these clients, and the nurses' station has too much stimulation. Option #4 should be decreased due to need to minimize stimulation. Option #5 is incorrect. Neurological assessment should be done more frequently than 8 hours; these should be done per hospital protocol or as prescribed for this diagnosis.
②

I CAN HINT: Refer to *Nursing Made Insanely Easy* for an EASY way to remember the priority care.

3.32

③ Option #3 is first priority. *Due to the major risk for complications with the tracheostomy from obstruction or extubation which could be life-threatening.*
① Option #1 is the second, since the client has a temperature with the decubitus. *There is a need for further assessment to determine if the temperature is from an infection in the decubitus or a pulmonary infection. If the decubitus is draining, there can be additional complications with the temperature from the insensible fluid loss. The vital signs need to be evaluated in addition to the hydration status.*
④ Option #4 would be the third client to assess since there is a need to evaluate status of appropriate fluid replacement. *The assessment would include IV site for no signs of infiltration or phlebitis, characteristics of the lips and mucous membranes, skin turgor, urine output and specific gravity.*
② Option #2 would be the last to assess. *The client has no assessments to indicate client is unstable. Discharge is in the AM which indicates this client would be the last client to assess immediately following evening shift report.*

3.33 ② Options #2 and #5 are correct. Pneumocystis jirovecii pneumonia (PCP) is not easily transmitted from an infected client to a healthy person. This pathogen is frequently dormant in the body and is reactivated when the client's immune system is significantly depressed. Standard precautions must be adhered to with the client. It is not necessary to follow droplet or airborne precautions. Therefore, options #1, #3, and #4 are not appropriate for this client.
⑤

3.34 Rationale: To administer a blood transfusion the nurse should follow the steps as listed to ensure safe identification, administration and observation of adverse reactions.

④ Record the client's vital signs.
⑤ Check the PRBC's for abnormal color, clumping, gas bubbles and expiration date.
② Verify the identifiers on the blood bag, ABO group, and compatibility against the client identifiers with another RN.
① Flush the intravenous tubing and line with normal saline solution.
③ Remain with the client and watch for signs of a transfusion reaction during the start of transfusion.

3.35 ①② Options #1 and #2 are correct. Insertion or removal of a central line provides an opportunity for air to enter the client's circulation. A recumbent position and the Valsalva's maneuver increases intrathoracic pressure and pressure in the central veins. Option #3 and #4 are incorrect. While in option #3 turning head away from the insertion site would make it easier to remove the catheter and decrease the risk of infection, it has no effect on preventing air embolism. Option #4 could result in an air emboli. Option #5 is incorrect. Coughing is not encouraged. Bearing down would be more appropriate for preventing an air embolus.

3.36 ②③ Options #2 and #3 are correct. A National Patient Safety Goal of The Joint Commission is to improve the safety and accuracy of patient identification. In order to achieve the goal, nurses must use at least two client identifiers when providing care, administering meds, procedure, treatment or any services. Two appropriate identifiers include the client's name and the medical record number. Options #1 and #5 are incorrect since the client can change rooms and beds; these have not been identified as acceptable identifiers. Option #4 is incorrect. This also has not been adapted as criteria for client identification.
I CAN HINT: Notice that options #1, #4, and #5 all focus away from the client, but options #2 and #3 focus on the client by reviewing a medical no. and name band. Refer to *Nursing Made Insanely Easy* for a review of the standard.

3.37 ①④⑤ Options #1, #4, and #5 are correct. All equipment should be checked to make certain it is working appropriately prior to applying to a client. Options #4 and #5 are correct. The alarm settings should be checked for appropriate functioning when the infusion is started, at the start of each shift, and when client is moved from one unit to another. Option #2 is incorrect. The client being repositioned in the bed does not mandate checking the alarm settings. If the alarm is triggered, however, with repositioning client in bed, then the settings should be verified at that time. Option #3 is incorrect since there is no need after the procedure. This should have been done prior to any procedure versus following the procedure.

3.38 ②③④⑥⑦⑧ Options #2 is correct. Clients who have a cardiac catheterization need to be monitored for potential complications with perfusion (i.e., pulses, color, temperature, etc.) to the lower extremity distal to the catheter insertion site, comparing the assessments to the unaffected lower extremity. Option #3, another priority for the nurse is to assess the arterial puncture site for bleeding and report to the health care provider. Apply pressure first to minimize blood loss if bleeding. Option #4 is correct. BUN and creatinine should be evaluated pre and post-procedure due to risk for renal damage from the contrast dye resulting in an elevated BUN and creatinine levels. Option #6 is correct. The client needs to be monitored for cardiac dysrhythmias following the procedure. #7 is correct. Since a stent was placed in the client, clopidogrel per protocol is important to decrease the risk of a cerebrovascular accident resulting from emboli being released into the arterial system. Option #8 is correct. Encourage oral fluids to flush dyes from the client following the procedure. Option #1 is incorrect. The client will need to remain in the bed with the affected extremity maintained straight. Ambulation is not included in plan immediately following procedure. Option #5 is incorrect. Intake and output need to be monitored per protocol which is more than per shift.
I CAN HINT: Apply the clinical judgment/

cognitive skill, take-action (first-do priority interventions), when providing care for a client following a cardiac catheterization.
NCLEX® Standard: Use precaution to prevent injury and/or complications associated with a procedure.

3.39 ①② ③ ④ Options #1, #2, #3, and #4 are correct. These are high in iron. Option #5 is not high in iron.

3.40 ① ③ ⑤ Options #1, #3, and #5 are correct options. Urinary incontinence is a significant contributing factor to falls, fractures, depression, and altered skin integrity, especially in older adult clients. There are six major types of urinary incontinence. These include: stress, urge, overflow, reflex, functional, and total incontinence. Part of the collaborative care for these clients include: teaching how to perform Kegel exercises daily, reviewing the importance of avoiding or decreasing the intake of caffeine, and reviewing the rationale for avoiding alcohol consumption. Specific medications may result in the stimulation of voiding. Vaginal cone therapy may be used to strengthen pelvic muscles for clients with stress incontinence. Option #2 is incorrect. While dicyclomine (Bentyl) may be used to decrease urgency for a client with a neurogenic or overactive bladder, if the client has a diagnosis of glaucoma this medication can increase intraocular pressure. The order should be verified due to inappropriateness of this order for a client with glaucoma. Option #4 is incorrect. The vitamin is not prescribed to decrease incontinence.

I CAN HINT: The key to this question is that the client has glaucoma along with the incontinence. Anticholinergic medications are contraindicated for these clients. The intake of alcohol or caffeine that results in relaxation can cause an increase in the urination. Notice in the stem of the question, if there is a medication, disease, lab value, age, clinical assessment finding, etc., there is a reason, so pay attention! This will most likely be your clue to assist in selecting the correct answer(s).

3.41 ① ④ ⑤ Options #1, #4, and #5 are correct. Dexamethasone (Decadron) is a corticosteroid. It is an anti-inflammatory and can result in an increase in fluid retention as indicated by option #1, weight gain and may result in option #5, the moist cough. Option #4 is correct since the medication may cause the client to be immunosuppressed. The client may present with an infection such as the sore throat as many of the other signs of infection may be masked. Option #2 is incorrect. These symptoms indicate a complication with hypoglycemia and the actual undesirable effect of this medication would be hyperglycemia. Remember that *"if the skin is hot and dry the blood sugar is high, but cool and clammy means they need some candy."* Option #3 is incorrect since the BP has decreased. The undesirable effect from this medication would be an elevation in the blood pressure.

3.42 Answer = <u>367</u> mg

Step 1: Convert pounds to kilograms.
1 kilogram equals 2.2 pounds (120/2.2 = 55kg).

Step 2: Determine total dose
(20 mg x 55 kg = 1,100mg)

Step 3: Determine amount for each dose
(1,100/3= 367mg)

3.43 ① ② ⑤ Options #1, #2, and #5 are correct. This cardiac sound is indicative of heart failure. These are clinical findings for a client with right-sided heart failure. Options #3 and #4 are not associated with S_3. S_4 would indicate a complication with hypertension, diplopia, etc.

I CAN HINT: An easy way to remember this is that there are 3 syllables in "heart failure" and there is a S_3 with this complication. Left sided heart failure presents with lung involvement and there is an "L" in left and in lungs to help you remember. Right sided heart failure is the "Rest of the body" which includes peripheral edema, ascites, and jugular vein distention. There are 4 syllables in "Hy-per-ten-sion" and this is assessed by a S_4. Signs and symptoms of hypertension may be headache, diplopia, etc. See how EASY this can be! Clinical decision-making is all about using the information we already have in our head. The key is to move information from short term to long-term memory, so it can be retrieved and used!!

3.44 ③ Options #3 and #5 are correct. The key in
⑤ the stem of the question is "undiagnosed abdominal pain." The Do's for this diagnosis include: maintain on bed rest, place in a position of comfort, assess hydration, assess intake and output, assess abdominal status: distention, bowel sounds, passage of stool or flatus, generalized or local pain, keep client NPO until notified otherwise. Option #1 is incorrect since the client should get nothing by mouth. Option #2 is incorrect. Do not apply heat to the abdomen. Cold applications may provide some relief or comfort. Option #4 is incorrect. Do not give narcotics for pain control before a diagnosis of appendicitis is confirmed, because this could mask signs if the appendix ruptures. The Do Not's for this diagnosis include giving nothing by mouth, do not put heat on the abdomen, no enemas, no strong narcotics, and no laxatives.

3.45 ① Options #1, #2, and #5 are correct. These are
② within the scope of practice for the UAP and
⑤ are also appropriate for this concept of fluid excess. Option #3 is not within the scope of practice for the UAP. Option #4 would be incorrect for this client. These foods are high in potassium and could lead to a cardiac dysrhythmia if client took a diet high in these foods. Even if these foods were appropriate for the client, it is not within the scope of practice for the UAP to teach the client.

I CAN HINT: There are two concepts that are necessary for success with this question. The first is to understand the signs of fluid excess which are outlined below. Just remember these are all elevated just like the fluid volume is increased. The second concept is to understand the scope of practice for the UAP which includes basic care that does not require assessment, teaching, analysis, clinical decision making, or providing care for a client with unexpected outcomes.

↑ pulse

↑ temperature

↑ blood pressure

↑ in edema

↑ in ascites

↑ in crackles in lungs

↑ swelling neck (jugular vein distention)

↑ in confusion, headache and seizures

3.46 ③ Options #3, #4, and #5 are correct. This
④ diagnosis requires standard/contact
⑤ precautions. Hand hygiene; personal protective equipment (gloves and gown) if in contact with client. Disposal of infectious dressing material into nonporous bag. Dedicated equipment for the client or disinfect after each use. Option #5 is correct since the equipment should not be shared with clients if one is in contact precautions. Option #1 is incorrect. These clients should not be placed with a client with Clostridium Difficile. Option #2 is incorrect since this is not a sporicidal. Hands should be washed with soap and water.

3.47 ② Options #2, #4, and #5 are correct regarding
④ informed consents. Option #2 does indicate a
⑤ voluntary consent with the signature. Option #4 is correct. This indicates client will be provided with appropriate information prior to signature. Option #5 is correct. Client should have an understanding of the risks involved prior to signing consent. Option #1 is not within the scope of practice of the nurse. Option #3 is not standard.

3.48

③ Assist client in the knee-chest position and administer oxygen. *The priority nursing action is immediately relieve the pressure on the umbilical cord and increase the oxygenation that is being delivered to the fetus. In order to relieve the pressure, the mother should be positioned in the knee-chest, Trendelenburg, or modified Sim's. Another action that may need to be implemented is to insert sterile, gloved fingers into the vagina on either side of the cord and apply gentle manual pressure to relieve the pressure of the presenting part of the cord.*
① Notify the health care provider. *The second step would be to notify the health care provider of the emergency.*
④ Increase the current IV flow rate. *It is important to hydrate client in case there is a need for an emergency cesarean delivery or vaginal delivery.*
② Put sterile saline soaks loosely around the exposed cord. *The exposed cord should be kept moist, but the other options are a priority in order to reduce risk to the fetus.*

3.49 ③ Option #3 is correct. A full bladder may alter the location of the fundus of the uterus to the right or left of the abdomen. Option #1 is incorrect, since nursing interventions should be implemented prior to reaching out to the health care provider. Option #2 is incorrect. This will not alter the position of the uterus. Option #4 is incorrect, since the client should be able to void without any invasive procedures.

3.50 ②③④⑤ Options #2, #3, #4, and #5 are correct. Undesirable effects of oxytocin in the mother include hypertension, tachycardia, and fluid excess. Undesirable effects of oxytocin with the fetus include late decelerations, decrease in variability, and changes in the fetal heart rate. Option #1 is incorrect, since this is within the defined limits for the mother's heart rate.

3.51 ④⑤ Options #4 and #5 are correct. Option #4 is indicative the fetus has passed meconium while still in utero and may result in fetal distress. Option #5 may indicate a prolapsed cord requiring further evaluation and/or intervention such as position changes and/or an emergency delivery. Option #1 does not require further evaluation, since the FHR is within desired limits and increase in variability indicates oxygenation. Option #2 does not require further evaluation, since these decelerations indicate head compression and do not indicate a complication. Option #3 is an expected finding.

3.52 ③⑤ Options #3 and #5 are correct. The diaper should be placed under the cord to prevent from getting contaminated with urine and allow the cord to air-dry. Option #5 is correct, since the cord should be cleaned several times a day using a cotton swab with alcohol. Option #1 is incorrect. The newborn should be bathed with a sponge bath to prevent infection. Tub baths are not recommended until the circumcision is healed. Option #2 is incorrect because this is a normal assessment for a newborn. Option #4 is not the standard of care for cord care. Antibiotic ointments are typically only used if there are signs of an infection.

3.53 ④⑤ Options #4 and #5 are correct. Positive symptoms for schizophrenia include alterations in speech, delusions, and hallucinations. Options #1, #2, and #3 are negative symptoms. Affect, alogia, avolition, anhedonia, and anergia represent the negative symptoms of schizophrenia.

3.54 The answer is 4 units/hour.

Step 1: Determine the number of units in each milliliter of fluid.

40 units   = 0.4 unit/mL
100 mL

Step 2: Multiply the units per milliliter by the rate of milliliters per hour.

0.4 unit x 10 mL/hour = 4 units

3.55 Place in chronological order the steps for starting an IV.

② Cleanse site thoroughly; re-cleanse if area is palpated prior to insertion.
⑤ Apply the tourniquet 4 to 6 inches above the site.
④ Apply gloves. *(Standard Precautions)*
③ Insert needle with bevel up at 15-degree to 30-degree angle. *(After there is a good blood return, release the tourniquet.)*
① Release tourniquet.
⑥ Cover the insertion site with a transparent dressing. *(Do not place tape directly over the insertion site. A sterile gauze may be applied if not using the transparent dressing. Then always label the site with time, date, catheter/needle size and initials of the nurse. Label the infusion container with time it was hung; rate of infusion; any medications added. Do not encircle the arm with tape; this can restrict circulation to the extremity.)*

3.56

④	Verify the client has signed the informed consent.
①	Review blood coagulation study results and make certain on the chart. *(Physician needs to make certain client will not have any complications with the procedure bleeding due to altered studies. Liver is a very vascular organ.)*
⑤	Instruct client to take a deep breath, exhale completely, and hold breath. *(This should be done immediately before needle insertion. This will immobilize the chest wall and decrease the risk for penetration of the diaphragm with the needle.)*
②	Position client on bed rest for 12 to 14 hours and on right side for 2 hours. *(This will apply pressure and decrease risk for bleeding.)*
③	Assess for right upper abdominal pain or referred shoulder pain; observe for tachycardia, hypotension. *(These are assessments for complications following the procedure. Other complications may include pneumothorax; development of bile peritonitis.)*

3.57

③	Wash hands.
⑤	Shake the inhaler.
④	Hold breath for 5 to 10 seconds and then exhale.
②	Activate the MDI when inhaling.
①	Breathe out through the nose.

3.58

④	An older adult client who is presenting with a new onset of incontinence and does not seem to be as oriented as yesterday. *(The older client with a new onset of incontinence and acute confusion is the most acutely ill client out of these four and need immediate attention.)*
③	A middle-aged client with pneumonia who has been on antibiotics for 24 hours and needs pain medicine to assist with coughing and deep breathing. *(Assessment needs to be made to determine how client is progressing with coughing and deep breathing and to assess characteristics of the pain.)*
②	A young adult client with asthma who has a scheduled dose of a steroid inhaler to be administered. *(Next priority due to the need to administer the scheduled dose of steroid inhaler as close to the schedule as possible.)*
①	A middle-aged client who is presenting with COPD and is sleeping up in a chair at night. *(Last priority due to this is an expected behavior due to the chronic condition of COPD.)*

3.59 ③ Options #3 and #4 are correct. During the
④ post-procedure period following a kidney transplant, it is important to assess vital signs for fluid overload such as weight increase, hypertension, tachycardia; signs of infection such as fever, dyspnea, incisional drainage and redness. Option #1 is incorrect. This is an expected finding for the first few days. Option #2 is incorrect. If there was an immediate complication, it would be hypertension. Option #5 is incorrect since a complication would result in hyperkalemia.

I CAN HINT: The focus of care is on the recipient of a kidney transplant. "**RIPE**" will assist you in organizing the clinical findings for recipient clients during the post-operative care for a kidney transplant.

Rejection—can occur within days; 3 months is most common time, but can be as last as 2 years; ↑ WBCs, ↑ fever; ↑ serum creatinine and BUN levels, ↑ BP; tenderness over graft site—early sign along with malaise.

Infection—shaking, chills, fever, tachycardia, leukocytosis, and tachypnea.

Psychological needs—Fear of rejection.
Electrolytes and fluid status.
Evaluate to analyze renal graft function.

3.60 ②③ Options #2 and #3 are correct. Delirium is an acute that is typically secondary to another physiologic process. Options #1, #4, and #5 are indicative of dementia which is more progressive.
I CAN HINT: The bottom line is that "Delirium" is acute and reversible. "Dementia" slowly progresses and is irreversible.

3.61 ②③④⑤ Options #2, #3, #4, and #5 are correct. These are high in potassium and should be limited in the diet when taking a potassium sparing diuretic such as spironolactone. Option #1 is not high in potassium.

3.62 ①②⑤ Options #1, #2, and #5 are correct. Option #1 is correct. Levothyroxine should be taken on an empty stomach before breakfast. Option #2 is correct. Do not change brands since they are not bioequivalent. Option #5 is important to report since this may indicate they are receiving too much of the medication. Option #3 is incorrect since this may indicate too much of the medication. This rapid weight loss is not an expected outcome. Option #4 is incorrect due to the HR identified in the option. The medication should be held if HR is > 100 bpm. The client does need to learn how to take the HR, but the second part of the statement is incorrect. The entire option must be correct for the answer to be right.

3.63 ②③ Options #2 and #3 are correct. A sore throat and fever may be signs of agranulocytosis, an undesirable effect from this medication. Option #1 is an expected finding due to the anticholinergic effects with this medication, but does not need further evaluation. Option #4 may also be an expected finding and does not need further evaluation. Option #5 is a result of the orthostatic hypotension that may occur with this medication. This is a concern, but due to rising quickly does not mandate further evaluation by the health care provider. *This can happen to us with no medication if we rise too quickly.*

3.64 ①④⑤ Options #1, #4, and #5 are correct. Option #1 is important due to the risk for hypertension with the corticosteroid. Option #4 is important due to the risk for developing hyperglycemia. Option #5 is important due to the risk of hypocalcemia resulting in fractures if client was to fall. Option #2 is incorrect because the client should eat these foods due to the risk of developing hypokalemia. Option #3 is incorrect because with the risk of the sodium being elevated, the client should not use salt.

3.65 ①②④ Options #1, #2, and #4 are correct. Option #1 will assist in minimizing the complication with esophagitis. Option #2 will assist with absorption of the medication. Option #4 will decrease the most serious adverse effects of esophagitis and ulceration. Option #3 requires notification of the heath care provider. This is not an expected finding. Option #5 is incorrect. If a dose is skipped, wait until the next day 30 min. prior to eating breakfast to take the dose.

CHAPTER 4
Pretest

We delight in the beauty of the butterfly, but rarely admit the changes it has gone through to achieve that beauty.
—Maya Angelou

✔ **About this test ...**

This 65-item test will help you begin to pinpoint your study needs.
FOR BEST RESULTS:

☞ Complete the entire Pretest. Do NOT look in the back of the book for the answers until you have completed the exam.

☞ Spend a few minutes analyzing the questions you have missed. Use the test worksheet and Category Analysis to help determine your study needs. Once you determine your weak area(s), spend the next hour studying this content using a good review book as a guide.

**REMEMBER THAT MISTAKES ARE A WAY OF GROWING—
BE GENTLE WITH YOURSELF!**

"The reason that angels can fly is that they take themselves so lightly."
—G. K. Chesterson

These activities are taken from the National Council of State Boards of Nursing, Inc. (2022). 2021 *RN Practice Analysis: Linking the NCLEX-RN® Examination to Practice*. Chicago: Author.

TOMORROW—

☞ Skip to the chapter in this book that evaluates questions in the area(s) of your biggest identified weaknesses—we like to think of these as areas for growth!

☞ Take the test from this chapter and note the questions that you missed. Spend the next hour studying this content. ETC! ETC! ETC!

As NIKE says, "Just do it!"
You are the only one who can pinpoint your own study needs.
This is an excellent way to begin.

Chapter 4: PRETEST

4.1 Which of these dietary selections are priority for the nurse to instruct the client to avoid when taking buspirone for an anxiety disorder?
① Chicken salad sandwich
② Grapefruit juice
③ Yeast rolls
④ Grilled cheese sandwich

4.2 A client with chronic kidney disease has received a hemodialysis treatment. Which clinical findings are important for the nurse to monitor for disequilibrium syndrome? **Select all that apply.**
① Hgb – 9.0 g/dL (5.59 mmol/L)
② Nausea
③ Headache
④ Vomiting
⑤ BUN 38 mg/dL (13.57 mmol/L)
⑥ Acute confusion

4.3 Which of these clinical findings for a client diagnosed with schizophrenia and is taking clozapine would require further evaluation by the health care provider? **Select all that apply.**
① Dry mouth
② Sore throat
③ Temperature—101°F (38.3°C)
④ Occasional feeling of being tired
⑤ Complaints of dizziness when rising quickly

4.4 During an in-service presentation, the nurse is reviewing the care of a client diagnosed with a pneumothorax and has a left-sided chest tube in place. Which nursing actions should the nurse include during the presentation? **Select all that apply.**
① Discuss the importance of reporting tidaling in the under-water seal chamber.
② Review rationale for milking chest tubes routinely.
③ Evaluate the characteristics and trend amount of drainage per protocol.
④ Maintain the water-sealed system at the level of the chest-tube insertion site.
⑤ Review that there needs to be an order regarding the amount of suction control.
⑥ Teach the importance of clamping the chest tube during transport.

4.5 When providing care for an older adult client with diabetes mellitus, which nursing actions will the nurse delegate to the unlicensed assistive personnel (UAP)? **Select all that apply.**
① Check the client's technique for drawing up insulin into the syringe.
② Check to make certain that the bath water is not too hot for the client.
③ Assist client with muscle cramps by applying a heating pad to lower extremities while in bed.
④ Remind client to wear shoes when walking to the bathroom.
⑤ Assist client with ambulating after assisting with clipping toe-nails.
⑥ Assist client as requested with washing hair.

4.6 What is the priority of care for an elderly client who has a prescription for metformin?
① Discuss the importance of taking metformin with digoxin.
② Evaluate the HbA1c prior to administering the order.
③ Monitor AST and ALT while taking metformin.
④ Notify the provider of care and question the appropriateness of this order.

4.7 Which clinical findings will the nurse need to immediately report to the health care provider for a client with pneumonia? **Select all that apply.**
① Potassium: 4.5 mEq/L (4.5 mmol/L)
② Hemoglobin: 12.8 g/dL (7.94 mmol/L)
③ Heart rate (HR): 114 bpm
④ Respiratory rate (RR): 32 breaths/min
⑤ WBC Count: 20,000 mm³ (20 x 10⁹/L)
⑥ Breath sounds: coarse rales bilaterally
⑦ BUN: 12 mg/dL (4.29 mmol/L)

4.8 Which statement made by the client indicates an understanding of how to use a metered-dose inhaler?
① "I will exhale immediately after inhaling the medication."
② "I will take my respiratory rate for 60 seconds after the medication."
③ "I will wait 2 minutes before taking the second dose of medication."
④ "I will pull the top of the medication canister while I take a deep breath."

4.9 The nurse has reviewed the SBAR report and is planning the care for a client who has undergone a craniotomy. Which nursing interventions need to be included in the plan of care? **Select all that apply.**
① Evaluate hourly neurological assessments.
② Evaluate urine output every 4 hours.
③ Maintain head of bed in the supine position.
④ Initiate seizure precautions.
⑤ Encourage coughing and suction endotracheal tube hourly.
⑥ Apply and maintain sequential or pneumatic compression devices.
⑦ Assess for pain using appropriate pain scale.
⑧ Measure Jackson-Pratt drain output per protocol.

4.10 Which of these nursing instructions from the licensed practical nurse (LPN) requires further intervention for a client with an arterial ulcer of the left lower extremity from peripheral arterial disease (PAD)?
① Instruct client to keep legs elevated as much as possible.
② Discuss the importance of not crossing legs.
③ Review the importance of quitting smoking.
④ Teach the importance of stopping activity when pain in the calf occurs and start again when pain has subsided.

4.11 Which of these clinical assessment findings would require the nurse to immediately follow up for a client with poorly controlled diabetes mellitus? **Select all that apply.**
① Respiratory rate – 32 breaths/min
② Heart rate – 128 bpm
③ pH – 7.40
④ Urine output – 150 mL/hour
⑤ Warm, dry, flushed skin
⑥ Potassium level – 5.6 mEq/L (5.6 mmol/L)

4.12 Which interventions could the nurse delegate to the unlicensed assistive personnel (UAP) for a client with pneumonia? **Select all that apply.**
① Assess breath sounds every shift.
② Assist client in using a bedside commode.
③ Encourage client to drink oral fluids.
④ Teach client to cough and deep breathe.
⑤ Assist with mouth care.
⑥ Remind client to remain on bed rest.

4.13 The client diagnosed with chronic kidney disease (CKD) with a right forearm graft has an unlicensed assistive personnel (UAP) providing nursing care. Which nursing actions require immediate intervention by the charge nurse? **Select all that apply.**
① The UAP provides a fruit tray with oranges, bananas, and strawberries for a snack.
② The UAP weighs client on same scales every morning and records weight.
③ The UAP uses the right arm for the blood pressure reading.
④ The UAP provides a salt substitute with the breakfast tray.
⑤ The UAP reports a new congested cough to the charge nurse.

4.14 Which statement made by the nurse indicates an understanding of cost effectiveness for a postpartum client requesting peripads, diapers, tucks, and Americaine spray prior to discharge?
① "I will be glad to get these supplies for you."
② "It would be much better if you would just stop and pick them up on your way home."
③ "I will be happy to get them for you and pull some extras for you to take home."
④ "What items do you need until you leave to go home?"

4.15 The nurse is admitting an older adult client in the Emergency Department who is presenting with epigastric pain, dyspnea, and syncope. Vital signs are: T: 97.4° F (36.33° C), HR: 126 bpm, RR: 30 breaths/min, BP: 86/52 mm Hg. Abdomen distended; peripheral pulses weak bilaterally. Lips and mucous membranes dry and pale. Serum sodium: 147 mEq/L (147 mmol/L). SaO_2 89% on 2L O_2 per nasal cannula. Which potential nursing actions will the nurse include in the plan of care for this client? **Select all that apply.**
① Monitor for widening pulse pressure and report.
② Elevate the head of the bed to the high-Fowler's position.
③ Administer bolus of 1000 mL 0.9 Normal Saline as ordered.
④ Initiate seizure precautions.
⑤ Administer oxygen via nasal cannula.
⑥ Ensure venous access for 2 large-bore 14-to-16-gauge peripheral lines.

4.16 Which nursing approach would be most appropriate for obtaining a specimen from a retention catheter?
① Disconnect the drain at the bottom of the draining bag and drain urine into a sterile container.
② Disconnect the tubing between the catheter and the drainage bag and drain urine into sterile container.
③ Clamp the drainage tube. When fresh urine collects, open the tubing and drain into a sterile container.
④ Use a sterile syringe and needle to obtain urine from the porthole.

4.17 Which documentation indicates the nurse has an understanding of the priority of care for a young child admitted with the diagnosis of Kawasaki disease?
① Positioned on the right side with the head of the bed elevated.
② Applied lotion to decrease skin discomfort.
③ Monitored intake and output hourly.
④ Instructed UAP to encourage child to drink Gatorade q 2 to 3 hours to replace electrolytes.

4.18 What statement indicates the client understands the collection of urine specimen for culture and sensitivity?
① "I will call the lab before I collect my urine."
② "I will drink several glasses of water before the urine is collected."
③ "I will call the nurse to help me with aseptic technique."
④ "I will discard my first voiding in the morning."

4.19 Which nursing observation would most likely indicate an early side effect of the elderly client taking digoxin?
① Confusion
② Bradycardia
③ Constipation
④ Hyperkalemia

4.20 Which assessment of the lungs by auscultation would the nurse expect to evaluate if a client has a left lower lobe consolidation?
① Absent breath sounds
② Bronchophony
③ Vesicular breath sounds
④ Wheezes

4.21 Which of these undesirable effects would the nurse teach a client who is being discharged on diphenhydramine for allergic rhinitis? **Select all that apply.**
① Diarrhea
② Dry mouth
③ Nonproductive cough
④ Rash
⑤ Urinary retention

4.22 Which neonatal assessment finding would the nurse report to the health care provider 1 hour after delivery?
① A caput succedaneum that crosses the suture lines.
② A resting heart rate of 140 and a respiratory rate of 40.
③ Head circumference—34 cm. Chest circumference—30 cm.
④ The umbilical cord has 2 arteries and 1 vein.

4.23 Which assessment indicates a neonate with an infection is not fully recovered?
① Heart rate of 150.
② Axillary temperature of 98.6°F (37°C).
③ Weight increase of 4 oz. (0.11 kg).
④ Resting respiratory rate of 65.

4.24 Which of these documentations regarding restraints made by the LPN would need immediate intervention by the charge nurse?
① Restraints applied from an order that was written 48 hours ago.
② Restraints removed 1 hour ago and client allowed to exercise one hand at a time.
③ Bilateral radial pulses strong with sensation and movement in both hands.
④ Client cooperating with procedure and asking about the length of time for wearing restraints.

4.25 A client with a pneumothorax has a chest tube connected to a water-seal chest tube drainage system in place. Identify the chamber by placing an X where continuous bubbling should occur.

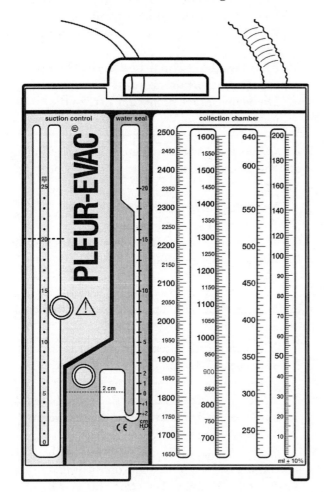

4.26 A client had profuse vomiting for 6 hours. Arterial blood gases note a pH—7.50; PaCO$_2$—40 mm Hg; and HCO$_3$—40 mEq/L (40 mmol/L). Which additional physical assessment finding would be most important for the nurse to report?

① Muscular twitching
② Kussmaul's respirations
③ Anuria
④ Irregular pulse

4.27 A client has a history of oliguria, hypertension, and peripheral edema. Current lab values include BUN—25 mg/dL (1.4 mmol/L); K—5.0 mEq/L (5.0 mmol/L). Which nutrients would be restricted in this client's diet?

① Protein
② Fats
③ Carbohydrates
④ Magnesium

4.28 What would be important for the nurse to include in a teaching plan for a child diagnosed with varicella? **Select all that apply.**

① Use aspirin for fever.
② Recommend bathing child in warm baths with a mild soap.
③ Isolate child until all the vesicles have crusted.
④ Instruct parents to keep fingernails short or apply mittens if necessary.
⑤ Provide quiet activities to keep child occupied.

4.29 The nurse is providing care for a client who is receiving intravenous (IV) therapy. The client begins presenting with a HR – 128 bpm, RR – 28/min, BP – 140/92 mm Hg, adventitious breath sounds, and a new congested cough. What nursing actions will be important to include in the plan of care? **Select all that apply.**

① Place client in the high-Fowler's position.
② Notify health care provider to recommend an increase in IV fluids.
③ Continue to monitor vital signs every shift.
④ Prepare to administer furosemide as prescribed.
⑤ Prepare to administer oxygen supplement as prescribed.
⑥ Reposition client every two hours.

4.30 Which action demonstrates an understanding of how to manage confidential information?

① Discuss this information with all of the nurse's colleagues.
② Document the information only on the client's flow sheet.
③ Review the information with those staff involved in the plan of care.
④ Share the information with nobody.

4.31 Which client would be assessed first after shift report?
① A client who had a lobectomy 24 hours ago with a chest tube inserted
② A post-operative larnygectomy client
③ A client with headaches of unknown origin
④ A client who is in Buck's traction

4.32 Which clinical finding would require the next dose of procainamide to be held?
① Premature ventricular contractions
② Occurrence of severe hypotension
③ Recurring paroxysmal atrial tachycardia
④ A sedimentation rate of 10

4.33 Which of these clients would be the highest risk for acquiring pneumonia during hospitalization?
① A post-operative client who is ambulating
② An infant in Bryant's traction who is frequently crying and screaming
③ A school-age child with diabetes mellitus
④ An immobile client with a spinal cord injury

4.34 A hospitalized client has been vomiting for three days with a low-grade temperature, and feels lethargic. Which nursing action is most appropriate in evaluating for fluid volume deficit?
① Obtain a urinalysis for casts and specific gravity.
② Determine client's weight and assess gain or loss.
③ Ask client to provide a 24-hour intake and output record.
④ Determine the quality of the skin turgor.

4.35 A client is placed on bed rest with an order to immobilize the right leg due to tenderness, increased warmth, and diffuse swelling. Which nursing action is most appropriate to maintain skin integrity?
① Apply a trapeze to client's bed.
② Assess bony prominence every 12 hours.
③ Apply granular spray to the bony prominence.
④ Turn client every 2 hours.

4.36 During the first 24 hours after a below-the-knee amputation, which nursing action would be most important?
① Notify the health care provider for a small amount of serosanguineous drainage.
② Elevate the stump on a pillow to decrease edema.
③ Maintain the stump flat on the bed by placing the client in the prone position.
④ Do passive range of motion TID to the unaffected leg.

4.37 Which measure would the nurse take in reducing the discomfort of gas pains in a one-day post-op client?
① Encourage a diet high in fiber.
② Assist with early ambulation.
③ Teach how to splint the abdomen with activity.
④ Position on right side.

4.38 What is the priority teaching for the mother of a school-age child with a piece of glass imbedded in the eye?
① "Put a loose eye patch over both eyes and have the child taken to an emergency room immediately."
② "Place pressure dressing to the injured eye and have the child taken to an emergency room."
③ "Remove the broken glass immediately from the eye to reduce the possibility of further trauma and apply Vaseline on the eyelid."
④ "Irrigate the injured eye with warm normal saline and apply a dressing to the eye."

4.39 What information would be priority for the LPN to report to the RN regarding a client who is 1 day post-operative for an appendectomy and is receiving hydromorphone?
① Client is requesting the pillow to assist with splinting when coughing.
② Client is slow to get out of bed due to being dizzy with quick movements.
③ Client's urine output was 270 mLs for an 8 hour shift from 400 mL's from previous 8 hour shift.
④ Client has hypoactive bowel sounds.

4.40 In which position would a nurse place a client who is in respiratory distress, extremely anxious, edematous, and cyanotic?
① Lithotomy position
② Low-Fowler's position
③ Sim's position
④ High-Fowler's position

4.41 A client has just been intubated in preparation for mechanical ventilation. What would be the first action to evaluate the effectiveness of the intervention?
① Assess lung sounds.
② Call for a stat chest x-ray.
③ Call for stat arterial blood gasses.
④ Suction the endotracheal tube.

4.42 A client has been complaining of sharp pain in the epigastric area and has an order for an antacid. Which statement made by the client indicates a correct understanding of when to take the antacid?
① "It is important to only take my medicine prior to bedtime."
② "By taking the medication before meals, I will decrease the side effects."
③ "I will take the medication one hour after meals."
④ "As I start to feel uncomfortable, I will take the medication."

4.43 The client needs an infusion of IV fluid at 40mL/hr. If the tubing set is calibrated at 15 gtt/mL, what is the drip rate?

Answer: _____ gtts/min

4.44 Which selection indicates compliance for a client with cardiac disease?
① Baked chicken, green vegetables, and fresh fruit
② Hot dog, cup of canned soup, and lettuce salad
③ Baked fish, baked apples, and avocado salad
④ Baked ham, rice, and fruit cup

4.45 An RN assigns the care of a new post-operative mastectomy client to an LPN. At the time of the assignment, the RN reminds the LPN not to take the blood pressure on the operative side. Later in the shift, the RN discovers the blood pressure cuff deflated, but still on the arm of the client's affected side. How would the RN handle the situation?
① Make a note to talk with the LPN in private after the shift is over.
② Call the LPN in for counseling to determine why directions were not followed.
③ Find the LPN and review the importance of not taking the blood pressure on the affected side.
④ Write up a report regarding the incident and place it in the LPN's personnel folder.

4.46 The staff nurse of an acute pulmonary unit is preparing notes that will be necessary for a shift report on assigned clients. What information is critical to communicate in a shift report on this unit?
① Laboratory work drawn on the client, arterial blood gas reports, nutritional intake, and vital signs for the shift.
② Any respiratory difficulty client experienced, tolerance to activity, sputum production, and significant variances in vital signs during the shift.
③ Name of the client's provider of care, date client was admitted, dietary intake and client's general condition.
④ Urinary output, PO and IV fluid intake, visits by attending provider of care, vital signs each time evaluated, any respiratory problems encountered.

4.47 An LPN is securing a Foley catheter on a female client. As the nurse walks in the room, the Foley drops on the floor. Which action would be the highest priority?
① Review aseptic technique with the LPN.
② Complete an incident report.
③ Get a new Foley catheter and assist LPN with the procedure.
④ Report the incident in the continuous quality improvement (CQI) report.

4.48 A provider has ordered timolol 1 gtt to both eyes bid. Point to the location of the eye where the medication will be placed.

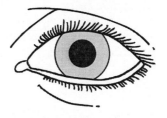

4.49 An elderly client is admitted to an inpatient psychiatric unit with an initial diagnosis of psychotic depression. What would be the priority nursing plan?

① Clarify perceptual distortions.
② Establish reality orientation.
③ Ensure client and milieu safety.
④ Increase self-esteem.

4.50 A client in an assisted living facility asks the nurse to sign as a witness for an advanced directive. What is the best intervention by the nurse?

① Notify the provider of care that the client needs a witness for the advanced directive.
② Politely decline the request by the client.
③ Sign the advanced directive as a witness.
④ Work with the client to find someone who is an unrelated third party.

4.51 A client diagnosed with a lower GI bleed has an order for 1 unit of packed red blood cells. What information is most important to be documented during this procedure?

① Vital signs prior to procedure
② Confirmation that the nurse alone verified the blood label information
③ The total volume that is to be infused
④ Vital signs before, during, and after procedure, date and time started and completed

4.52 Which of these clients would be seen immediately after report?

① A client who is 10 hours postpartum and presents with fundus midline and 1 cm above the umbilicus.
② A client who is 18 hours postpartum with a T—100.1°F (37.8°C), and has lochia rubra as a discharge.
③ A client who is 30 hours postpartum with a T—101.2°F (38.4°C), and has dark vaginal drainage.
④ A client who is 48 hours postpartum and is awakened during the night several times to urinate and noted that gown and bedding were wet from profuse diaphoresis.

4.53 What would be the plan of care for a client who has a blood sugar of 200 mg/dL (11 mmol/L) at 7:00 AM?

① Increase the PM dose of NPH insulin.
② Increase the AM dose of regular insulin.
③ Have the client wake up at 3:00 AM and evaluate the blood sugar.
④ Decrease the PM dose of NPH insulin.

4.54 Which nursing action represents the best technique to set up a sterile field?

① Place all supplies as close to the edge as possible.
② Wear gown and gloves at all times.
③ Set up the field above waist level.
④ Open supplies with sterile gloves.

4.55 During the shift report, a client's ventilator alarm is activated. Which action would the nurse implement first?

① Notify the respiratory therapist.
② Check the ventilator tubing for excess fluid.
③ Deactivate the alarm and check the spirometer.
④ Assess the client for adequate oxygenation.

4.56 What nursing intervention would be implemented within an hour prior to surgery?

① Administer an enema.
② Verify that the signed consent form is on chart.
③ Perform preoperative shave and scrub.
④ Evaluate for food or medication allergies.

4.57 A school-age client presents to the pediatric unit with symptoms of a headache, photosensitivity, stiff neck, and temperature 102.2° F (39°C). Which nursing plan of care is the priority?

① Provide safety teaching to family.
② Decrease environmental stimuli.
③ Implement seizure precautions.
④ Implement droplet precautions using a surgical face mask.

4.58 Which response by the client indicates an understanding of how to collect a 24-hour urine specimen?

① "I will discard the first morning voided specimen, and then collect the urine for 24 hours into one container."
② "I will start collecting all of the urine into one container after 8:00 AM and continue until 8:00 PM tonight."
③ "I will place urine specimens in a separate container."
④ "I will notify the nurse so a call can be made to the lab to start this test."

4.59 Which fluid would be the most appropriate for a client receiving furosemide and digoxin?
  ① Milk
  ② Gatorade
  ③ Orange juice
  ④ Water

4.60 One hour after a bronchoscopy is completed on a client, which nursing observation would indicate a complication?
  ① Depressed gag reflex
  ② Sputum streaked with blood
  ③ Tachypnea
  ④ Widening pulse pressure

4.61 What is most important for the nurse to include in the plan of care for a child presenting with mumps? **Select all that apply.**
  ① Apply a sterile gown, gloves, and mask prior to entering the room.
  ② Apply a surgical face mask when providing care to the client.
  ③ Apply sterile gloves when providing care to the client.
  ④ Wear gloves when starting an IV.
  ⑤ Place client in a negative-pressure room.
  ⑥ Apply a N95 mask on when entering the client's room.

4.62 An older adult client begins choking while eating dinner. Organize the steps in chronological order when performing the Heimlich maneuver. **All options must be used.**

① Thrust upward 6-10 times.
② Position nurse's thumb toward client, above the waist and below the rib cage wrapping one arm around the client.
③ Assess by asking client if he is choking.
④ Position self behind client.
⑤ Form a fist with one hand.
⑥ Other arm should be wrapped around the client placing that hand on top of the nurse's fist.

4.63 The nurse is assessing the emotional support available to an adolescent client who is starving herself. Which question would be most important for the nurse to ask in the assessment interview?
  ① "What do you consider your ideal weight?"
  ② "How does your eating habit change when you are around other people?"
  ③ "What happens at home when you express opinions that are different from those of your parents?"
  ④ "What do you think about your present weight?"

4.64 Which symptoms might alert the nurse to an alcohol problem in a client hospitalized for a physical illness?
  ① Depression, difficulty falling asleep, decreased concentration.
  ② Elevated liver enzymes, cirrhosis, decreased platelets.
  ③ Tremors, elevated temperature, complaints of nocturnal leg cramps, complaints of pain symptoms.
  ④ Flu-like symptoms, diarrhea, night sweats, elevated temperature, decreased deep tendon reflexes.

4.65 An elderly client with terminal cancer requests that the nurse give him a second dose of Morphine, so he "can get it over with." What is the nurse's next action?
  ① Give the client Morphine to help the client out of misery.
  ② Call the provider of care for an order for the extra dose.
  ③ Ask the client to read their Living Will document before the nurse makes a decision.
  ④ Gently refuse as this is beyond the nurse's scope of practice.

Category Analysis–Pretest

1. Pharmacology
2. Physiological Adaptation
3. Pharmacology
4. Physiological Adaptation
5. Management of Care
6. Pharmacology
7. Physiological Adaptation
8. Pharmacology
9. Physiological Adaptation
10. Basic Care and Comfort
11. Reduction of Risk Potential
12. Management of Care
13. Management of Care
14. Management of Care
15. Physiological Adaptation
16. Basic Care and Comfort
17. Basic Care and Comfort
18. Safety and Infection Control
19. Pharmacology
20. Physiological Adaptation
21. Pharmacology
22. Health Promotion
23. Health Promotion
24. Management of Care
25. Physiological Adaptation
26. Physiological Adaptation
27. Basic Care and Comfort
28. Safety and Infection Control
29. Reduction of Risk Potential
30. Management of Care
31. Management of Care
32. Pharmacology
33. Health Promotion
34. Physiological Adaptation
35. Basic Care and Comfort
36. Reduction of Risk Potential
37. Basic Care and Comfort
38. Reduction of Risk Potential
39. Pharmacology
40. Physiological Adaptation
41. Physiological Adaptation
42. Pharmacology
43. Pharmacology
44. Basic Care and Comfort
45. Management of Care
46. Management of Care
47. Safety and Infection Control
48. Pharmacology
49. Psychosocial Integrity
50. Psychosocial Integrity
51. Phamacology
52. Health Promotion
53. Reduction of Risk Potential
54. Safety and Infection Control
55. Physiological Adaptation
56. Management of Care
57. Safety and Infection Control
58. Basic Care and Comfort
59. Pharmacology
60. Physiological Adaptation
61. Safety and Infection Control
62. Reduction of Risk Potential
63. Psychosocial Integrity
64. Psychosocial Integrity
65. Management of Care

Chapter 4: ANSWERS & RATIONALES

Directions

1. Determine questions missed by checking answers.
2. Write the number of the questions missed across the top line marked "item missed."
3. Check category analysis page to determine category of question.
4. Put a check mark under item missed and beside content.
5. Count check marks in each row and write the number in totals column.
6. Use this information to:
   - identify areas for further study.
   - determine which content test to take next.

We recommend studying content where most items are missed—then taking that content test.

Number of the Questions Incorrectly Answered

Pretest	Items Missed																									Totals
C Management of Care																										
O Safety and Infection Control																										
N Health Promotion and Maintenance																										
T Psychosocial Integrity																										
E Physiological Adaptation: Fluid Gas																										
N Reduction of Risk Potential																										
T Basic Care and Comfort																										
Pharmacology and Parenteral Therapies																										

Answers & Rationales

4.1 ② Option #2 is correct. Grapefruit juice increases serum levels and effect; ingestion of large amounts of grapefruit juice is not recommended. Options #1, #3, and #4 are incorrect. There is no reason for these foods to be avoided.
NCLEX® Standard: Review pertinent data prior to medication administration (e.g., potential interactions).

4.2 ②③④⑥ Disequilibrium Syndrome is caused by too rapid a decrease of BUN and circulating fluid volume. It may result in cerebral edema and increased ICP (confusion); headache, seizures, nausea, and vomiting. Other problems may include blood loss, hypotension, sepsis, hepatitis B and C. Option #1 is not a sign of disequilibrium syndrome. Anemia (Decrease in hemoglobin) is a result of blood removal during dialysis. Client already has anemia from decrease in erythropoietin secretion. Option #5, BUN is elevated and the cause of this syndrome is from a too rapid decrease of BUN versus an increase in the lab value.
I CAN HINT: Apply the clinical judgment/cognitive skill, recognize cues (system-specific assessments). The topic, clinical findings (cues) of disequilibrium syndrome, focuses on the syndrome which include neurological findings.
NCLEX® Standard: Manage the care of a client receiving hemodialysis.

4.3 ②③ Options #2 and #3 are correct. A sore throat and fever may be signs of agranulocytosis, an undesirable effect from clozapine (Clozaril). Option #1 is an expected finding due to the anticholinergic effects with this medication, but does not need further evaluation. Option #4 may also be an expected finding and does not need further evaluation. Option #5 is a result of the orthostatic hypotension that may occur with this medication. This is a concern, but due to rising quickly does not mandate further evaluation by the health care provider. This can happen to us with no medication if we rise too quickly.
NCLEX® Standard: Evaluate client response to medication (e.g., therapeutic effect, side effects, adverse effects).

4.4 ③⑤ Options #3 and #5 are correct. The presentation should include the importance of monitoring the drainage characteristics. Review hourly and mark level on the collection chamber. Assess output in comparison to previous hour. Identify if there has been a trend with an increase or decrease in output. Note when the chamber is half full. Option #5 is correct. Option #1 is incorrect, since this an expected finding. Option #2, milking chest tubes routinely is not appropriate since it can increase pleural pressure. Option #4 is incorrect. Equipment for drainage should all be kept below the chest-tube insertion site. Option #6 is incorrect. Chest tubes should not be clamped except to assess for leak in the system per protocol.
I CAN HINT: Apply the clinical judgment/cognitive skill, take-action (first-do priority interventions, when providing care for clients with a chest tube in place.
NCLEX® Standard: Monitor and maintain devices and equipment used for drainage (e.g., surgical wound drains, chest tube suction, etc.).

4.5 ②④⑥ Options #2, #4, and #6 are correct. The older adult client may have changes in perfusion and not feel the hot water resulting in a burn. Diabetes mellitus may cause peripheral neuropathy which can result in numbness to the extremities causing the client not to recognize that the bath water is too hot. Option #4 is correct. The UAP's scope of practice does allow reminding the client to wear shoes to prevent injury to feet. Option #6 is correct. Option #1 is not within the scope of practice for the UAP. Option #3 is incorrect because it would be unsafe for a diabetic client who may have a neuropathy. Option #5 is incorrect because while the UAP is able to ambulate, the toenails should not be clipped by the UAP.
I CAN HINT: Apply the clinical judgment/cognitive skill, take-action (first-do priority interventions, when delegating care for clients with diabetes mellitus.
NCLEX® Standard: Assign and supervise care of client provided by others (e.g., LPN/VN, assistive personnel, other RNs).

4.6 ④ Option #4 is correct. As a client ages the kidney perfusion decreases. Metformin may result in a major complication with lactic acidosis. This should not be routinely administered to the geriatric client due to potential renal complications.
I CAN HINT: Renal function declines with age, along with a lot of other systems! The result is that many medications may lead to renal toxicity. This is the reason so many drug-drug interactions and undesirable effects with renal toxicity occur with the elderly client. This strategy will assist you in answering many of these type of questions related to the geriatric client. Option #1 is incorrect. If digoxin is taken with metformin, then digoxin may increase metformin concentrations. Option #2 does need to be monitored, but with the age of the client and the potential risk with lactic acidosis, option #4 is still a priority. HbA1c was most likely elevated for metformin to be ordered. It does need to be monitored while client is taking the medication. Option #3 is incorrect. For this option to be correct, it would need to read *"monitor renal function tests."* This medication is eliminated almost entirely unchanged by the kidneys.

4.7 ③ ④ ⑤ ⑥ The clinical findings that require immediate reporting support the concept of alteration in oxygenation. The elevated HR and RR reflect a sympathetic response to the tissue's increased oxygen requirements. Elevations in RR may also result from impaired gas exchange or acid-base imbalances. Option #5 is correct due to the pneumonia and will require antibiotic therapy. Increased WBC count is often seen with generalized inflammation. Option #6 is correct since this may progress to labored breathing as secretions become more consolidated. Options #1, #2, and #7 are within the defined reference range and do not require immediate reporting.
I CAN HINT: Apply the clinical judgment/cognitive skill, analysis of cues, to the disease process of pneumonia or the concept of alteration in oxygenation.
NCLEX® Standard: Recognize signs and symptoms of client complications and intervene. Manage the care of the client with impaired oxygenation.

4.8 ③ Option #3 is correct. The client should wait for 2 minutes prior to taking the second dose of medication. Option #1 is incorrect. The client should hold the breath as long as possible and then exhale through pursed lips. Option #2 is incorrect because pulse rate versus the respiratory rate should be monitored, since the medication may result in tachycardia. The key in this option is that it reads 60 seconds. The rate of the RR is important; however, it is important to assess the breath sounds to evaluate the effectiveness. Option #4 is not the correct procedure. The client should push the top of the medication canister while taking a deep breath.

4.9 ① ④ ⑥ ⑦ ⑧ Option #1 is correct. Hourly neurological assessments are indicated because frequent neurological exams will increase the likelihood of early detection and treatment of increased intracranial pressure. Option #4 is correct. Due to the craniotomy, there is a risk for seizures, so precautions are important to include in the plan of care. Option #6 is correct due to the immobility following the surgery. This increases risk of a venous thromboembolism, so prevention is important to include in the plan of care. Option #7 is correct. Pain can affect hemodynamic status and neurological stability. Assessment of pain with the client with altered mental status should be performed using a Behavioral Pain Scale. There are several versions of behavioral pain scales. These scales include non-verbal cues such as increased heart rate, blood pressure and respiratory rates. They also include grimacing, restlessness, and agitation. Option #8 is correct. Measuring Jackson-Pratt drain output is indicated for evaluation of post-operative blood loss. Option #2 is incorrect. This should be done every hour for early detection of endocrine disorders such as Diabetes Insipidus or Syndrome of Inappropriate Antidiuretic Hormone (SIADH). Option #3 is incorrect because of risk of increasing ICP. Recommended position is elevation of head of bed to 30 degrees. Option #5 is contraindicated due to risk of increasing intracranial pressure. It is important to maintain endotracheal tube patency, but suctioning does not need to occur hourly.
I CAN HINT: Apply the clinical judgment/cognitive skill, generate solutions (first-do priority plans), when developing a plan of care for the client who is receiving post-operative

care for a craniotomy.
NCLEX® Standard: Managing the care of a client with alteration in cerebral perfusion.

4.10 ① Option #1 is the correct answer since the nurse would need to intervene because this is not the Standard of Practice for this condition. Elevating legs would be appropriate for venous insufficiency. The other options are appropriate for PAD.

4.11 ① Option #1 needs immediate follow up.
② Tachypnea indicates a compensatory action
④ for the diabetic ketoacidosis (DKA) in the
⑤ attempt to decrease the CO_2 to compensate
⑥ for the metabolic acidosis from the DKA. The breath may also be acetone with a fruity smell. The HR option #2) may be increased due to the fluid deficit from the increase polyuria (option #4). Option #5 is due to the hyperglycemia. Option #6 is correct. This elevation in potassium is dangerous and can result in cardiac dysrhythmias. The potassium is high due to the attempt to correct the acidosis. Option #3 is not correct. It is within the normal reference range.
I CAN HINT: Apply the clinical judgment/cognitive skill, recognize cues, to the disease process of Diabetic Ketoacidosis. Memory strategy for option #5: *"Hot and dry your blood sugar is high. Cold and clammy, you need some candy!"* There are numerous concepts involved with this one disease process, but you CAN do this. You are mastering these concepts as you work through this book. We are proud of you!
NCLEX® Standard: Recognize signs and symptoms of client complications and intervene.

4.12 ② These correct options are within the scope of
③ practice for the UAP and appropriate for this
⑤ medical condition.
I CAN HINT: Apply the clinical judgment/cognitive skill, take-action (first-do priority interventions), when delegating care for clients with alteration in oxygenation such as pneumonia.
NCLEX® Standard: Assign and supervise care of client provided by others (e.g., LPN/VN, assistive personnel, other RNs).

4.13 ① Options #1, #3, and #4 are correct. Options #1
③ and #4 are correct because each of these
④ selections are high in potassium. Clients with CKD are unable to excrete potassium which may result in dysrhythmias. Option #3 is correct. This will result in too much pressure on the graft; charge nurse needs to intervene. Options #2 and #5 do not require immediate intervention, since these are included in the standard of care for clients with CKD.
I CAN HINT: Apply the clinical judgment/cognitive skill, take-action (first-do priority interventions), when providing care for a client with chronic kidney disease with a right forearm graft.
NCLEX® Standard: Recognize limitations of others and intervene.

4.14 ④ This option is the most diplomatic response and considers cost effectiveness. Many insurance companies view extra supplies on the day of discharge as stockpiling, and the client may be stuck with the bill. While some companies may still pay the entire bill as presented, many are becoming dollar-wise and view each bill with a critical eye. Options #1 and #3 do not consider cost effectiveness. Option #2 is an inappropriate response.

4.15 ③ Option #3 is correct. This client is presenting
④ with clinical findings of a GI bleed. The client
⑤ is at the stage of progressive shock, requiring
⑥ an immediate plan of care. Fluid resuscitation with the bolus of 1000 mL of 0.9 Normal Saline will assist with fluid replacement. Option #4 is correct. Due to the elevated serum sodium which can occur from fluid deficit, client is at risk for seizures. Seizure precautions are important to initiate for safe and effective care. Option #5 is correct. Oxygen needs to be administered via nasal cannula to assist in maximizing circulating oxygen levels due to the oxygenation saturation and blood pressure further decreasing. Option #6, due to the decrease in intravascular volume from the bleed, the nurse needs to ensure venous access with 2 large-bore (14-16 gauge) peripheral lines for IV medication and fluids. Option #1 is incorrect. The pulse pressure would narrow for this client presenting in shock. The widening occurs with increased intracranial pressure. Option #2 is contraindicated due to the risk of lowering the BP and further compromising perfusion. The correct position would be to place client flat or no greater than 30 degrees; the knees and feet may even need to be elevated to assist in perfusing the major organs.

I CAN HINT: Apply the clinical judgment/cognitive skill, (generate solutions), to the client who is experiencing hypovolemic shock. **NCLEX® Standard:** Manage the care of a client with alteration in hemodynamics, tissue perfusion, and/or hemostasis.

4.16 ④ This represents the appropriate process in collecting a "sterile" urine specimen. Options #1 and #2 open a closed system which allows bacteria to be introduced. Option #3 is incorrect information.

4.17 ③ Option #3 is correct. Kawasaki's disease is the leading cause of heart disease in children. I&O are important assessments for any client with heart disease. Option #1 is incorrect. This would be more of a priority for a child with tracheoesophageal fistula (TEF). Option #2 is important but not a priority. Option #4 could lead to complications with heart disease due to fluid and sodium excess.

4.18 ③ Aseptic techniques decrease the possibility of contamination with organisms. Options #1, #2, and #4 are incorrect. Option #1 is incorrect; there is no need to call lab prior to collecting the specimen. Option #2 is not specific to this urine for culture and sensitivity. Option #4 would be appropriate if the client was collecting a 24-hour urinalysis.

4.19 ① The elderly are particularly prone to digoxin-induced confused states which can occur in the presence of subtoxic digoxin levels and without other signs of toxicity. Option #2 occurs as a late side effect. Options #3 and #4 are incorrect.

4.20 ② Option #2 is correct. Bronchophony may be auscultated with a consolidation.
Option #1 = prolapsed lung. Option #3 = majority of the lung fields. Option #4 = asthma.

4.21 ② ⑤ Options #2 and #5 are correct. Dry mouth and urinary retention are anticholinergic symptoms that may occur when taking this medication. Option #1 is incorrect since the undesirable effect would be constipation, not diarrhea. Options #3 and #4 may be the reason for taking this medication (rash may be from allergen).

4.22 ③ Option #3 should be reported. The head circumference should be 2 cm larger than the chest circumference. 4 cm larger is not normal and requires further assessment. Options #1, #2, and #4 are normal clinical findings.

4.23 ④ The normal respiratory rate of a neonate is 30 to 50. Tachypnea is a sign of sepsis or hypoxia with a neonate. Option #1 is incorrect because it is within the normal range. Option #2 is not significant. Option #3 is incorrect. Neonates normally experience between a 5–10 percent loss of weight within the first few days of life.

4.24 ① Option #1 is correct. The LPN did not follow the standard of care for a client for the use of restraints. There should be an order written every 24 hours. Options #2, #3, and #4 do not require immediate intervention by the charge nurse, since these are consistent with safe care for clients using restraints.

4.25

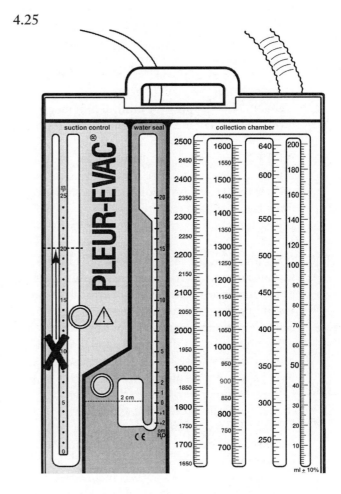

4.26 ① Metabolic alkalosis results in neuromuscular excitability. Alkalosis causes calcium to bind with albumin making less available for contraction of smooth skeletal muscle leading to muscle cramps and twitching.

4.27 ① A decreased production of urea nitrogen can be achieved by restricting protein. These metabolic wastes cannot be excreted by the kidneys. Options #2 and #3 decrease the non-protein nitrogen production; therefore, these foods are encouraged. Option #4 is incorrect.

4.28 ③ ④ ⑤ Option #3 is correct. The standard of care is to isolate affected children from others until vesicles have crusted – this is one priority. Airborne and contact precautions should be implemented; Standard precautions as needed. Options #4 and #5 will lessen pruritus and prevent scratching. Option #1 is incorrect. Acetaminophen and/or ibuprofen for fever. Aspirin has been linked to Reyes syndrome when administered for varicella. Warm baths and mild soap are not included in the plan. Cool baths with no soap are appropriate. Skin care to decrease itching includes antihistamines, antipruritic, calamine lotion, paste of baking soda, cool baths.
I CAN HINT: Apply the clinical judgment/ cognitive skill, (generate solutions), to the client who has a diagnosis of varicella.
NCLEX® Standard: Apply principles of infection prevention (e.g., hand hygiene, aseptic technique, isolation, sterile technique, universal/standard enhanced barrier precautions).

4.29 ① ④ ⑤ ⑥ It is important for you to understand clinical findings of fluid overload to answer this question appropriately. Fluid overload can result in tachypnea, adventitious breath sounds, and a congested cough. Link this to the pathophysiology of fluid excess and develop a mental image. Option #1 will assist in optimal lung expansion to support the clinical findings. Option #4 is correct. A diuretic will assist in removing the excess fluid. Option #5 is correct. An oxygen supplement is important for this client due to excess fluid. Option #6 is important due to the risk for skin breakdown from fluid excess. Option #2 is incorrect. This client does not need extra fluids. Option #3 is incorrect; these need to be assessed more frequently per protocol.

I CAN HINT: Apply the clinical judgment/ cognitive skill, (generate solutions), to the client who is experiencing alteration in oxygenation.
NCLEX® Standard: Recognize changes in client condition and intervene as needed.

4.30 ③ This information must be respected and remain confidential. Under the Invasion of Privacy, it states that the client has the constitutional right to be free from publicity and exposure to public view. Option #4 does not benefit the client in any constructive way.

4.31 ② The maintenance of a patent airway for a postoperative larnygectomy client would be a priority. Options #1, #3, and #4 would not be a priority to a potential airway issue.

4.32 ② Option #2 is correct. Severe hypotension or bradycardia are signs of adverse reaction with this medication. Options #1 and #3 are not typically adverse effects from this medication. Option #4 is within the defined limits.

4.33 ④ Clients who are immobilized from a spinal cord injury are high risk for developing pneumonia. Options #1 and #2 are not high risk. A postoperative client who is ambulating and has no direct insult to the respiratory system is not high risk. The infant is in traction, but is frequently expanding the lungs with the crying. Option #3 is a concern, but not a priority to Option #4.

4.34 ② The daily weight is the best way to evaluate for fluid volume deficit. Options #1, #3, and #4 provide information regarding the fluid volume level, but are not the best actions for evaluation.

4.35 ④ Turning client at frequent intervals is one of the most effective methods of preventing the development of skin breakdown caused by pressure, friction, or shearing forces. Option #1 encourages independent moving, but does not relieve pressure. Option #2 is an incorrect standard of practice. Skin inspection should be carried out at least once every 8 hours. Option #3 does not offer any prevention.

4.36 ② Elevation after surgery will minimize edema and optimize venous return. This would not be done for more than 24 hours due to the potential development of a contracture. Option #1 is not correct because some bloody drainage is expected. The nurse should outline the drainage and assess again in 5 minutes. Options #3 and #4 contain incorrect information.

4.37 ② Ambulation increases the return of peristalsis and facilitates the expulsion of flatus. Option #1 should not be encouraged until the bowel sounds have returned. Option #3 does nothing to increase peristalsis, but may make the client more comfortable. Option #4 doesn't provide anything.

4.38 ① The objective is to minimize eye movement in order to prevent further injury. Options #2, #3, and #4 would lead to further injury.

4.39 ③ Option #3 is correct. Since an undesirable effect from hydromorphone (Dilaudid) may be urinary retention, this option is demonstrating a downward trend with the urine output over the last 8 hours. This clinical finding should be reported to the RN to alert the nurse for a need to do further assessments. Option #1 is an appropriate action for a client who is one day post-op. The client needs to cough and deep breathe in order to decrease the risk of developing alteration in gas exchange. There is no need for the LPN to report this finding. Option #2 is an appropriate behavior; there is no reason to report this to the RN. This is a safe action and will minimize the risk of being dizzy. Option #4 is an expected finding from the anesthesia, and does not need reporting at this time.

4.40 ④ This allows optimum pulmonary expansion. Sitting decreases the venous return to the heart which assists in lowering the ventricle's output and pulmonary congestion. Options #1, #2, and #3 do not enhance ventilation.

4.41 ① Option #1 helps establish if there is equal, bilateral lung expansion. Intubation of the right mainstem bronchus would cause decreased or absent sounds in the left lung. Option #2 is not the appropriate first action. Waiting for this result will cause a delay in adjusting tube placement. Option #3 will also cause a delay in adjusting tube placement. Option #4 is not diagnostic.

4.42 ③ Antacids are the most effective after digestion has started but prior to the emptying of the stomach. Option #1 will not be beneficial because they must be taken several times a day to be effective. Option #2 contains incorrect information. Option #4 is incorrect because antacids are used to prevent pain through protecting the gastric mucosa.

4.43 Answer: $\underline{10}$ gtts/min.
First convert 1 hour to 60 minutes to fit the formula.

Then set up a fraction. Place the volume of the infusion in the numerator. Place the number of minutes in which the volume is to be infused as the denominator.

$$\frac{40 mL}{60 \text{ min}}$$

To determine X, or the number of drops per minute to be infused, multiply the fraction by the drip factor. Cancel units that appear in both the numerator and denominator.

$$X = \frac{40 \text{ mL}}{60 \text{ min.}} \times \frac{15 \text{ gtt}}{mL}$$

$$X = \frac{40 \times 15}{60 \text{ min.}}$$

$$X = \frac{60}{6} \quad X = 10 \text{ gtts/min.}$$

On the NCLEX®, you may have a box for your answer. Put only the number in the box.

4.44 ① This option is low both in sodium and fat. Option #2 contains selections (hot dog and canned soup) high in sodium. Option #3 is incorrect due to the avocado salad which is high in fat. Option #4 includes baked ham which is high in sodium.

4.45 ③ The problem needs to be taken care of now. If the LPN continues to make mistakes in client care, then a counseling report should be done. An LPN is expected to understand the importance of this requested procedure. Options #1, #2, and #4 are not appropriate at this time.

4.46 ② This option lists critical information that is significant to the safety and quality of the client's care. Other items are important, but not a priority to #2.

4.47 ③ This indicates the action of a client advocate and dealing with the immediate situation. Option #1 would not be done in front of a client. Options #2 and #4 are not addressing the immediate problem.

4.48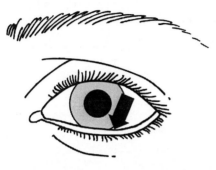

4.49 ③ The initial nursing priority for all psychiatric clients is to ensure their safety and the safety of all members of the milieu. Options #1, #2, and #4 are extremely important, but secondary to safety issues.

4.50 ④ An advanced directive needs to be witnessed by two individuals that are unrelated to the client. The two individuals will need to witness the client signing the advanced directive. Option #1, there is no reason to call the provider of care unless the client has any additional medical questions. Option #2 is not acting in the best interest of the client. Option #3, the nurse does not need to sign because it is considered a conflict of interest.

4.51 ④ Option #4 is correct. Option #1 is not as inclusive as #4. Option #2, blood should be verified with another nurse. Option #3 should be actual volume versus projected amount since the infusion may need to be discontinued prior to total amount being infused.

4.52 ③ Option #3 is correct. This client is presenting with infection. Options #1, #2, and #4 are expected findings. Option #1 is a correct finding. At approximately 12 hours, the fundus may be palpated at 1 cm above the umbilicus. Every 24 hrs the fundus should descend approximately 1 to 2 cm. By the sixth postpartum day, the fundus should be halfway between the symphysis pubis and the umbilicus. By the tenth day, the uterus should lie within the true pelvis and should not be palpable. Option #2 is also an expected finding. If temp, was above 101 and lochia rubra was brown or had a foul odor, then this would be a complication. Option #4 is also an expected finding. While it would be imperative for the nurse to go in and provide physical care due to the discomfort from the diaphoresis, it still would not be a priority over Option #3 which is a postpartum complication with infection.

4.53 ③ It is important to evaluate the 3:00 AM blood sugar to determine if the hyperglycemia is from the somoygi effect. Options #1 and #4 will be adjusted after knowing if the AM blood sugar is the accurate reading or a rebound response to a low blood sugar at 3:00 AM. Option #2 is incorrect.

4.54 ③ Sterile fields should be set up above the waist. Option #1 will not maintain sterility. Option #2 is incorrect because gowns are not always necessary. Option #4 is incorrect because supplies can be opened with bare hands, but touched inside the package with sterile gloves.

4.55 ④ The priority intervention is to assess the client's airway. Option #1 is done only if the nurse is unable to determine the problem. Option #2 would be appropriate after the client assessment. Option #3 contains inappropriate information. The alarm should not be deactivated or silenced.

4.56 ② The surgical consent should be verified that it is on the chart prior to going to surgery. Notice, it does not read that the consent needs to be signed or obtained. This should have already been done. In some clinical situations the consent has been signed, but for some reason does not get put on the chart. This is just going through the check offs to make certain the form is on the chart. OR will not accept the client without a signed consent. Options #1, #3, and #4 should be done prior to one hour before surgery..

4.57 ④ Option #4 is correct precautions for these symptoms of meningitis. Infection droplet precautions are priority for providing safe care. Options #1, #2, and #3 are important to include in the plan of care, but not priority over option #4.
I CAN HINT: Apply the clinical judgment/ cognitive skill, (generate solutions), to the client who is presenting with assessments of meningitis.

NCLEX® Standard: Apply principles of infection prevention (e.g., hand hygiene, aseptic technique, isolation, sterile technique, universal/standard enhanced barrier precautions).

4.58 ① The initial specimen is to remove the residual urine prior to the collection. Options #2, #3, and #4 contain incorrect information.

4.59 ③ This will assist in restoring potassium which is depleted through diuresing. Option #1 is inappropriate since it does not have any potassium to assist in correcting the depletion. Option #2 is too high in sodium, and it counteracts the effectiveness of giving furosemide. Option #4 is ineffective in restoring the potassium.

4.60 ③ After a bronchoscopy, the client should be assessed for symptoms of respiratory distress from swelling due to the procedure. Signs of respiratory distress include tachypnea, tachycardia, respiratory stridor, and retractions. Option #1 does occur and could become a complication if the client is given fluids before reflex has returned. Option #2 is common for a few days after a bronchoscopy. Option #4 is not associated with the procedure, but is a sign of increased intracranial pressure.

4.61 ② Option #2 is correct precautions for mumps.
④ This organism requires droplet precautions. Option #4 is correct for any client when starting an IV due to blood. Option #1 is appropriate for an immunocompromised client, but not necessary for a client with mumps. Option #3 is appropriate if performing an invasive procedure, providing central line care, etc. Options #5 and #6 are for airborne precautions that include organisms such as TB, smallpox, etc.
I CAN HINT: Apply the clinical judgment/cognitive skill, (generate solutions), to the client who is presenting with mumps which requires droplet precautions.
NCLEX® Standard: Apply principles of infection prevention (e.g., hand hygiene, aseptic technique, isolation, sterile technique, universal/standard enhanced barrier precautions).

4.62

③	The first step is to assess by asking client if he is choking.
④	The second step is to position self behind client.
⑤	The third step is to form a fist with one hand.
②	The fourth step is to position nurse's thumb toward client, above the waist and below the rib cage wrapping one arm around the client.
⑥	The fifth step is wrap other arm around the client placing that hand on top of the nurse's fist.
①	The sixth and last step is to thrust upward 6–10 times.

4.63 ③ This is the question that identifies the ability of parents to support the emotional needs of their children as separate human beings. Options #1, #2, and #4 are important questions to ask during the assessment, but are not directly related to the issue of emotional support.

4.64 ③ When a client is admitted to a general medical, surgical, or critical care unit for another physical problem, the nurse may become the case finder and must be alert for subtle symptoms of an alcohol-related problem. The client who has several complaints of pain that do not appear related to the admissions problem requires a further investigation. Tremors, elevated temperature, and pain may be indicative of an alcohol-related problem. Option #1 is more indicative of a dysphoric or depressed, medically ill client. Option #2 could warrant further exploration of alcohol use. Option #4 is more indicative of withdrawal from narcotics or an infective problem such as tuberculosis.

4.65 ④ Option #4 is the only correct answer. Options #1 and #3 are outside the nurse's legal scope of practice. Option #2 is also outside the provider of care's scope of practice although the provider should be apprised of the situation.

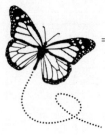

Notes

CHAPTER 5
Management of Care

Let whoever is in charge keep this simple question in her / his head - NOT how can I always do the right thing Myself but how can I provide for this right thing always to be done.
— FLORENCE NIGHTINGALE

✔ Clarification of this test ...

Note this percentage has decreased to 15–21% with the revised NCLEX-RN®. The minimum standards include performing and directing activities that manage client's care such as: the provision of care within the legal scope of practice, practicing in a manner that is consistent with the code of ethics for RNs, client rights, confidentiality, establishing priorities, ethical practice, legal rights and responsibilities, collaboration with an interdisciplinary team, quality improvement, referrals, resource management, informed consent, staff education, and supervision.

- Practice in a manner consistent with the nurses' code of ethics.
- Provide care within the legal scope of practice.
- Maintain client confidentiality and privacy.
- Organize workload to manage time effectively.
- Use approved terminology when documenting care.
- Receive, verify, and implement health care provider orders.
- Prioritize the delivery of client care based on acuity.
- Provide and receive hand off of care (report) on assigned clients.
- Collaborate with multi-disciplinary team members when providing client care (e.g., physical therapist, nutritionist, social worker).
- Verify the client receives education and client consents for care and procedures.
- Advocate for client rights and needs.
- Initiate, evaluate and update client plan of care.
- Recognize limitations of self and others and utilize resources.
- Utilize resources to promote quality client care (e.g., evidence-based research, information technology, policies, and procedures).

Continued ➡

- Perform procedures necessary to safely admit, transfer, and/or discharge a client.
- Provide education to clients and staff about client rights and responsibilities.
- Assess the need for referrals and obtain necessary orders.
- Delegate and supervise care of client provided by others (e.g., LPN/VN, assistive personnel, other RNs).
- Provide resources to minimize communication barriers.
- Practice and advocate for cost effective care.
- Integrate advance directives into client plan of care.
- Manage conflict among clients and health care staff.
- Participate in performance improvement projects and quality improvement processes.
- Report client conditions as required by law (e.g., abuse/neglect and communicable diseases).
- Recognize and report ethical dilemmas.

Adapted from: © National Council of State Boards of Nursing, Inc. (NCSBN). (2022). 2021 *RN Practice Analysis: Linking the NCLEX-RN® Examination to Practice*. Chicago: Author.
Adapted from: © National Council of State Boards of Nursing, Inc. (NCSBN). (2023) *Next Generation NCLEX® NCLEX-RN® Test Plan. Chicago*: Author.

Chapter 5: MANAGEMENT OF CARE

5.1 What plan is most important the nurse to include in the nursing care for clients with the following diagnoses: Gonorrhea, Hepatitis C, and Meningococcal Meningitis?
① Notify public health officials about these infections.
② Place client in contact precautions.
③ Place client in standard precautions.
④ Review with client and family the purpose of using a positive pressure room.

5.2 The nurse manager is conducting a quality improvement process to assure there is no breach in client confidentiality. Which of these nursing actions would require a performance improvement action plan for the nurse?
① Provides report for the nurse on the next shift at the bedside.
② Logs off the computer one time at the end of the day prior to leaving the workstation area.
③ Refuses to take an image of the client with phone.
④ Refuses to provide information when roommate inquires as to client's progress.

5.3 A nurse receives an end-of-shift report. Which assessment findings require immediate follow-up by the nurse?
① A client who has a right femur fracture, is in Russel's traction, and is presenting with a new onset of confusion.
② A client with gastroenteritis and has a blood pressure of 102/68 mm Hg, urine specific gravity – 1.028.
③ An infant with a heart rate of 178 bpm while the nurse is attempting to start an IV.
④ A client who has received digoxin and has a heart rate of 62 bpm.

5.4 A client has peritoneal dialysis prescribed due to acute renal failure following a multiple trauma accident. What action is important to implement when the nurse is not confident with how to initiate this procedure?
① Advise that procedure be assigned to a more experienced nurse.
② Notify health care provider and refuse assignment.
③ Review procedure in the policy manual.
④ Start dialysate slowly and assess for any discomfort.

5.5 The nurse has a licensed practical nurse (LPN) and unlicensed assistive personnel (UAP) on the team. Which client would be most appropriate to assign to the LPN?
① A client with a renal calculus and requires all urine to be strained.
② A 2-day post operative client who requires ambulation every 4 hours.
③ A 3-week post client with a cerebrovascular accident who requires repositioning every 2 hours.
④ A client with a tracheostomy who requires suctioning.

5.6 The nurse has a registered nurse (RN), licensed practical nurse (LPN) and unlicensed assistive personnel (UAP) on the team. Which client would be most appropriate to assign to the RN?
① A client who requires vital signs every 3-4 hours.
② A post-operative appendectomy who requires an abdominal dressing change.
③ A client who had an asthma exacerbation in Emergency Department and has been admitted in room.
④ A client with Mysathenia Gravis and needs assistance with a bath.

5.7 Which interventions will the nurse implement when providing care to an older adult client who appears malnourished and is wearing clothes that are soiled? **Select all that apply.**
① Encourage admission to a hospital for monitoring.
② Document interactions between client and caretaker.
③ Report suspected client neglect to proper authorities.
④ Ask caretaker if client is being abused.
⑤ Evaluate client access to necessities.

5.8 Which of these infants in the newborn nursery will the nurse assess first following shift report?
① A 14-hour-old neonate with RR-45 breaths per minute and irregular.
② A 24-hour-old neonate who has a bulging anterior fontanel when crying.
③ A 24-hour-old neonate from a mother with diabetes who is lethargic.
④ A 48-hour-old neonate with a HR- 160 bpm when quiet.

5.9 Which client is priority for the nurse to follow-up immediately following shift report?
① A laboring client 7 cm dilated with an occasional early deceleration.
② A laboring client presenting with a board like abdomen with sharp pain.
③ A laboring client presenting with an increase in variability.
④ A client presenting with one variable deceleration, FHR – 156 bpm.

5.10 Which of these nursing actions by the LPN/VN require immediate intervention from the charge nurse?
① Covers the newborn's head with a cap.
② Administers eye drops and vitamin K.
③ Bathes a newborn with a temperature of 96.8° F.
④ Fosters parent-newborn attachment.

5.11 Which nursing intervention is most appropriate to delegate to the unlicensed assistive personnel (UAP) for a client with a serum sodium of 148 mEq/L who has been vomiting for 12 hours?
① Restrict PO water intake.
② Evaluate effectiveness of diuretic.
③ Provide oral hygiene every 2-4 hours.
④ Provide a snack of crackers and cheese.

5.12 The nurse is assigned to take care of three clients in the neurological intensive care unit and does not think this is a safe assignment. What would the nurse implement first in this situation?
① Accept the assignment, and then make an appointment with nurse manager to discuss.
② Document concerns prior to accepting the assignment.
③ Explain to the charge nurse the concern with the unsafe assignment.
④ Refuse the assignment.

5.13 Which nursing action by the unlicensed assistive personnel (UAP) requires immediate intervention by the nurse?
① The UAP refuses to feed the client who just returned from a bronchoscopy.
② The UAP would not get the client up to the bathroom following a cardiac catheterization.
③ The UAP maintained a client on the right side following a liver biopsy.
④ The UAP placed the client with a head injury in the supine position for AM care.

5.14 Which of these clinical assessment findings for a client with esophageal bleeding requires immediate intervention by the nurse?
① The abdomen is soft and nontender in all four quadrants.
② The nasogastric tube is draining coffee ground drainage.
③ The hemoglobin is 12 mg/dL and the hematocrit is 36%.
④ The vital signs are: T— 98.9°F (37.17°C) HR—114 bpm, RR—20/min, BP—92/60.

5.15 What action would the nurse implement first after overhearing two UAPs discussing a client in the elevator?
① Report the two UAPs to their manager.
② Document the conversation heard on the elevator and submit to Chief Nursing Office (CNO).
③ Ask to speak to the UAPs in privacy and explain that they are violating client's confidentiality.
④ Notify the Quality Assurance Director about the breach of confidentiality.

5.16 Which of these clients are appropriate to assign the LPN/VN when working on the Pediatric unit?
① A 6-year-old client with increased intracranial pressure (IICP)
② An 8-year old client with Hepatitis B with elevated liver enzymes
③ A 10-year-old client with sickle cell crisis
④ A 12-year-old client with pneumonia

5.17 Which of these nursing actions would the nurse delegate to an unlicensed assistive personnel (UAP) on a medical nursing unit? **Select all that apply.**
① Assisting a client to ambulate on the second post-operative day.
② Bathing a client experiencing respiratory distress.
③ Educating a client about the importance of deep breathing and coughing to prevent post-op pneumonia.
④ Reminding a client to use an incentive spirometer (IS) every 1 to 2 hours while awake.
⑤ Setting up lunch trays for clients who have orders for regular meals.

5.18 Which of these antidepressant medication orders should the nurse question for an elderly client?
① Amitriptyline
② Haloperidol
③ Sertraline
④ Aripiprazole

5.19 Which of these nursing actions reflect the ethical principle of justice?
① The nurse administers a blood transfusion to a young adult client with leukemia who consented to the transfusion against the wishes of the family, who are all Jehovah Witnesses.
② The nurse establishes a plan to ambulate the post-op client as ordered by the provider of care even when the client would prefer staying in bed all day due to discomfort.
③ The nurse provides the same caring approach along with the nursing interventions for both the client who is the CEO of his company and a client who is homeless.
④ The nurse notifies the health care provider regarding a client that is not receiving any outcomes from the pain medication and has an alteration in the sensation in the foot with a cast.

5.20 Which of these nursing actions by the LPN would require the RN to intervene with due to the violation of the Privacy Rules outlined by HIPAA? **Select all that apply.**
① Discussing the client's condition during a telephone conversation with an individual who has provided the nurse with the client's code information.
② Refusing to share any information with a family member who is out of town.
③ Answering questions about a client's condition for the client's son.
④ Reviewing client's condition and medical information outside the client's room in rounds.
⑤ Photocopying client's lab reports for the medical team to have during rounds.

5.21 The nurse assessed a trend in the prevalence of falls among older clients in a Rehab Unit. The nurse documented the findings and collaborated with the unit manager to develop and implement a new policy using a *Fall Risk Indicator and Risk for Injury* Reference. Which of these plans would include this process?
① Advocacy
② Case Management
③ Collaboration
④ Quality Improvement

5.22 Which of these actions by the nurse demonstrates ethical practice for a nurse working on a Rehabilitation Unit?
① Discusses the inappropriate behavior only with the nurse who was seen taking part of a client's narcotics for personal use versus discarding it as per protocol.
② Encourages a client to take a walk to the recreation room, and explains the reason is so the health care provider will have some privacy to discuss the bad results of the biopsy.
③ Explains an answer to a client's question to the best of the nurse's ability due to limited knowledge about the medical condition.
④ Notifies the health care provider that a client has refused the chemotherapy treatment and wants to discontinue the treatment.

5.23 What would be the priority plan for a young child's parents that are Jehovah Witness who clearly state they do not want to make a decision that might kill their child, but are unable to give permission to administer blood due to hemorrhaging from an accident?
① Contact case management while administering fluids to maintain BP.
② Consult the ethics committee while administering fluids to maintain BP.
③ Call the hospital attorney while administering fluids to maintain BP.
④ Realize that this is the family's religious belief and support their decision.

5.24 A client is admitted with a kidney stone. The client is moaning in pain and vomiting. ABGs are: pH—7.54; PaO_2—78 mm Hg; PCO_2—26 mm Hg; and HCO_3—25 mEq/L (25 mmol/L). What is the nursing priority?
① Administer pain medication.
② Administer albuterol.
③ Administer an antiemetic.
④ Prepare for intubation.

5.25 Which of these clients would the nurse see first after report?
① A middle-aged client with liver failure and an INR of 3.0 who is complaining of IV site leaking.
② A middle-aged client who is complaining of shortness of breath.
③ An older client with Type II diabetes mellitus who is complaining of feeling weak and shaky.
④ An elderly client who is scheduled for surgery.

5.26 The nurse has not received training in the use of a new type of wound-drainage machine, but the charge nurse assures the nurse that it is easy to operate. What is the next action?
① Let client demonstrate how the device functions.
② Notify the charge nurse that the nurse has not been checked off in the use of this equipment.
③ Read the instruction manual and accept care of the client.
④ Care for the client, but call for help whenever there is a question about the machine's functioning.

5.27 Which of the following clients would be best to delegate to the LPN (licensed practical nurse)?
① A client who needs to be taught administration of enoxaparin.
② A client who has hypertension and is being managed with IV enalapril.
③ A client with potassium level of 3.0 mEq/L (3.0 mmol/L) and needs oral potassium replacement.
④ A client who is on a nitroglycerin drip and has complaints of chest pain.

5.28 During the admission physical, the nurse notes multiple bruises on a client, particularly on the breasts, back, and arms. When the nurse asks the client how the bruises occurred, the client begins to cry and states, "I fall down a lot." The nurse suspects domestic abuse. What is the priority nursing action?
① Do a referral to case management.
② Contact the health care provider for guidance.
③ Ask the client if anyone is hurting her.
④ Contact law enforcement.

5.29 The nurse is caring for a client with end stage COPD. The client has an advanced directive that specifies no ventilator. The client is in acute respiratory distress and states, "I need some relief. I want the machine!" The spouse states, "No, we are not doing that again!" What is the priority nursing action?
① Notify the health care provider (HCP) that the client has rescinded the advanced directive, but that the spouse is in disagreement.
② Prepare for intubation and mechanical ventilation.
③ Inform the spouse that the client has a legal right to change their mind about the advanced directive.
④ Administer anti-anxiety medication and call respiratory therapy to give the client a breathing treatment.

5.30 A client has pulled out the IV and Foley and has climbed out of bed. When attempting to get the client back into bed, the client begins to shout and tries to punch the nurse. What is the priority nursing action?
① Tell the client to stop in a strong, confident voice.
② Call security.
③ Run out of the room.
④ Restrain the client.

5.31 What is the priority nursing action for the manager to initiate on a medical unit for a nurse who is frequently late for work even after a verbal warning?
① Notify Human Resources about this problem and ask for advice.
② Ask the nurse why this behavior of being frequently late for work continues.
③ Give the nurse a written warning informing the nurse of the plan for termination if this behavior occurs again within the next three months.
④ Terminate the nurse effective immediately.

5.32 What is the priority nursing action for a client's angry spouse who comes to the nurses' station shouting and demanding that his wife be seen by a health care provider (HCP) immediately?
① Contact security because of the potential of injury to staff.
② Contact the client's HCP and inform the spouse of the situation.
③ Check on the client to see what is needed.
④ Ask the spouse to sit down and try to talk with the client.

5.33 What is the priority nursing action for a client who was admitted with GI bleeding and has removed the IV, and is insisting on signing self out of the hospital against medical advice?
① Give the client the AMA paper to sign and help gather client's belongings.
② Encourage the client to stay in the hospital until client is more stable, but do not prohibit client from leaving.
③ Call security to prevent the client from leaving the hospital room.
④ Tell the client not to leave the hospital since it is prohibited until client is discharged by the HCP.

5.34 What is the priority nursing intervention for an estranged wife and current girlfriend who are loud, disruptive at the client's bedside, and arguing about who is to blame for the overdose?
① Ask them to leave until the client is able to communicate.
② Call security to escort them out.
③ Tell the girlfriend to leave, but allow the estranged wife to stay.
④ Close the door to the room and let them finish the argument.

5.35 Which of these assignments would be appropriate for the unlicensed assistive personnel (UAP) to perform?
① Give a bed bath to a newly admitted client with chest pain.
② Evaluate a client's tolerance to activity while ambulating.
③ Document a client's intake and output.
④ Feed a client who has had a CVA and a history of aspiration.

5.36 A nurse from the oncology unit is floated to the ICU. Which assignment is most appropriate for the oncology nurse?
① A newly admitted client with respiratory failure on a CPAP machine.
② A post-operative client who needs two units of blood transfused before being transferred to the surgical unit.
③ A client with sepsis who has been on the ventilator for 5 days.
④ A client who has post-op delirium and is removing his tubes and attempting to climb out of bed.

5.37 What would be the first action for the nurse who has received a health care provider's (HCP's) order that reads: "100 mL D_5W with 80 mEq (80 mmol) of KCL to infuse in 1/2 hour"?
① Assess urine output.
② Ensure the patency of the IV line.
③ Request an order for Lidocaine to be added to the IV.
④ Check the accuracy of the order.

5.38 The nurse is caring for a client with Type 1 diabetes who is being treated with insulin glargine. The MAR reads 10 units SubQ twice daily. What is the priority nursing action?
① Check the client's glucose level.
② Administer the medication as prescribed.
③ Provide the client with a 15g carbohydrate snack.
④ Verify the appropriateness of the order.

5.39 A client with chronic lung disease is admitted to the acute pulmonary unit with: respiratory rate of 50; pulse of 140 and irregular; skin pale and cool to touch; client confused as to place and time. Orders are: oxygen per nasal cannula at 4L/minute, bed rest, soft diet and pulmonary function tests in the AM. What is the best sequence of nursing activities?
① Place in semi-Fowler's position, begin the oxygen, have someone stay with the client, then notify the health care provider regarding the current status of the client.
② Begin the oxygen, call the nursing supervisor, keep the bed flat to maintain blood pressure, and stimulate client to take deep breaths.
③ Call the nursing supervisor, discuss with the family if the client has experienced this problem before, offer the client sips of clear liquids.
④ Advise respiratory therapy of the client's problem, place the client in semi-Fowler's position, and begin the oxygen.

5.40 The nurse arrives for the day shift and receives the assignments around 7:30 AM. The assignment includes:
- A man with a diagnosis of rule-out MI who is on a monitor and having 4–6 premature beats per hour.
- An elderly client who is confused and has constant urinary dribbling.
- A client with pneumonia who is presenting with an increase in the confusion and a temperature of 104°F (40°C) at 6:30 AM.
- A client with diabetes mellitus who experienced a restless night and 7:00 AM serum glucose was 170 mg/dL (9.44 mmol/L).

Which client is a priority and how would the nurse plan the care?
① The client with pneumonia has priority; the client's condition should be assessed immediately.
② The elderly client is probably wet and uncomfortable and should be taken care of first. Then obtain a stat blood glucose to determine the diabetic client's current serum glucose level.
③ The client with cardiac symptoms should be assessed immediately as the monitor indicates cardiac irritability. Then the temperature on the client with pneumonia should be reassessed.
④ The client with diabetes should be seen immediately to assess for evidence of hyperglycemia. Then the client with pneumonia should be assessed for patency of airway.

5.41 After the nurse administered Lidocaine from a verbal order for a cardiac client who experienced numerous premature ventricular contractions, the health care provider entered the order for procainamide into the electronic medical order instead of Lidocaine. What would be the priority nursing action?
① Request a meeting with the health care provider when making rounds.
② Notify health care provider; discuss the order, and request a change in order if it is appropriate.
③ Discuss situation with the manager and ask if she/he could call health care provider regarding the situation.
④ Complete an incident report.

5.42 At 5:00 PM, the nurse on the evening shift opens the nurses' notes and discovers that the last entry was at 9:00 AM. The day nurse did not complete the charting and did not sign the nurses' notes. What is the priority nursing action?
① Leave a note on the front of the chart for the day nurse to make a late entry and begin charting on the line below the last entry on the nurse's notes.
② Leave enough space for the day nurse to complete the charting when the day nurse comes in the next morning.
③ Not chart anything until the day nurse returns to complete the charting for the care delivered that morning.
④ Call the day nurse and ask about the care the day nurse gave that morning so the evening nurse can complete the chart.

5.43 Which assignment would be appropriate for the Labor and Delivery (L&D) nurse who will be working for one shift on the Medical Surgical unit?
① A toddler with croup
② A young adult with malignant hypertension
③ A middle-aged client with unstable angina
④ An older adult client with heart failure

5.44 Which of these clients with spinal cord injury (SCI) would be assessed immediately following shift report?
① A client with a C6 SCI presenting with partial paralysis of hands, arms, and lower body
② A client with a T6 SCI presenting with a BP 170/68, severe headache, and HR—48 bpm
③ A client with a L1 SCI presenting with paralysis below the waist
④ A client with a C4 SCI presenting with paralysis below the neck and is on ventilator

5.45 After establishing IV access, what is best for the nurse to document immediately after the procedure?
① The type of catheter used and number of venipuncture attempts.
② The type of IV fluid hung and equipment used.
③ The date, time, venipuncture site, type and gauge of catheter, and IV fluid hung.
④ Type, amount, and flow rate of IV fluid, condition of IV site.

5.46 Which of these clients would need to be triaged first?
① A client who is taking NSAIDs for arthritic pain, experiencing epigastric pain, HR—90 bpm.
② A client who has a decline in the cranial nerve #1, reporting a problem with presbyscusis and presbyopia.
③ A client with thin skin, alteration in depth perception, and episodes of incontinence.
④ A client with fixed, dilated pupils, and is asystole.

5.47 Which would be the most appropriate to assign to the LPN?
① A client who is being discharged and needs new diabetic teaching.
② A client who is a new admission with chest pain.
③ A client who is receiving chemotherapy.
④ A client who has the diagnosis of Myasthenia Gravis.

5.48 Which would have the highest priority when caring for a terminally ill client during the final stage of dying?
① Encourage family to discuss legal matters with an attorney.
② Provide privacy for the client and his family to spend time together.
③ Keep client sedate.
④ Encourage family to limit visiting hours, so they can rest.

5.49 Which of these clients would be priority to assess after shift report?
① The husband of a cardiac client who indicates that the IV pump is alarming and his wife is not receiving the appropriate amount of medication.
② A cardiac client who is presenting with multifocal, trigeminal premature ventricular contractions on the ECG monitor.
③ A post-op appendectomy client 2 days ago; T—102°F (38.9°C); HR—104 bpm; and Respirations—30 breaths/min and is complaining of chest discomfort when coughing.
④ A newly admitted client with gastroenteritis: T—100°F (37.8°C); HR—100 bpm; and Respirations—20 breaths/min and a BP—114/76.

5.50 After the nurse receives report, which of these clients would be priority for the nurse to assess first?
① A client with COPD who is experiencing some shortness of breath with exertion.
② A client who had a CVA and has been hospitalized for 1 week.
③ A client who had a laminectomy 2 days ago and is complaining of pain.
④ A client with diabetes who is diaphoretic, with nausea, and is vomiting.

5.51 Which assignment would be most appropriate to assign to the pregnant nurse?
① A client with HIV
② A client with a cervical radium implant
③ A client with syphilis
④ A client with cytomegalovirus (CMV)

5.52 After the nurse receives shift report, which of these clients would be priority for the nurse to assess?
① A 30-year-old female client refusing to take cimetidine before breakfast.
② A 40-year-old male client scheduled for a cholecystectomy and complaining of chills.
③ A 50-year-old female client with right-sided weakness, asking to go to the bathroom.
④ A 60-year-old male with an NG tube who had a bowel resection 2 days ago.

5.53 Which sequence is correct when providing care for a client immediately prior to surgery?
① Administer preoperative medication, client signs operative permit, determine vital signs.
② Check operative permit for signature, advise client to remain in bed, administer preoperative medication.
③ Remove client's dentures, administer preoperative medication, client empties bladder.
④ Verify client has been NPO. Client empties bladder; family leaves room.

5.54 The nurse observes that a fire has started in the client's room. Which action would be the first nursing action?
① Confine the fire to the client's room.
② Extinguish the fire.
③ Pull the fire alarm.
④ Rescue the client.

5.55 Which room assignment is most appropriate for an adult male client who has sustained a second degree burn over 10% of the body?
① A semi-private room with a male client undergoing chemotherapy.
② A semi-private room with a male client who is three days post abdominal surgery.
③ A semi-private room with a male pediatric client.
④ A semi-private room with a male client admitted for chest pain.

5.56 What would be included in the documentation for a client who has returned from surgery with a new, fine, reddened rash noted around the area where Betadine prep had been applied prior to surgery?
① The time and circumstances in which the rash was noted.
② Explanation to client and family the reason for rash.
③ Notation on an allergy list and notification of the health care provider.
④ Application of corticosteroid cream to decrease inflammation.

5.57 The charge nurse demonstrates an understanding of appropriate delegation when which client assignment is made to the LPN?
① A psychotic client
② A client receiving chemotherapy
③ A client in Buck's traction
④ A client receiving a blood transfusion

5.58 A client with active multi-drug resistant TB is admitted to the unit and placed in the negative pressure room. The client is insistent upon smoking and states "If I can't smoke, I will sign myself out of the hospital against medical advice!" What would be the priority nursing action?
① Allow the client to leave because it is the client's right.
② Notify security and the charge nurse since this represents a public health hazard.
③ Permit the client to smoke in his room to protect the community.
④ Confiscate the client's cigarettes.

5.59 A client with bacterial endocarditis is being discharged home on IV antibiotics through a PICC line. Which statement by the client indicates the need for further teaching?
① "I will need antibiotics for at least the next six weeks."
② "I will be able to have lab drawn through the PICC line."
③ "I need to keep the occlusive dressing over the insertion site and cover it with plastic when I shower."
④ "I should check my blood pressure on the arm with the PICC line at least once a day."

5.60 Which of these clients would be most appropriate to discharge early in order to have a bed for a new client that is being admitted from the Emergency Unit?
① A client who had a cholecystectomy 4 days ago. Currently has active bowel sounds, is taking po fluids with no problems, and has an abdominal drain.
② A client who had an epidural bleed and is currently lethargic. Vital signs: HR—62 bpm; BP—160/92 mm Hg; Respirations—26 breaths/min; and Temperature—99.4°F (37.4°C).
③ An elderly client with some acute confusion and a new onset of incontinence.
④ A one-day post thyroidectomy client who has been stable and is now presenting with an increase in hoarseness.

5.61 A client who has an allergy to Penicillin has an order to receive ceftriaxone. What would be the priority of care for this client?
① Question the order.
② Administer the drug as ordered.
③ Call the pharmacy.
④ Ask the client if they have a history of any hypersensitivity to ceftriaxone or any other cephalosporin drug.

5.62 What would be the priority nursing action for the spouse of a client with dementia who confides in the nurse a concern about being able to handle the client following discharge from the hospital?
① Make a case management referral.
② Reassure the spouse that management of the husband's care can be done at home.
③ Notify the health care provider (HCP) that the client needs long-term care placement.
④ Tell the spouse that the client will improve after being discharged and returns home.

5.63 There is an order to administer 1000 mL. 0.9 NS over 10 hours. The tubing calibration factor is 10 drops/mL. To deliver this, set the infusion at _____ gtts/min.

5.64 One of the clients is a male admitted with dehydration. The client has an IV infusing at 150 mL/hr. The client's vital signs are: BP—82/98; HR—36; and RR—6. The pulse oximeter reads 87%. The client is in acute distress, coughing up pink, frothy sputum. What would be the first nursing action?
① Raise the head of the bed.
② Apply oxygen at 4 L/min.
③ Inform the provider of care.
④ Slow the IV rate.

5.65 There is a shortage of rooms, and the nurse must assign two clients to the same room in order to accommodate the newly admitted client. Which of these clients would the nurse assign to the same room?
① A 25-year-old female who is one day post-operative hysterectomy and an 80-year-old female who is confused and agitated.
② A 35-year-old male who is two days post-operative cholecystectomy and a 40-year-old male with pain due to fibromyalgia.
③ A 40-year-old female who has gastroenteritis and occasional vomiting with a 45-year-old female who is receiving corticosteroids for nephrotic syndrome.
④ A 50-year-old male with a MRSA infection and a 55-year-old female client with a Clostridium difficile infection.

Answers & Rationales

5.1 ① Option #1 is correct. The most important plan is to notify public health officials regarding the communicable diseases. Other observations that must be reported to the public health officials include abuse/neglect, and gunshot wounds. Option #2 is incorrect. Hepatitis C would require contact precautions but these precautions are not consistent with each of the diseases. The entire option must be correct for the answer to be correct. While standard precautions must be included for each of these medical conditions (option #3), it is not the most important over option #1. Other infection prevention precautions must also be included with these communicable diseases. Option #4 is incorrect for these clients; positive pressure room is appropriate for immunocompromised clients.
I CAN HINT: Apply the clinical judgment/cognitive skill, generate solutions (first-do priority plans), for infection prevention and reporting client conditions as required by law. Note, each option gave a type of infection prevention precautions, but the correct answer was about reporting these infections.
NCLEX® Standard: Report client conditions as required by law (e.g., abuse/neglect, communicable disease).

5.2 ② Option #2 is correct. Remember to log off before you walk off. Confidentiality is one priority when documenting electronically. This nurse requires a performance improvement action plan. Options #1, #3, and #4 are correct plans and do not require a performance improvement action plan for the nurse.
I CAN HINT: Apply the clinical judgment/cognitive skill, take-action (first-do priority interventions), for safe and effective care. When you read the question, focus on the nursing action that is incorrect.
NCLEX® Standard: Participate in quality improvement processes.

5.3 ① Option #1 is correct. The immobilized client with a long bone fracture is at risk for a fat emboli which can become impacted in the pulmonary and other microvasculature beds (i.e., brain). This new onset of the altered mental status may be a result of the emboli. This is a medical emergency. Option #2 is a concern due to the low blood pressure and increased specific gravity. This is secondary to fluid volume deficit from the gastroenteritis but is not priority to the emergency in option #1 with the new onset of confusion. Option #3 is most likely a result from the IV needle insertion. Option #4 is not a priority. The HR remains in the normal range; the outcome is an improved stroke volume and cardiac output, so the HR does not have to beat so fast.
I CAN HINT: Apply the clinical judgment/cognitive skill, analysis of cues (analysis). After comparing each option, the immediate concern is the client at risk for a fat embolit.
NCLEX® Standard: Provide and receive hand off of care (report) on assigned clients. Prioritize delivery of care.

5.4 ③ Option #3 is correct. Self-directed learning is an important characteristic of a nurse. Nurses learn daily; never implement a procedure if not confident with the process. Option #1 is incorrect. The only way the nurse is going to get experience is by learning and implementing the procedure. Option #2 is not appropriate if there is a policy manual outlining the process. Option #4 is incorrect and would be unsafe without reviewing the procedure.
I CAN HINT: Apply the clinical judgment/cognitive skill, take-action (first-do priority interventions), with a new assignment. The nurse must always understand the procedure.
NCLEX® Standard: Utilize resources to enhance client care (e.g., policies and procedures, evidenced-based research, etc.).

5.5 ④ Option #4 is correct. It is within the scope of practice for the LPN to suction the client with a tracheostomy. The procedure requires data collection prior to and evaluation following the procedure. It is within the scope of practice for the UAP to strain urine, assist with ambulation, and reposition the client (options #1, #2, and #3).
I CAN HINT: Apply the clinical judgment/cognitive skill, take-action (first-do priority intervention), when delegating. *Nursing Made Insanely Easy*, by Manning and Rayfield will assist you in remembering this concept for the

scope of practice for the UAP.
NCLEX® Standard: Assign and supervise care of client provided by others (e.g., LPN/VN, assistive personnel, other RNs).

5.6 ③ Option #3 is correct. This client is the most unstable and requires ongoing management from the RN. This asthma exacerbation can result in hypoxia. Options #1 and #4 are within the scope of practice for the UAP. Option #2 is within the scope of practice for the LPN/VN.
I CAN HINT: Apply the clinical judgment/cognitive skill, take-action (first-do priority intervention), when delegating.
NCLEX® Standard: Assign and supervise care of client provided by others (e.g., LPN/VN, assistive personnel, other RNs).

5.7 ② Options #2, #3, and #5 are correct; these review
     ③ assessments of neglect. Option #1 is incorrect
     ⑤ because there are not obvious complications mandating hospital admission. Option #4 is incorrect because the caretaker may be the one who is being neglectful.
I CAN HINT: Apply the clinical judgment/cognitive skill, take-action (first-do priority intervention), with suspected elder neglect and abuse.
NCLEX® Standard: Report client conditions as required by law (e.g., abuse/neglect, communicable disease).

5.8 ③ Option #3 is correct. Fetal insulin production was stimulated in the uterus due to maternal hyperglycemia. Hypoglycemia may frequently occur in the first few hours of life, secondary to the use of energy to establish respirations and maintain body heat. Options #1, #2, and #4 are expected findings for the neonate. The normal RR – 30-50 breaths/min, the anterior fontanel will bulge when crying, and the 48-hour-old neonate can be expected to have a HR between 110-160 bpm when quiet
I CAN HINT: Apply the clinical judgment/cognitive skill, analysis of cues (analysis), when providing care for the neonate. An understanding of how to safely assess the normal newborn and the newborn from a mother with diabetes mellitus are important for answering this question appropriately.
NCLEX® Standard: Prioritize delivery of client care. Provide care for the newborn.

5.9 ② Option #2 is correct and supports the diagnosis of an abruptio placenta which is an emergency and requires immediate follow-up and intervention. Options #1 and #3 do not require immediate assessment. Option #1 indicates head compression, and option #3 indicates good oxygenation. Option #4 is a normal FHR and the one variable deceleration indicates cord compression, so ongoing assessment will be required to monitor any trending with additional variable decelerations.
I CAN HINT: Apply the clinical judgment/cognitive skill, analysis of cues (analysis), when providing care to the client in labor.
NCLEX® Standard: Prioritize delivery of client care. Provide care for the client in labor.

5.10 ③ Option #3 is correct. The newborn's temperature is too low. The protocol for the bath is a temperature of 97.7 °F or higher. The LPN/VN needs to understand that this is unsafe care. Options #1, #2 and #4 include appropriate safe care and do not require immediate intervention from the charge nurse.
I CAN HINT: Apply the clinical judgment/cognitive skill, take-action (first-do priority intervention), for newborn care.
NCLEX® Standard: Recognize limitations of others and intervene. Recognizing Unsafe Care of Health Care Professionals and Intervene as Appropriate. Provide care for the newborn.

5.11 ③ Option #3 is correct due to elevated sodium level. The normal range for sodium is 135-145 mEq/L (135-145 mmol/L). The sodium is elevated for this client. The client may be dehydrated due to the vomiting, so option #3 is important for the UAP to provide oral hygiene. Option #1 is incorrect because fluid restriction would be inappropriate for a client who is vomiting with an elevated sodium level. Option #2 is incorrect. Evaluation is not in the scope of practice for the UAP and diuretic is inappropriate. Option #4 is incorrect. These foods are high in sodium.
I CAN HINT: The key to success with this question is fluid and electrolyte mastery and an understanding of delegation.
NCLEX® Standard: Assign and supervise care of client provided by others (e.g., LPN/VN, assistive personnel, other RNs). Manage the care of the client with a fluid and electrolyte imbalance.

5.12 ③ Option #3 is correct. The first step the nurse needs to take is to notify the charge nurse the concern with the assignment due to the fact that adequate care will be difficult for this number and type of clients. Option #1 is incorrect due to the risk and patient safety. Option #2 is incorrect. While documentation is the second step, this should be done after option #3 has been implemented. It states that there is a "safe harbor" clause in the Nursing Practice Act preventing the nurse from losing the license should a poor outcome result from the assignment. Option #4 is incorrect. This will make client care more strained resulting in more errors and increase risk to clients.

NCLEX® Standard: Report unsafe care of health care personnel and intervene as appropriate (e.g., substance abuse, staffing practices, improper care).

5.13 ④ Option #4 is correct. The client with a head injury should not be in the supine position due to the risk of increasing the intracranial pressure. The HOB should remain at least 45°. Options #1, #2, and #3 do not require immediate intervention, since these all represent the standard of care for the specific clients.

NCLEX® Standard: Report unsafe care of health care personnel and intervene as appropriate (e.g., substance abuse, staffing practices, improper care).

5.14 ④ Option #4 is correct. The HR is above normal range and BP is low which may indicate hypovolemic shock. Option #1 is an expected finding. Option #2 would not be unexpected for this client. Option #3 does not require additional intervention.

NCLEX® Standard: Prioritize delivery of client care.

5.15 ③ Option #3 is correct. This is a violation of HIPPA. The two UAPs need to be confronted and behavior corrected. Option #1 is incorrect. They can be reported to their manager, but the priority remains to speak to them first. The same with option #4; the UAPs need to be informed with an action plan to correct behavior.

NCLEX® Standard: Maintain client confidentiality/privacy.

5.16 ④ Option #4 is correct. This client is most stable with altered oxygenation. Option #1 is not correct due to the necessary ongoing assessments required for IICP. Option #2 is not correct due to risks involved with elevated liver enzymes. Option #3 is in a crisis and needs immediate intervention and ongoing assessments.

I CAN HINT: The lowest acuity and older child are the keys for answering this question appropriately. Refer to the book, *Nursing Made Insanely Easy*, by Manning & Rayfield to further review the concept of delegation to the LPN/VN.

5.17 ① ④ ⑤ Options #1, #4, and #5 are correct. These assignments are all within the legal scope of practice for the UAP. Refer to "*Bart*" in the book, *Nursing Made Insanely Easy*, in order to assist in remembering this concept. A quick I CAN Hint: "BART" will assist you in remembering the actions the UAP can implement within their scope of practice. A UAP can Bathe clients who are stable, Ambulate clients who are stable, conduct Routine tasks, and Tasks that do not require clinical decision making. Option #2 is incorrect because client is in distress, and the UAP will not have the knowledge to know the importance of discontinuing the procedure for this client. The procedure should not actually even be started when a client is in distress. Option #3 is incorrect because teaching is not within the legal scope for UAPs.

5.18 ① Option #1 is correct. To begin down the path of success for answering this question, you must first know which of these drugs include antidepressants. The two antidepressants in these options include Amitriptyline and Sertraline. Amitriptyline has the most anticholinergic and sedating side effects of these two antidepressants. There may be pronounced effects on the cardiovascular system (hypotension) which may result in falls. This medication order should be questioned due to the risk to the client for injury from the falls. Option #2 is incorrect since it is an antipsychotic medication. Option #3 is a useful antidepressant due to the decrease in undesirable effects in comparison to the traditional tricyclic antidepressants. It has one of the shortest half-life of the currently marketed serotonin reuptake inhibitors. In other words, there would be no need to question this order. Option #4 is incorrect since it is an antipsychotic medication.

5.19 ③ Option #3 is correct. This is an example of justice which reflects fair treatment in matters related to physical and psychosocial care and use of resources. There should be no difference in the quality of care for any individual based on economics or professional accomplishments. Option #1 is incorrect. This is an example of autonomy which allows the client to make personal decisions, even those decisions that may not be in the client's own best interest. Option #2 is incorrect. This is an example of beneficence which is the care that is in the best interest of the client. Option #4 is incorrect. This is an example of nonmalefiscence which is prevention of harm or pain as much as possible during treatment.

5.20 ③ Options #3, #4, and #5 are correct answers.
④ These demonstrate inappropriate
⑤ dissemination of client information as outlined by HIPAA. These would require intervention by the RN since these actions demonstrate a violation in the Privacy Rules. Option #1 does not require intervention since the individual has the client's code information. Option #2 does not require intervention since this is appropriate practice.

5.21 ④ Option #4 is correct. Quality Improvement includes activities such as assessing opportunities and developing plans/policies for improving the quality of nursing practice. Identifying an increase in the trend of falls and implementing a policy focused at improving the assessment and prevention of falls among the older clients fulfills the focus of quality improvement. Option #1 is incorrect since advocacy refers to the nurse's responsibility to act on behalf of the client. Option #2 is incorrect since this refers to the coordination of care to minimize costs and fragmentation. This also assists with the improvement in outcomes and quality. Option #3 is incorrect. While the nurse did collaborate with the unit manager, this plan goes beyond collaboration to assessment and policy development based on high-volume risks.

5.22 ④ Option #4 is the correct answer. This demonstrates respect for the client autonomy, even if the decision may not be in the client's own best interest. Option #1 is incorrect. Taking narcotics from a client demonstrates unethical practice. Most employers have protocols for reporting of witnessed theft or conduct that is unprofessional. The nurse needed to report this behavior to the manager due to unethical practice. Option #2 is incorrect. This action is a violation to client confidentiality. The nurse shared the fact the client had a biopsy and also that there were bad results from the biopsy. Option #3 is incorrect. The nurse violated veracity (truth telling); the nurse should have indicated the truth which was a lack of knowledge regarding the answer to the question, and would be happy to go and find out the correct information.

5.23 ③ Option #3 is correct. The child is a minor and cannot make own medical decisions. By contacting the hospital attorney there can be a decision made by the court to allow the life-saving administration of blood in this circumstance. This will also support the family who is unable to make the decision due to the support system. Option #1, while case management can be supportive, and there is a need for the ethic committee to meet and give their opinion it is essential to have a legal opinion regarding the treatment. Option #4 is incorrect. It clearly indicates the family is in a dilemma, and in this situation would welcome medical and/or legal support.

5.24 ① Option #1 is correct. The ABGs indicate respiratory alkalosis, uncompensated. By relieving the client's pain, the respiratory rate should decrease and should stop blowing off the CO_2. Option #2, the albuterol, is not a standard of practice for the clinical presentation. Option #3, an antiemetic can be administered after the pain medication. Option #4, there is no indication that client should be intubated.

5.25 ② The priority assessment will be option #2 (possible hypoxia), followed by option #3 (possible hypoglycemia), option #1 (bleeding due to increased PT/INR) and finally option #4. Each of these clients need to be seen by the nurse.

5.26 ② Option #2 is the correct choice. A nurse should not use new equipment until there has been training in the use and documentation that the nurse can safely use the equipment. Options #1, #3, and #4 could put the nurse in legal jeopardy.

5.27 ③ Option #3 is correct. Option #1, LPNs do not do initial teaching, and the options #2 and #4 are unstable situations.

5.28 ③ Option #3 is correct. Options #1 and #2 are using the provider to make a nursing judgment. Option #4 would be appropriate if the client admits that she is being physically harmed and is willing to involve the legal system. Whether or not the client admits that abuse is occurring, careful documentation of bruising and the client's response is important.

5.29 ① Option #1 is correct. The client has a right to rescind the advanced directive. The nurse needs a HCP's order to reverse the Do Not Resuscitate order on the chart, and the HCP needs to know about the conflict between the client and spouse. Option #2 is dependent upon the HCP's order. Option #3 would be best handled by the HCP. Option #4 could provide relief to the client, but could also suppress the client's respirations and postpone their wishes.

5.30 ① The first nursing action would be option #1. The client is out of control and at risk of harming self and the nurse. That might be enough to enable the client to regain control. Option #2, security then needs to be called. Option #3 is inappropriate. Option #4, restraints should be used only as a last option and requires a health care provider's (HCP's) order.

5.31 ③ Option #3 is correct. The manager is responsible for responding to employee problems. This is not the role of the Human Resources Department as stated in option #1. The nurse has already had a verbal warning, so the next step is a written warning. Option #2 is incorrect. Asking why nurse is late does not resolve the problem. A written warning (Option #3) precedes termination (Option #4).

5.32 ① Safety is the priority in this situation. Contacting security will decrease the risk of injury to staff. The spouse appears to be out of control. Contacting the HCP in option #2 will not take care of the immediate problem. Leaving the scene (Option #3) to check on the client could increase the risk of injury to staff. Option #4, asking the spouse to sit down and talk may not be possible due to spouse's level of agitation.

5.33 ② Option #2 is the best choice. The client has not been involuntarily committed and has every right to leave the facility. Option #1 is encouraging the client to leave. Options #3 and #4 may be considered as false imprisonment.

5.34 ① Option #1 should be attempted first. If they refuse to leave, then option #2, call security to escort them out of the building. Options #3 and #4 are not appropriate.

5.35 ③ Option #3 is the correct answer. Documenting vital signs and I&O are within the UAP's scope of practice. Option #1 is not appropriate to give a bed bath to a newly admitted client with chest pain. Option #2 is not within the UAP's role. The client in Option #4 is at high risk for aspiration and needs to be fed by a licensed care giver.

5.36 ② Option #2 is correct. The client is stable enough to be transferred to the surgical unit, and the oncology nurse frequently administers blood products. Option #1 is a newly admitted client and therefore requires very close monitoring and may not be stable. Option #3, care of a ventilator client is not in the usual scope of practice for the oncology nurse. Option #4, a client with delirium needs frequent and close assessment to determine if the treatment is working.

5.37 ④ Option #4 is correct. Potassium chloride must be diluted and administered at a rate not to exceed 10mEq/hr (10 mmol/hr) for adults with a serum potassium level > 2.5 mEq/L (2.5 mmol/L) or if serum potassium is < 2 mEq/L (2 mmol/L) the rate is not to exceed 20 mEq/hr (20mmol/hr). Checking the accuracy of the order would be the first action. Options #1 and #2 are correct after the order has been corrected. Option #3, Lidocaine, should not be added to this IV.

5.38 ④ Option #4 is correct since glargine (Lantus) is administered one time a day versus twice daily. Option #2 is incorrect since the order is inappropriate, the nurse needs to focus on collaborating with the HCP to revise the order, so it is safe. While it is important to monitor the client's glucose (Option #1), this option does not answer the question. The question is evaluating the understanding for "safe medication administration." *Remember, the key to successful testing is to focus on what the question is asking.* Option #3 is not correct for this question. There is no indication in the stem of the question that the client is experiencing hypoglycemia which would then indicate a need for the nurse to administer a carbohydrate.

5.39 ① The health care provider's orders do not address the seriousness of the client's condition. The health care provider should be notified immediately. However, the client should not be left alone. Options #2, #3, and #4 do not address the seriousness of the client's immediate needs.

5.40 ① The sickest client is the client with pneumonia, and the client's needs should be addressed first. This client has an increased temperature, which may indicate his pneumonia is getting worse; the confusion may be indicative of hypoxia. The client status should be evaluated immediately. Option #3, premature beats of 4–6 per hour are benign and not unusual for a cardiac client. Option #2, the elderly client may be uncomfortable, but the respiratory status of the client with pneumonia is priority. Option #4, a serum glucose of 170 mg/dL (9.44 mmol/L) is abnormally high and should be addressed. The respiratory status of the pneumonia client, however, remains the highest priority.

5.41 ② During emergency situations, verbal orders should be entered into the electronic medical record and signed. The nurse must notify the health care provider and explain the order. If the nurse did hear this order correctly, then a new order should be requested from the health care provider. Option #1 is incorrect since the nurse would be waiting for the health care provider to make rounds, and this needs to be completed as soon as possible. (Not later!) Options #3 and #4 are incorrect. Option #3 is asking another nurse to intervene which is nurse avoidance. Option #4 is incorrect, since this may not be necessary if the nurse did hear the verbal order correctly.

5.42 ① The best way to handle the situation is to begin charting on the line below last entry, and have the day nurse make a late entry for the omitted information. Options #2, #3, and #4 would be illegal.

5.43 ② Option #2 is correct. The L&D nurse provides care for clients with pregnancy induced hypertension. These assessments and plans of care would correlate with the nurse's skills. Options #1, #3, and #4 would not be appropriate for this nurse. L&D nurses do not routinely provide care for children. Options #3 and #4 require an understanding of cardiology.

5.44 ② Option #2 is correct. This is an emergency and requires immediate intervention. The client is presenting with assessments of autonomic dysreflexia. Options #1, #3, and #4 are expected findings for the level of SCI.

5.45 ③ Option #3 is the most correct answer. Options #1 and #2 are appropriate but not as inclusive as option #3. Option #4 should be included in the once-per-shift documentation. This question states "after establishing IV access."

5.46 ① Option #1 is correct. This client is presenting with symptoms of a bleeding ulcer with the history of the NSAIDs and the location of the pain and elevated heart rate. Options #2 and #3 are normal findings and do not need to be triaged. In option #4, the client is dead.

5.47 ④ Option #4 is most stable. Option #1 is incorrect because it requires initial teaching. The LPN can reinforce teaching, but it is currently not in the scope of practice to do the initial teaching. Option #2 would require initial assessment. LPNs can do ongoing assessment, but it is not in the scope of practice to complete the initial assessment. Option #3 would require IV management and specialized assessment skills, so it is not a priority to option #4.

5.48 ② A priority is to provide privacy. Options #1 and #3 are inappropriate at this time. Option #4 is partially correct about rest, but incorrect regarding the limiting of visiting hours.

5.49 ② Option #2 is correct. The cardiac client is the most unstable and is presenting with cardiac irritation which requires immediate assessment. Option #1 is not life-threatening. This can wait for an assessment. Option #3 is incorrect. This client may be experiencing some pneumonia and may require some revision in the plan of care, but does not mandate immediate assessment following report. Option #4 is dehydrated, but is not in any acute situation that would mandate immediate assessment over the priority client that is presenting with trigeminal premature ventricular contractions.

5.50 ④ The diabetic client is presenting with hypoglycemia. This can be dangerous. Option #1 may be expected with COPD. Options #2 and #3 are not priorities to option #4.

5.51 ① An HIV client would not present a risk to the pregnant woman if she does not come in contact with the body secretions. Options #2, #3, and #4 could result in teratogenic effects to the fetus.

5.52 ② Option #2 is correct. The client is scheduled for surgery and has a sign of infection (chills)! Option #1 does not give any indication of any complications or any specific information about the client to indicate he would be a priority. Option #3 does not require a nurse. This client does need assistance, but the RN is not required for this client. Option #4 is high risk for potential complications, but none are indicated at this time. Option #2 has already developed a complication.

5.53 ② The operative permit must be signed prior to the client receiving his preoperative medication. The client is considered incapacitated after receiving a narcotic. Option #1, administer the medication prior to the permit being signed, is incorrect. Option #3 is incorrect because medication was given before emptying bladder which leads to a risk for falls. Option #4 is important information, but it is unnecessary for the family to leave the room.

5.54 ④ Option #4 is correct. Rescuing the client is always the priority. "RACE" will assist you in remembering fire safety. R = rescue client; A = activate an alarm; C = confine the fire; and E = extinguish the fire.

5.55 ① Both clients have lost major protective mechanisms and are at risk for infection. Options #2 and #3 are incorrect due to the infection risk they pose. Option #4 is incorrect due to the need to decrease stimulation to conserve oxygen, and does not need the same isolation precautions.

5.56 ③ Option #3 is correct. Any suspected reaction to drugs should be reported to the health care provider, and noted on the list of possible allergies. Option #1 would be noted, but is not as high a priority as option #3. Option #2 would be important to implement, but would not be a priority over option #3. Option #4 does not address the fact that the rash is new and occurred following the Betadine prep.

5.57 ③ This client is the lowest acuity out of the group and requires the least specialized care. The scope of practice would allow the LPN to care for this client. Options #1, #2, and #4 require care from the RN which is out of the LPN's scope of practice.

5.58 ② Option #2 is correct. This represents a public health hazard. Infection prevention standards will require notification of security to keep the client in the negative pressure room until the health department determines the best course of action. Option #1 would endanger the community, option #3 is not a possible action due to smoke free facilities, and option #4 could endanger the nurse if it angered the client.

5.59 ④ Option #4 indicates a need for further teaching. Blood pressure should not be taken on the arm with a PICC line. The other options indicate effective teaching.

5.60 ① Option #1 is correct. This client is the most stable out of the four clients. Option #2 is incorrect since the client is lethargic and BP is elevated. Option #3 needs ongoing evaluation for a urinary tract infection. Elderly clients presenting with acute confusion along with incontinence may have an infection. Option #4 is not appropriate to discharge since the hoarseness may indicate a complication from laryngeal edema.

5.61 ④ Option #4 is correct. There is a possibility for cross-sensitivity between penicillin and cephalosporins. Asking the client about the previous use of a cephalosporin may indicate that there is no problem with cross-sensitivity. Option #1, the nurse should then call the provider of care to question the order and inform the provider about the client's previous use of cephalosporins. Options #2 and #3 are incorrect because they do not address the issue with the allergy in the stem of the question. This would be unsafe practice.

5.62 ① Option #1 is the best choice. The case manager can work with the spouse to determine what resources are available in the community and make needed referrals. Options #2 and #4 are giving false reassurance. Option #3, this is not the staff nurse's role to inform the provider of care that the client needs long-term care placement.

5.63 <u>17</u> drops/minute

Step 1: Volume to be infused =
Volume (mL) 1000 mL

Step 2: Time for the infusion =
Time (min) Convert hr to min
$\frac{60 \text{ min}}{1 \text{ hr}} = \frac{x \text{ min}}{10 \text{ hr}}$
10 hrs = 600 min

Step 3: What is the drop factor on the IV tubing?
10 drops/ mL

Step 4: Equation
1000 mL x 10 gtt/mL = $\frac{10{,}000 \text{ gtt}}{600 \text{ min}}$ = 17 gtts/min

5.64 ④ Option #4 is correct. The first action is to decrease the IV rate. All of these actions need to be taken. The client is most likely in pulmonary edema due to fluid overload. The next action would be to raise the head of bed, option #1, then apply oxygen, option #2. At that point, the provider of care needs to be notified for orders, option #3.

5.65 ② Option #2 is correct. Both of these clients would require ongoing pain assessment, pain management interventions, and there is no indication of an infection with either client. Option #1 is incorrect. The developmental needs are very different, and with a 25-year-old client most likely having numerous visitors, this may cause the agitation and confusion of the older client to be increased. Another concern with option #1 is that the option does not say if this is a new onset of confusion. If it did state "new onset of confusion," this could be a sign of infection. This assignment then would not be appropriate for this client who had surgery one day ago. Of course, we NEVER want to read into the options or the questions, so with the information available you can problem solve this option correctly by understanding the differences in the developmental stages. Option #3 is incorrect since the 40-year-old is presenting with vomiting and an infection, and the client taking corticosteroids may be immuno-compromised. Option #4 is in direct violation of the standard of practice for these clients. Based on the standards of care for these clients, they should not be in the same room.

CHAPTER 6
Safety and Infection Control

> You must be the change you wish
> to see in the world.
> — GHANDI

✔ Clarification of this test …

This percentage has increased to 10–16% on the new NCLEX-RN®. These minimum standards include performing and directing activities that manage client care such as: ensuring proper identification, applying principles of infection prevention, protecting client from injury due to (falls, electrical hazards), applying ergonomic principles, safe equipment use, accident & error prevention, handling hazardous and infectious materials, incident reports, use of restraints, disaster planning, emergency response plan & home safety.

- Apply principals of infection prevention (e.g., hand hygiene, aseptic technique, isolation, sterile technique, universal/standard enhanced barrier precautions).
- Properly identify client when providing care.
- Protect client from injury.
- Assess client care environment.
- Facilitate appropriate and safe use of equipment.
- Educate client on safety issues.
- Verify appropriateness and accuracy of a treatment order.
- Assess client for allergies and intervene as needed.
- Use of ergonomic principles when providing care.
- Follow procedures for handling biohazardous materials.
- Educate client and staff regarding infection prevention measures.
- Promote staff safety.
- Follow requirements when using restraints.
- Follow security plan and procedures (e.g., newborn security, violence, controlled access).
- Participate in emergency planning and response.
- Report, intervene, and/or escalate unsafe practice of health care personnel (e.g., substance abuse, improper care, staffing practices).
- Acknowledge and document practice errors and near misses.

Adapted from: © National Council of State Boards of Nursing, Inc. (NCSBN). (2022). 2021 *RN Practice Analysis: Linking the NCLEX-RN® Examination to Practice*. Chicago: Author.

Adapted from: © National Council of State Boards of Nursing, Inc. (NCSBN). (2023) *Next Generation NCLEX® NCLEX-RN® Test Plan. Chicago*: Author.

Chapter 6: SAFETY AND INFECTION CONTROL

6.1 What clinical situation would the charge nurse intervene with due to the LPN/VN not following the appropriate standard of practice?
　① The LPN/VN reinforces the instruction with a client who has Hepatitis A that this can be transmitted through infected food handlers.
　② The LPN/VN puts on gloves to administer an injection with a client who has Hepatitis B.
　③ The LPN/VN discusses the need to avoid sexual activity for a client with Hepatitis A.
　④ The LPN/VN puts on a gown and mask prior to giving a bath to a client with Hepatitis B.

6.2 A school-age client presents to the pediatric unit with symptoms of a headache, photosensitivity, stiff neck, and temperature 102.2° F (39° C). Which is priority for the nurse to include in the of plan of care for this client?
　① Provide safety teaching to family.
　② Decrease environmental stimuli.
　③ Implement seizure precautions.
　④ Implement droplet precautions using a surgical face mask.

6.3 A client has been receiving Ceftriaxone for the past 5 days in the treatment of a serious infection. The nurse notes the client has developed profuse watery diarrhea and is complaining of moderate abdominal cramping. Further assessment reveals BP - 92/62 mm Hg; Heart rate 102 bpm. Based on these assessments what actions should the nurse implement? **Select all that apply.**
　① Obtain a stool specimen for a Clostridioides difficile test.
　② Post a sign on the client's door alerting to imposed Protective Precautions.
　③ Perform hand hygiene with a soap and water after client contact.
　④ Use clean gloves for any contact with client or client environment.
　⑤ Encourage the client to increase their intake of oral fluids.

6.4 A client has been admitted with high fever, headache, shortness of breath and pulmonary congestion. Upon testing positive for COVID 19, what actions should be taken by the nurse?
　① Don gown, N-95 mask, goggles, and gloves prior to and during client contact.
　② Instruct the family that visitors are not allowed in the client's room for 5 days.
　③ Use sterile gloves for any direct client contact procedures.
　④ Dispose of personal protective equipment (PPE) for other reuse in a common disposal unit outside the client's room.

6.5 A nurse is instructing the family of a client who has tested positive for COVID 19 on the application of personal protective equipment (PPE). Which instructions are most appropriate for the nurse to include in the plan of care?
　① Don an N-95 mask, goggles, gloves, and sterile gown prior to entering the client's room.
　② Wash hands with an alcohol-based foam prior to donning appropriate personal protective equipment PPE and client contact and wash hands again upon removing personal protective equipment (PPE) and exiting the room.
　③ Don an isolation gown and clean gloves prior to entering the client's room and place in receptacle inside the room.
　④ Wash hands with soap and water, dry, and apply sterile gloves, mask, and gown prior to entering the client's room.

6.6 Which clinical situation would the Registered Nurse intervene with due to not following the appropriate standard of practice?
　① A student nurse exits a client room and enters another without using an alcohol-based hand cleanser.
　② An LPN prepares for administration of a client's medications by using a computer on wheels positioned outside the client's room.
　③ A UAP obtains a client's vital signs using a disposable blood pressure cuff maintained on the client's bedside table.
　④ A registered nurse disinfects a telemetry unit with EPA-approved disinfectant upon removing from client use.

6.7 An infant has been admitted with respiratory syncytial virus (RSV) pneumonia. What is an appropriate aspect of parent teaching that the nurse should include in the plan of care?
① Mask and gown should be worn when holding the child.
② Limit close contact to the face of the child.
③ Wash all toys with 25 % chlorine bleach.
④ Keep other children at home from school.

6.8 Which LPN/VN will need further instruction regarding wearing the appropriate personal protective equipment (PPE)?
① The LPN/VN wears a gown and gloves when entering the room for a client with Clostridium Difficile.
② The LPN/VN wears an N95 mask for a client with tuberculosis.
③ The LPN/VN wears sterile gloves when bathing an infant with Respiratory Syncytial Virus (RSV).
④ The LPN/VN wears a surgical face mask when providing care for an infant with pertussis.

6.9 What would be important for the nurse to include in a teaching plan for a child diagnosed with varicella? **Select all that apply.**
① Use aspirin for fever.
② Recommend bathing child in warm baths with a mild soap.
③ Isolate child until all the vesicles have crusted.
④ Instruct parents to keep fingernails short or apply mittens if necessary.
⑤ Provide quiet activities to keep child occupied.

6.10 What is priority for the nurse to include in the teaching plan for a client being discharged with a prescription for haloperidol?
① Discuss with client that it is expected to experience a skin rash when taking medication.
② Review the importance of monitoring serum glucose when taking haloperidol.
③ Explain importance of removing throw rugs at home and reason for taking benztropine.
④ Discuss the reason client should not eat any smoke, pickled, or aged foods.

6.11 Which clinical findings indicate a complication with an allergic reaction for client who is receiving a transfusion of a unit of packed red blood cells? **Select all that apply.**
① Lower back pain
② Chills
③ Urticaria
④ Pruritus
⑤ Wheezing

6.12 What is the priority to teach a client who is taking methylprednisolone after being discharged from the hospital?
① Advise to limit foods high in potassium such as oranges, potatoes, etc.
② Advise to limit dairy products.
③ Advise to put on a face mask when in public and with large crowds.
④ Advise to expect a sore throat when taking this medication.

6.13 Which client would be most appropriate to assign as a roommate for a client recovering from a renal transplant?
① A client with methicillin-resistant staph aureus (MRSA).
② A client admitted with diarrhea of unknown origin perhaps from food poisoning.
③ A client admitted with systemic lupus erythematous.
④ A client recovering from herpes zoster.

6.14 What is the priority for an elderly client who has Alzheimer's disease and wanders the halls of the nursing unit during the day?
① Assess client's gait to determine balance and steadiness.
② Encourage client to watch television in the room.
③ Administer prn lorazepam as prescribed to calm client.
④ Only allow client to wander in the unit with the assistance from an unlicensed assistive personnel.

Chapter 6: SAFETY AND INFECTION CONTROL

6.15 What nursing actions indicate the nurse understands how to safely provide care for a client with herpes zoster? **Select all that apply.**
  ① The nurse who hasn't had chickenpox or vaccine should not be assigned to the client.
  ② The nurse puts on sterile gloves when entering the client's room.
  ③ The nurse puts on a gown when entering the client's room.
  ④ The nurse only puts on gloves when starting an IV.
  ⑤ The nurse maintains the client in isolation precautions for the duration of visible lesions.

6.16 What is the correct order for the nurse to remove the personal protective equipment (PPE) following the care for a client in isolation? Organize the steps in chronological order. **All options must be used.**

① Mask
② Gloves
③ Goggles/Face Shield
④ Gown

6.17 Two Rehab nurses are preparing to transfer a client from the bed to the chair. Which of these nursing actions would the nurse implement to assure a safe transfer for the client?
  ① Instruct client to depend on the nurse whenever possible during the transfer.
  ② Position bed in highest position if client is able to tolerate.
  ③ Position chair so client is moving toward the strong side.
  ④ Instruct client to pivot prior to standing.

6.18 What is the priority of care for the Rehab nurse prior to administering atenolol as prescribed?
  ① Verify the identity of the client by asking the client to state first name.
  ② Verify the client's name and room number with the medication order.
  ③ Scan the hospital code along with the medication name and compare to wrist bracelet.
  ④ Verify the full name of the client and medical record number on the wrist bracelet with appropriate documentation.

6.19 Which of these actions by the older adult, who is being discharged from Rehab with a cane following a fall, indicate the client understands how to safely use the cane?
  ① The client places the cane on the affected side to provide support to that side.
  ② The client advances the cane simultaneously with the opposite affected lower limb.
  ③ The affected lower limb assumes the first full weight-bearing step on level surfaces.
  ④ The client places the cane on the unaffected side and moves before the affected lower limb.

6.20 Which of these nursing actions indicate an understanding of how to safely provide care for a client with Vancomycin-Resistant Enterococci (VRE)?
  ① The nurse puts on a mask and gown when entering the client's room.
  ② The client's roommate is located > 2 feet (61 cm) from the client.
  ③ The client will remain in isolation until there are three negative cultures from infection site 1 week apart.
  ④ The nurse will wear an N95 respirator when providing care for client.

6.21 A client arrives in ER with a chief complaint of very dark urine and swelling around the eyes. Client's blood pressure is 160/92 and is complaining of fatigue. In taking the client's history, what would be most important for the nurse to ask?
  ① "Have you had a recent strep infection?"
  ② "Have you had a recent staph infection?"
  ③ "Have you been camping recently?"
  ④ "Is anyone else in your home sick?"

6.22 What would be the priority of care for the nurse to implement when drawing blood cultures on a client with acute renal failure (ARF) on dialysis who has a temporary access catheter and spikes a temperature of 104°F (40°C)?
   ① Draw a sample from the dialysis catheter.
   ② Obtain 2 culture bottles from the same stick.
   ③ Use alcohol and Betadine to prep the skin.
   ④ Wait until the cultures are drawn to start the antibiotics.

6.23 What is the priority nursing action for a client in airborne precautions with the diagnosis of active tuberculosis who is refusing to eat or make eye contact?
   ① Limit contact with the client to reduce the risk of transmission of infection.
   ② Place a "No Visitors" sign on the door to give the client privacy.
   ③ Request a psychiatric consult because the client is obviously depressed.
   ④ Spend extra time with the client to assess the client's emotional status.

6.24 In order to best prevent infection in the NICU, the nurse would implement what nursing action?
   ① Use meticulous hand washing technique.
   ② Wear sterile gowns and gloves when in direct contact with an infant.
   ③ Administer ordered antibiotics.
   ④ Avoid contact with the infant unless absolutely necessary.

6.25 A client is admitted to the Emergency Department with complaints of abdominal pain and bloody diarrhea. The client has been traveling and eating in restaurants for the past week. What would the nurse implement first?
   ① Be certain blood cultures and a CBC are obtained.
   ② Institute IV therapy and IV antibiotics.
   ③ Obtain a stool specimen for culture and WBCs.
   ④ Administer antidiarrheal medication.

6.26 The teacher sends a first grader to see the school nurse. The child's eyes are red, and there is a small amount of purulent discharge. The nurse phones the parent and the parent says, "My child has been on antibiotic eye drops for 24 hours." What would the nurse implement?
   ① Permit the child to return to the classroom, but encourage frequent hand washing.
   ② Tell the parent the child must stay out of school until all the symptoms are gone.
   ③ Tell the teacher to prevent contact with other children and encourage frequent hand washing.
   ④ Demand the parent pick up the child immediately.

6.27 What is the priority of care for the nurse to implement after finding an elderly client on the floor during AM nursing rounds?
   ① Document that client fell out of bed due to side rails being low and place the description of the incident in the client's chart and on the medical record.
   ② Advise the supervisor on night shift to complete the incident report prior to leaving since supervisor was in charge on the previous shift.
   ③ Complete the incident report at the end of day, when nurse is less busy, and can think in a logical manner, so the provider of care can review it on the medical records.
   ④ Complete an incident report including an objective description of the incident and actions taken to safeguard the client, as well as assessment and treatment of injuries.

6.28 The nurse is changing a dressing on an infected abdominal wound with Penrose drains and a large amount of purulent drainage. What is the best way to perform this procedure?
① Obtain clean gloves and dressings, remove the soiled dressing, and use another pair of clean gloves to dress the wound.
② Use clean gloves to remove the soiled dressings, change to sterile gloves and use sterile dressings to cover the wound.
③ Use the sterile gloves to remove the dressing, obtain clean gloves and sterile dressing to reapply to the wound.
④ Initiate protective isolation, utilize only sterile gloves when removing the dressing, and reapply using sterile technique.

6.29 What observations indicate a potential risk and need modification for a client with dementia secondary to Alzheimer's disease who is being cared for by family at home? **Select all that apply.**
① There is a nightlight between the client's bedroom and the bathroom.
② Throw rugs on hard wood floor in front of the entry door and sinks.
③ Client wears nonskid shoes when up and walking in the home.
④ The client only wears glasses when attempting to read fine print.
⑤ Protective door handle covers opening to the outside.

6.30 A client with a necrotizing spider bite is to perform dressing changes at home. Which statement made by the client indicates a correct understanding of aseptic technique?
① "I need to buy sterile gloves to redress this wound."
② "I should wash my hands before redressing my wound."
③ "I should not expose the wound to air at all."
④ "I should use an over-the-counter antimicrobial ointment."

6.31 During the insertion of a central venous pressure monitor device, the tip brushes the underside of the sterile field. Which nursing action is most appropriate?
① Wipe the tip with alcohol before connecting to system.
② Notify the physician of the occurrence, so an antibiotic can be given.
③ Back-flush catheter for several seconds before connecting.
④ Obtain a new monitor device, and prepare for a second attempt.

6.32 During the post-op period for a cardiac client, the graduate nurse is providing dressing care for the client receiving total parenteral nutrition (TPN) through a single-lumen percutaneous central catheter. Which of these observations would require intervention by the charge nurse to review the standard of practice with the graduate nurse?
① The client is weighed daily per hospital protocol.
② The client has a mask on during dressing changes over the TPN site.
③ The client's dressing is changed daily using standard precautions.
④ The nurse discards a bag of TPN after it was hanging only 24 hours and hangs a new bag.

6.33 The nurse is changing the dressing on a client with a large abdominal wound. There are two Penrose drains in place. What is the priority information for the nurse to include when recording this procedure?
① Condition of the surrounding tissue, time necessary to change the dressing, the type of dressing used.
② Client's tolerance of the procedure, time the dressing was changed, amount of wound drainage.
③ Client's response to the dressing change, status of Penrose drains, type of drainage from Penrose drains.
④ Time dressing was changed, description of the wound, color and amount of drainage from Penrose drains.

6.34 While assessing the incision of a 2-day post-operative client, a shiny pink open area is noted with underlying visible bowel. What would be the priority nursing action?
① Cover gaping area with sterile gauze soaked in normal saline.
② Reapply sterile dressing after cleaning with peroxide.
③ Pack opened area with sterile ¾-inch (19 mm) gauze soaked in normal saline.
④ Apply Neosporin ointment and cover with Tegaderm dressing.

6.35 An older client has been recently diagnosed with Clostridium difficile following hospitalization for an elective surgery. Which of these nursing actions by the LPN requires further intervention by the charge nurse?
① The nurse places the client in a private room.
② The nurse refuses to share the dynamap and stethoscope with the nurse providing care for another client.
③ The nurse cleans hands with the hand antibacterial foam that is outside the client's room.
④ The nurse disposes the infections dressing material into the nonporous bag.

6.36 Which nursing implication is important regarding spinal anesthesia?
① The client should be adequately hydrated in order to prevent hypotension after anesthesia is established.
② The client must be NPO at least 12 hours prior to the initiation of the anesthesia to decrease the risk of aspiration.
③ Assess the client for any allergies to Betadine or iodine preparations.
④ Determine the specific gravity of the urine and prepare the client for a central line.

6.37 Which of these plans is most important for reducing the risk of falling for an elderly client admitted to the medical unit?
① Provide the client with long pajama bottoms and assist with tying them around waist, so they do not drag on the floor.
② Place the phone and personal items on the dresser in the client's room.
③ Provide client with a bed alarm if received sleeping medicine within 10 hours.
④ Verify bed alarm works every 24 hours.

6.38 To evaluate the adverse reactions from antibiotic therapy in a client with a post-operative infection and receiving ceftriaxone sodium IVPB every day, what would the nurse monitor?
① Surface of the tongue
② Hemoglobin and hematocrit
③ Skin surfaces in skin folds
④ Changes in urine characteristics

6.39 When irrigating a draining wound with a sterile saline solution, which sequence is most appropriate for the nurse to follow?
① Pour solution, wash hands, and remove soiled dressing.
② Wash hands, prepare sterile field, remove soiled dressing.
③ Prepare sterile field, put on sterile gloves, and remove soiled dressing.
④ Remove soiled dressing, flush wound, wash hands.

6.40 To protect a post heart transplant client from potential sources of infection, what is the priority nursing intervention?
① Keep client in total isolation.
② Limit participation in unit activities.
③ Adhere to and monitor strict hand-washing techniques.
④ Monitor vital signs, especially temperature, every 2 hours.

6.41 Which instruction is correct regarding the colletion of a specimen from a 4-year-old suspected of having pinworms?
① Collect the specimen 30 minutes after the child falls asleep at night.
② Save a portion of the child's first stool of the day, and take it to the physician's office immediately.
③ Collect the specimen in the early morning with a piece of scotch tape touched to the child's anus.
④ Feed the child a high-fat meal; then save the first stool following the meal.

6.42 What is the priority of care for a young adult client who was found unconscious with several empty medicine bottles at side with a breath that smelled like alcohol and BP—120/72, HR—64 bpm, R—10/min and shallow, T—97.8°F (36.6°C)?
① Keep client on a backboard and apply neck brace.
② Have respiratory therapy paged for ventilation support.
③ Call poison control for instructions and set up charcoal infusion.
④ Obtain the empty medicine bottles from the EMTs and notify the ER provider.

6.43 Which observation indicates a mother needs further teaching regarding protecting the newborn from infection?
① Wipes base of umbilical cord to keep dry and folds diaper so urine does not get on cord.
② Positions the diaper below the umbilicus.
③ Does not wash her hands prior to handling the newborn.
④ Applies sterile gauze with petroleum jelly to the circumcision.

6.44 What is the priority plan of care to promote client safety when they are receiving internal radiation therapy?
① Restrict visitors who may have an upper respiratory infection.
② Assign only male care givers to the client.
③ Plan nursing activities to decrease nurse exposure.
④ Wear a lead lined apron whenever delivering client care.

6.45 What is the priority nursing intervention to promote safety in the environment for a client with a marked depression of T cells?
① Keep a linen hamper immediately outside the room.
② Use sterile linens.
③ Provide masks for anyone entering the room.
④ Discard any standing water left in containers or equipment.

6.46 Which nursing observation indicates a major complication in a client who suffered a thermal injury two weeks ago?
① Increased heart rate and elevated blood pressure.
② Temperature of 100.6°F (38.1°C) and decreased respiratory rate.
③ Increased heart rate and decreased respiratory rate.
④ Increased respiratory rate and decreased blood pressure.

6.47 Which statement concerning the transmission of head lice is most important for the nurse to teach?
① Head lice occur primarily in lower socioeconomic groups.
② Transmission is airborne through insect vectors.
③ Infestation is reduced in cold weather.
④ Transmission is most common where there are crowded living conditions.

6.48 Prior to the insertion and after contact with a vascular access device for a client, what is the priority of care?
① Apply on a mold mask and goggles.
② Educate client regarding the procedure.
③ Initiate scrupulous hand hygiene.
④ Initiate vigorous friction to central catheter hubs with betadine prep x 10 seconds.

6.49 How should the nurse administer the DPT immunization to a 6-month old?
① By mouth in three divided doses.
② As an IM injection into the gluteus maximus.
③ As an injection into the vastus lateralis.
④ As a Z track injection into the deltoid.

6.50 Which action is necessary to maintain asepsis during a sterile dressing change?
① After scrubbing for the procedure, hold your elbows close to your body.
② Unused sterile dressing tray can be used for the next client if used within 15 minutes.
③ If you splash a liquid on the sterile field, start over again.
④ If you drop a dressing, leave it until you have completed the procedure.

6.51 Which statement made by a parent indicates a correct understanding of poison prevention at home?
① "We store gasoline for the lawn mower in the garage."
② "All our medications are kept in their original containers."
③ "We keep all our cleaning products in the bathroom."
④ "I keep most of our medications in my purse."

6.52 Which clinical finding is priority to report prior to administering gentamycin IV piggyback?
① Temperature—101.2°F (38.4°C)
② Intake 65 mL in one hour
③ BUN—29 mg/dL (10.4 mmol/L), creatinine—2.1 mg/dL (186 μmol/L)
④ WBC—12,000/mm^3

6.53 What is the appropriate nursing action for the client on the first post-operative day after a cholecystectomy who has 375 mL of dark serosanguineous fluid draining from the gastric tube?
① Notify the provider of care immediately.
② Prepare for a blood transfusion.
③ Document information in notes.
④ Replace fluid to prevent dehydration.

6.54 A school-aged child is being treated for Hepatitis A which was diagnosed two weeks ago. The client plans to return to school this week with a provider of care's permit. What plan for client's return is appropriate?
① Isolating client from the other children.
② Talking with the provider of care about the reason for return so soon.
③ No specific health requirements are necessary.
④ Not allowing participation in any sports.

6.55 What is the priority nursing action to teach the client and close associates to prevent the spread of Hepatitis A?
① Wash their hands every time they go to the bathroom.
② Refuse to use any blood products.
③ Teach drug addicts never to share their used needles.
④ Always use condoms during sexual intercourse.

6.56 Which measure would be explained to the staff to maintain safety while using the defibrillator?
① Remain clear of the bed when using the defibrillator.
② Check the defibrillator every 24 hours.
③ Ask staff not to leave the defibrillator plugged in.
④ Do not defibrillate over the electrodes.

6.57 What would be the priority plan of care for an elderly client with diabetes, hypertension, BUN—23 mg/dL (8.2 mmol/L); creatinine—2.1 mg/dL (186 μmol/L); who is scheduled for a CAT scan with and without contrast?
① Hydrate well prior to the procedure.
② Monitor BP before and after procedure.
③ Make client NPO six hours prior to procedure.
④ Recommend to provider that the scan is only done without contrast.

6.58 A client with renal cancer will be discharged home with a central venous catheter in place. Which of the following statements made by the client indicates a correct understanding of aseptic technique?
① "I should not take showers."
② "I must wash my hands after changing the dressing."
③ "I can reuse my equipment from the day before."
④ "I must wash my hands before changing the dressing."

6.59 At a health screening clinic, an adult male client's total plasma cholesterol level is reported to be 200 mg/dL (5.17 mmol/L). Based on this assessment, which nursing action is most appropriate?
① Refer the client to a physician for appropriate medication.
② Ask the client to lie down immediately.
③ Encourage the client to follow a low-fat diet.
④ Recheck the cholesterol level in two years.

6.60 The health care provider orders wrist restraints for an elderly client pulling at the Foley catheter. The client refuses to allow the nurse to put the restraints on arms. What is the priority nursing intervention?
① Chart the refusal, remove the restraints, and check the client frequently.
② Apply a vest restraint rather than wrist restraints.
③ Obtain the assistance of the UAP to apply the wrist restraints.
④ Administer client PRN for pain and apply restraints after client is asleep.

6.61 A client receiving patient-controlled analgesia (PCA) complains of no pain relief. Which is the safest action by the nurse?
① Check the programming of the pump for correctness.
② Replace the pump with a new one. Have the old one checked.
③ Report the pump dysfunction to the charge nurse.
④ Replace the pump. Send the old one to soiled utility.

6.62 Workplace violence especially in the ER Department is an increasing safety issue. Which are the best plans to reduce this type of violence? **Select all that apply.**
① Provide fast service to remove clients from ER as soon as possible.
② Provide hospital security in the ER department.
③ Maintain communication with clients in the waiting room.
④ Allow providers of care to carry guns.
⑤ Educate admitting staff regarding communication and caring.

6.63 What would be the priority discharge instructions for a client with hemiplegia from a stroke who is being discharged home with use of a cane?
① Rent a hospital bed with an overhead frame, so that the client can get up easily without falling.
② Remove throw rugs and other obstacles on the floor as canes can easily slip.
③ Build a ramp for easy access to the outside.
④ Insert handrails in the shower and beside the toilet for easy use.

6.64 The female client gets out of the bed and a cervical implanted radiation device falls to the floor. What is the nurse's best action?
① Call the hazardous materials department to remove the device immediately.
② Have the client take a shower and return to bed.
③ Remove the device from the room, so that the client will not be harmed.
④ Call the provider of care to inform of the situation.

6.65 What is the priority action if the hospital area becomes filled with smoke from a fire?
① Remove the clients from the smoke.
② Sound the fire alarm.
③ Use fire extinguisher to put out the fire.
④ Contain fire to prevent the spread to other clients.

Answers & Rationales

6.1 ④ Option #4 is correct. The LPN/VN does not need to wear a mask when giving a bath to a client with Hepatitis B. Hepatitis B requires contact and standard precautions which do not require a mask. The nurse needs to intervene, since the LPN/VN does not understand the standard of practice for this client as evidenced by the application of the mask. Options #1, #2, and #3 are correct practice for these clients and do not require intervention by the charge nurse.
I CAN HINT: Apply the clinical judgment/cognitive skill, take-action (first-do priority interventions). The topic focuses on principles of infection prevention with a focus Hepatitis B. The standard of practice for Hepatitis is standard and contact precautions.
NCLEX® Standard: Report and intervene unsafe practice of health care personnel (e.g., improper care, staffing practices); Apply principles of infection prevention.

6.2 ④ Option #4 is correct. he client is presenting with assessment findings for meningitis. Droplet precautions should be priority to include in the plan of care by applying a surgical facemask when 3-6 feet from the client to assist with infection prevention. Options #1, #2, and #3 should also be included in the plan, but are not the priorities over infection prevention.
I CAN HINT: Apply the clinical judgment/cognitive skill, (generate solutions), to the client who is presenting with assessment findings of meningitis. You first need to understand the client's clinical findings and analyze these to support the medical condition of meningitis. Refer to the book, *Nursing Made Insanely Easy*, by Manning, L. & Rayfield, S. for an easy strategy to master the nursing care for clients with meningitis.
NCLEX® Standard: Apply principles of infection prevention. Manage the care of a client with alteration in hemodynamics, tissue perfusion, and hemostasis.

6.3 ① Option #1 is correct. Cephalosporin antibiotics
③ have a broad spectrum of activity, easily
④ changing the gastrointestinal mycobiome
⑤ allowing for the proliferation of pathogens such as C.Diff. C.diff colonization results in foul-smelling diarrhea and abdominal cramping that often progresses in severity. Previously known as Pseudomembranous colitis, C.Diff superinfections can quickly lead to dehydration requiring fluid resuscitation especially in the elderly. Stool analysis is required to confirm C.Diff colonization. A physician's order is required however the astute nurse can collect the specimen to hasten the process. Option #3 is correct. Hand hygiene after direct client contact or contact with the client's environment should include hand hygiene with soap and water if any transmittable microbes are suspected. Option #4 is correct. Use of clean non-latex gloves is required with direct client contact as precaution to reduce the risk of microbial spread. Option #5 is correct. Diarrhea presents a threat to fluid and electrolyte balance regardless of cause. This is evident by the client's HR and BP. Increasing fluid intake will help reduce the risk of dehydration especially in children and the elderly. Option #2 is incorrect. Contact Precautions are the correct transmission-based precautions for C.Diff. Protective precautions are standards of practice for clients who are immunosuppressed.
I CAN HINT: Apply the clinical judgment/cognitive skill, take-action (first-do priority interventions) for a client presenting with an infection and is presenting with fluid deficit.
NCLEX® Standard: Apply principles of infection prevention. Manage the care of the client with a fluid and electrolyte imbalance.

6.4 ① Option #1 is correct. Infections caused by SARS-CoV-2 (coronavirus or COVID 19) require Airborne Precautions. Personal protective equipment(PPE) for direct client care for Airborne precautions include gowns, goggles, gloves, and an N-95 mask or respirator. Option #2 is incorrect. At the outset of the COVID pandemic, visitors were restricted due to the limited knowledge the novel virus. Increased knowledge surrounding transmission, treatment, and prevention of spread of the virus as well as vaccine development have allowed visitation policies to be amended. Visitors continue to be limited as to number and times of day in some cases and Airborne Precautions maintained by all who enter the client's room. Option #3 is incorrect. Sterile gloves are required for invasive procedures but not for all client care procedures. Clean gloves are required as part of PPE for Airborne Precautions. Option #4 is incorrect. All soiled linen and refuse from a client requiring transmission-based precautions should be disposed of in a dedicated, designated disposal bag, container, and area.
I CAN HINT: Apply the clinical judgment/cognitive skill, take-action (first-do priority interventions) for a client presenting with an infection.
NCLEX® Standard: Apply principles of infection prevention.

6.5 ② Option #2 is correct. These measures are correct as they incorporate handwashing prior to and after visiting. Hand hygiene remains a dominate force in preventing the transmission of infectious disease. Option #1 is incorrect. While these measures are correct for caregiver personal protective equipment (PPE), visitors have the option of N-95 mask or surgical mask for visiting. N-95 is suggested for anyone who is immune compromised. Option #3 is incorrect. COVID 19 transmission guidelines are Airborne Precautions. Option #4 is incorrect. Sterile gloves are not required in Airborne Precautions.
I CAN HINT: Apply the clinical judgment/cognitive skill, (generate solutions), to the client who is presenting with COVID 19.
NCLEX® Standard: Educate client and staff regarding infection prevention measure.

6.6 ① Option #1 is correct. Hand hygiene after exiting a client's room and before entering another client's room is a breach of standard precautions designed to protect all clients from the spread of hospital acquired infections. Options #2, #3, and #4 are correct standards of practice and do not require intervention by the Registered Nurse. Option #2 is incorrect. Computer on Wheels have become an excellent method of safe effective administration of client's medications by checking the EHR MAR closely prior to entering the client environment. The Computer on Wheels could be taken into the room but would require careful decontamination upon leaving the patient environment. Leaving the Computer on Wheels just outside the individual client's environment supports best practice medication administration and standard enhanced barrier precautions. Option #3 is incorrect. Use of disposable equipment, including blood pressure cuffs, thermometers, and stethoscopes, supports standard enhanced barrier precautions as well as transmission-based infection measures. Option #4 is incorrect. Any equipment used inside the client's environment must be carefully decontaminated prior to reuse, especially one that has had the close contact that telemetry units have to the client.
I CAN HINT: Apply the clinical judgment/cognitive skill, (generate solutions), to the clinical situation that is violating the standard of practice for standard enhanced barrier precautions to provide safe care.
NCLEX® Standard: Report and intervene unsafe practice of health care personnel (e.g., improper care, staffing practices); Apply principle of infection prevention.

6.7 ② Option #2 is correct. Due to RSV being a respiratory infection and being transmitted by direct contact the standard of practice requires contact precautions. Parents should not have direct contact with their child's face like kissing. Option #1 is incorrect. Masks are not required for contact precautions. Option #3 is not included in the standard of practice for these clients. RSV can be destroyed on toys by first cleansing with detergent and water and then applying a one-to-ten dilution of regular (5.25%) bleach and water (e.g., one cup of bleach to nine cups of water). Option #4 is not included in the standard of practice.
I CAN HINT: Apply the clinical judgment/cognitive skill, (generate solutions), to the clinical situation that is violating the standard of practice for standard enhanced barrier precautions to provide safe care.
NCLEX® Standard: Report and intervene unsafe practice of health care personnel (e.g., improper care, staffing practices); Apply principle of infection prevention.

6.8 ③ Option #3 is correct. RSV requires contact and standard precautions. Sterile gloves are not included in the standard of practice for this type of transmission-based precautions. The LPN/VN requires further instruction regarding best nursing practice for clients with RSV. Options #1, #2, and #4 do not require further instruction since these are included in the standard of practice for the specific medical conditions. Option #1 is included in contact precautions. Option #2 is included in airborne precautions. Option #4 is included in droplet precautions.
I CAN HINT: Apply the clinical judgment/cognitive skill, (generate solutions), for the infant with RSV.
NCLEX® Standard: Apply principles of infection prevention. Educate client and staff regarding infection prevention measures.

6.9 ③ Options #3, #4, and #5 are correct statements.
④ Varicella can be transmitted via airborne or
⑤ contact. Option #1 is incorrect. Research has connected administering aspirin to a child with varicella high risk for developing Reye's syndrome. Option #2 is incorrect. Mild soap should not be used.
I CAN HINT: Apply the clinical judgment/cognitive skill, (generate solutions), for the child with varicella. Refer to the book, *Nursing Made Insanely Easy*, by Manning, L. & Rayfield, S. for an easy strategy to master the nursing care for clients with varicella.
NCLEX® Standard: Apply principle of infection prevention. Educate client, family, and/or staff regarding infection prevention measures.

6.10 ③ Option #3 is correct. Due to the risk of the undesirable effect of extrapyramidal effects, clients may be at risk for falls. Benztropine is a centrally acting anticholinergic drug used for Parkinson's Disease to decrease the tremors and ease dystonia. This medication will assist in improving client's gait and balance. Therapeutic effects are seen with this medication within 2-3 days after initiation of therapy. Option #1 is incorrect. First generation antipsychotic medications do not experience the undesirable effect from a skin rash. Option #2 is incorrect. Option #4 is incorrect but would be appropriate if the question was asking about MAO inhibitors.
I CAN HINT: Apply the clinical judgment/cognitive skill, (generate solutions), for the client taking haloperidol. "STANCE" in the book, *Pharmacology Made Insanely Easy*, by Manning and Rayfield will provide an easy strategy for mastering undesirable effects for the medications in the 3 generations of antipsychotic medications.
NCLEX® Standard: Protect client from injury (e.g., falls).

6.11 ③ Options #3, #4, and #5 are correct. These
④ clinical findings occur with the release of
⑤ histamine that is released with an allergic reaction. Options #1 and #2 can occur if a hemolytic reaction was to occur from the transfusion.

6.12 ③ Option #3 is correct. The strategy to answering this question is to understand that corticosteroids cause immunosuppression. This places the client at a high risk for infection. Placing a mask on client may assist in decreasing the risk of infection. Option #1 is not correct. The potassium may be decreased with the use of steroids and would require a diet high in potassium. Option #2 is not correct. Calcium may be decreased with these medications, and will require additional support with calcium intake. Option #4 is not correct. Symptoms of infection should not be expected, but should be reported.

6.13 ③ Option #3 is correct. The strategy for answering this question correctly is to recognize this client who is recovering from a renal transplant will be immunocompromised and very high risk for infection. This will assist in determining what room mate would be best for this client. Option #3 is the client who is not going to transmit an infection to this client recovering from a renal transplant.

6.14 ① Option #1 is the correct answer. The strategy is to focus on the safety for this client. This elderly client is high risk for falls. Option #2 is not correct; it does not address the fact the client wanders the halls. Option #3 may result in falls due to the medication. Option #4 is not correct, since this is unrealistic.

6.15 ① ③ ⑤ Option #1 is correct. Nurses who have not had chickenpox or the vaccine should not provide care for this client due to the risk of transmission. Option #3 is correct. The precautions used for this organism include standard/airborne/contact precautions. Part of contact precautions includes gown, gloves, and as needed mask and goggles. Option #5 is a correct statement. Option #2 is incorrect, Option #4 is incorrect, since gloves are part of the isolation precautions for this infectious agent. It would violate the standard of care if the nurse ONLY put on gloves for this client when starting an IV.

6.16

② Gloves: *The first step would be to extend arms and slowly peel one glove downward, turning it inside out. With the ungloved hand, slide a finger under the inside portion of the remaining glove, turning inside out, and discard.*
③ Goggles/ face shield: *The second step in this process is to remove the goggles/face shield by grasping the ear pieces or headband to remove.*
④ Gown: *The third step is to remove the gown by unfastening the neck, then the waist ties; pull gown forward away from the body, folding it inside out and rolling it into a bundle for disposal.*
① Mask: *The fourth step is to remove the mask by only touching the ties. It is important the front of the mask is not touched.*

6.17 ③ Option #3 is correct. During a transfer from the bed, always remember "*Strong side leads*." Option #1 is incorrect. The client should be advised how to assist when possible versus depending on the nurse. Option #2 is incorrect since the bed should be lowered to the lowest position to decrease the risk for falls. Option #4 is incorrect since the client should be standing first and then pivot.

6.18 ④ Option #4 is correct. The 2009 National Patient Safety Goals mandate reviewing and using a minimum of two client identifiers. This goal is to prevent medication errors and optimize the delivery of safe care to the clients. Option #1 is not a complete answer. While asking a client who is alert and coherent to state name is correct, the new National Patient Safety Goals mandate using a minimum of two client identifiers prior to administering the medication. Option #2 is incorrect. While it is imperative to verify the name of the client prior to administering a medication, the room number is not an acceptable client identifier. Option #3 is incorrect. If the hospital has a bar coding system, then it may be correct to scan the medication label and the client's wrist bracelet; however, not the hospital code and this would not be a priority over option #4.

6.19 ② Option #2 is correct. The client should advance the cane simultaneously with the opposite affected lower limb to promote safety and prevent from falling. Option #1 is incorrect since the cane should be placed on the unaffected side to provide support to the opposite lower limb. Option #3 is incorrect since the unaffected lower limb should assume the first full weight-bearing step on level surfaces. Option #4 is incorrect even though the first part of the answer is correct regarding placing the cane on the unaffected side, it should be moved simultaneously with the opposite affected lower limb not before the affected lower limb.

6.20 ③ Option #3 is correct. Until there are three negative culture reports from infectious site (1 week apart), the client will remain in standard/contact precautions. Option #1 is incorrect since there is not a need for a mask unless there is an anticipation of splashing of body fluids. The gown would be correct if in contact with contaminated material. Hand hygiene and gloves are definitely part of these precautions for this infectious agent. Option #2 is incorrect; CDC recognizes situations may occur necessitating the roommates. If this becomes necessary, then the guidelines are that clients should be located > 3 feet (91.4 cm) apart from each other. It is also imperative that protective attire is changed and hand hygiene is performed between contact with clients in the same room, regardless of the disease status. Option #4 is incorrect for this client. This N95 respirator is necessary for clients with tuberculosis (TB) who are in airborne precautions.

6.21 ① Option #1 is correct. The client is showing symptoms of APSGN (acute post-streptococcal glomerulonephritis). Other symptoms for APSGN may include: oliguria, proteinuria, orthopnea, bibasilar rales, weight gain; an elevation in the serum BUN and creatinine; decrease in the creatinine clearance; hematuria, increased urine specific gravity; hyperkalemia, hypermagnesemia, dilutional hyponatremia if urine output is decreased. Throat culture will be positive for streptococcus infection. Options #2, #3, and #4 do not directly relate to the client's symptoms.

6.22 ④ Option #4 is correct. Starting an antibiotic prior to obtaining the culture can alter the results. Option #1, staff nurses and lab personnel do not use the dialysis catheter to obtain blood samples. Option #2, when cultures are ordered x 2 they should be drawn from 2 different sites. Option #3, clorhexadine is the preferred skin prep.

6.23 ④ Option #4 is the correct answer. It is important to further assess the emotional state to determine the cause of the behavior. It may be that when the nurse does additional assessment that the nurse learns the behavior is from some inappropriate concerns regarding isolation, and it can be improved with specific knowledge. In reality, there is a lot of different emotional concerns that the client may be experiencing. The key is for the nurse to assess, in order to unlock the appropriate plan to provide support for the client. Options #1 and #2 could worsen the situation. Option #3 is a possible correct answer, but the nurse should first assess the situation.

6.24 ① Option #1 is correct. The best method to reduce the risk of infection is hand washing. Option #2 is not usually necessary, Option #3 will not prevent infection. Option #4 could cause harm to the infant and result in failure to thrive.

6.25 ③ Option #3 is the priority action. This will determine the necessity of antibiotic use. Option #4, if this is bacterial gastroenteritis, antidiarrheals are contraindicated. Option #1 is not a priority over option #3.

6.26 ① If the child has been under treatment for 24 hours, the child should no longer be contagious, so option #1 is correct. Option #2 is not necessary as symptoms can last for several days after treatment begins. Option #3 is not practical to prevent contact among children in a classroom, and option #4, there is no need for the child to be picked up immediately. Hand washing is the best method to reduce the spread of infection.

6.27 ④ Option #4 is correct. The nurse should complete an incident report including an objective description of the incident and actions taken to safeguard the client, as well as assessment and treatment of injuries. This report should be included as soon as possible and within 24 hours of the incident. These are considered confidential and are not shared with the client (nor does the nurse inform the client that one has been completed.) These incident reports should not be in the chart of the client nor in the medical record. A description of the incident should be documented in clear concise and factual language in the client's record. This report should be forwarded to the risk management department after being reviewed by the nurse manager. Option #1 is incorrect, since the nurse is not certain as to the reason the client fell out of bed, and the report should not be placed in the client's chart nor in the client's medical record. The report should include a factual description of the incident and injuries incurred, avoiding any assumptions as to the cause of the incident. Option #2 is incorrect. The incident report should be completed by the person who identifies that an unexpected event has occurred. Option #3 is incorrect since the report should be completed as soon as possible and within 24 hours of the incident.

6.28 ② Sterile gloves and dressings are used in the application of dressings to wounds. Option #4 is incorrect because protective isolation is not appropriate for this client. Sterile gloves are not necessary for removing the soiled dressings.

6.29 ② ④ Options #2 and #4 are correct. Throw rugs should be removed since they can lead to falls. If the client has glasses, these should be worn on a routine basis. These can assist in the prevention of falls. Option #1 is not an answer since this is not a risk. This is a good practice to assist the client to see when going to bathroom. Option #3 will decrease the risk for falls, option #5, the protective door handle covers will prevent the client from going outside and wandering outdoors unattended.

6.30 ② The hallmark of asepsis is hand washing. Option #1 is incorrect because the question addresses medical aseptic technique, not sterile procedure. Option #3 is not necessary. Option #4 is incorrect because the client should use only prescribed medications on the wound.

6.31 ④ Contamination of equipment mandates new equipment be employed. Options #1 and #3 are not adequate because the catheter is still contaminated. Option #2 may be appropriate later, but obtaining a new monitoring device is a priority.

6.32 ③ Option #3 is correct. The technique should be surgical aseptic technique versus standard precautions. Typically, based on hospital protocol, the dressing is changed every 48 to 72 hours. This would require further intervention by the charge nurse to review the standard of practice with the graduate nurse. Option #1 would not require intervention by the charge nurse. Option #2 would be considered part of the standard of practice for this procedure, and would not require intervention due to lack of understanding. Option #4 would not require further intervention since this is included in the standard of care for toal parenteral nutrition. Solutions hanging for 24 hours should be discarded and a new bag of solution should be hung.

6.33 ④ The information in option #4 best describes the essential information that should be charted after a dressing change for a wound of this type. Options #1, #2, and #3 contain important information. However, the information in option #4 is more important.

6.34 ① Evisceration is treated immediately by application of sterile gauze soaked in sterile normal saline followed by notification of the physician. Options #2, #3, and #4 are not correct responses to this complication.

6.35 ③ Option #3 is correct because the charge nurse needs to explain to the LPN that this antibacterial foam has alcohol in it which does not kill the spores from Clostridium difficile. Hand washing with soap and water are the preferred nursing action to prevent infecting other clients. Option #1 is correct practice for a client with Clostridium difficile, and does not need intervention by the charge nurse. While the private room is the priority plan for this client, if there are no other rooms, the clients can be put in a room together with Clostridium difficile. The nurse, however, will need to change PPE and perform hand washing in between client care since they can be growing different spores. Option #2 is also correct practice and requires no further intervention. Equipment should be dedicated for the client or disinfected after each use. Option #4 is also correct practice, and does not require any further intervention by the charge nurse.

6.36 ① It is important that the client be well hydrated to prevent hypotensive problems after the spinal anesthesia is initiated. Option #2 is unnecessary. Option #3 is not necessary as iodine dyes are usually not used. Option #4 is irrelevant to the procedure.

6.37 ③ Option #3 is correct. Clients should have a bed alarm in place for the first 24 hours of their hospital stay based on their unit protocol and client population. After the first 24 hours, then the need to continue with the alarm will be based on the following: confusion, impulsive, impaired mobility, recent fall, and/or sleeping med within 10 hours. Option #1 is incorrect since they can become loose after being in bed and sleeping. It would be much better to provide clients with capri-length pajama bottoms versus having long bottoms that can cause falls. Option #2 is incorrect. It is not the most important plan for fall prevention in comparison to option #3. Even if the dresser was closer to client, it still would not be the priority over #3. Option #4 is incorrect since the alarm should be verified every shift for safe care.

6.38 ① Long-term use of ceftriaxone can cause overgrowth of organisms such as Candida albicans; therefore, monitoring of the tongue and oral cavity is recommended. Options #2, #3, and #4 do not reflect a problem with this medication.

6.39 ② Hand washing should be done prior to beginning any procedure—especially irrigating a wound. Options #1, #3, and #4 are in the incorrect sequence.

6.40 ③ One of the most important nursing strategies with a client who is immunosuppressed is adherence to, and monitoring hand-washing of self and others to prevent transmission of sources of infection. Option #1 is not necessary although a private room might be helpful. Option #2 would allow the client to further withdraw and limit their opportunities for corrective milieu experiences. Option #4 is more often than necessary unless there is a temperature elevation.

6.41 ③ Pinworms crawl outside the anus early in the morning to lay their eggs. This specimen should be collected early in the morning before the child awakens. Option #1 is not the optimum time for collecting the eggs and may result in a false negative test. Option #2 is incorrect because pinworms are rarely found in the stool. Option #4 is incorrect protocol for this test.

6.42 ④ Option #4 is correct. The bottles will likely determine the next step in the emergency treatment. Option #1 is incorrect. There is nothing in the stem of the question indicating a risk for a neck injury. Option #2 may be the second step. Option #3 is premature since the bottles are a mystery until they are examined.

I CAN HINT: This question is evaluating your understanding of the general principles for poison control. A way to help you remember this is by using the mnemonic "**SIRES**":

Stabilize the client's condition. Assess condition and provide respiratory support, IV access.

Identify the toxic substance. Obtain history and retrieve any available poison. Notify HCP.

Remove the substance to decrease absorption. Shower or wash off radioactive substance.

Antidotes: for heroin or other drug overdose. Ingested substances: lavage, absorbents (activated charcoal), or cathartics.

Eliminate the substance from client's body.

Support client both physically and psychologically.

6.43 ③ Proper hand washing is a priority in preventing infection. Options #1, #2, and #4 are correct and do not indicate a need for further teaching.

6.44 ③ The principles for radiation safety include: time, distance, and shielding. The nurse should decrease the time spent at a close distance to the client. Option #1 is incorrect because all visitors must keep distance from the client. Option #2 is incorrect since radiation is as harmful to males as to females. Option #4 is used when the nurse has to spend any length of time at close distance with the client—not for routine care.

6.45 ④ Water should not be allowed to stand in containers, such as respiratory or suction equipment, because this could act as a culture medium. Option #1 is incorrect because the protocol for handling soiled articles is accomplished within universal/standard precautions guidelines using double biohazard bags. Option #2 is incorrect because sterile linens are used for clients who are burned or immuno-compromised. Option #3 is not protocol unless the client or visitor has an active pulmonary infection.

6.46 ④ Increased respiratory rate and decreased blood pressure may indicate burn wound sepsis—a life-threatening complication of thermal injury. Options #1, #2, and #3 should be investigated further, but alone do not represent significant compromise.

6.47 ④ Crowded living conditions where there is sharing of clothing and physical closeness increases the likelihood of transmission. Option #1 is incorrect because head lice occur in all socio-economic levels. Option #2 is incorrect because lice are transmitted by close contact. Option #3 is incorrect because weather is not a deterrent although more cases are seen in the winter in some areas due to the sharing of hats.

6.48 ③ Option #3 is correct. When answering questions about preventing Central Line (CVC) Associated Blood Stream Infection (CLABS) with insertion and maintenance—
I CAN HINT: Follow the "SAVE" Precautions. This is an easy way to remember the care. Scrupulous hand hygiene: Prior to insertion & before & after contact with vascular access device. Aseptic Technique- During CVC catheter insertion & care. Vigorous friction to central catheter hubs with alcohol prep x 15 seconds & allow to air dry – whenever a break to the connection is made with administering medication, obtaining a blood sample, flushing, changing tubing/port, or adding a device. Ensure CVC lumen patency. Positive pressure cap must be used on all CVC lumens, including PICC's. (Maximum Clear Access cap). Flush each lumen with 20 mL (2 pre-filled 10 mL syringes) preservative free NS after each medication or every 12 hours if lumen not in use or infusion rate <25 mL/hr. Do not force flush a line. CVC flush technique: 1. Flush line. 2. Disconnect syringe. 3. Clamp lumen. Change injection cap if unable to clear all blood from port after blood samples (do not leave blood in access cap).

6.49 ③ Because the muscle mass of an infant is small, the intramuscular injection should be given in the lateral aspect of the thigh (vastus lateralis). Option #1 is incorrect since the injection is not administered PO. Option #2 is incorrect because the gluteus does not have enough muscle mass. Option #4 is not necessary, and the deltoid is an incorrect area for this method of administration.

6.50 ④ To maintain a sterile field, all items in that field must remain sterile. Leave the contaminated dressing until the procedure is completed. Option #1 is incorrect because elbows are held away from the body. Option #2 is incorrect because sterile materials can be used only for one client; and if unused, must be discarded, or re-sterilized. Option #3 is unnecessary because a liquid can be covered with a sterile towel.

6.51 ② All medications should be kept in their original container and out of reach. Options #1, #3, and #4 are not appropriate safety measures to prevent accidental poisonings.

6.52 ③ Option #3 is important to report since gentamycin can be nephrotoxic. Options #1 and #4 are indications of an infection which is the reason for administering the antibiotic. Option #2 is a normal clinical finding.

6.53 ③ Option #3 is correct. The amount of drainage for the first post-operative day is approximately 300 to 500 mL. It is important to keep accurate records of the output. Options #1, #2, and #4 are incorrect.
I CAN HINT: If you did not know the drainage amount, then you could have clustered options #2 and #4 together, since these both address too much drainage.
Option #2 indicating the need to prepare for a blood transfusion is implying the client is bleeding or low in blood volume. Option #1 also indicates there is a problem if the provider of care has to be notified. Critical reasoning is not just effective for clinical decision making, but is also great for test taking strategies!

6.54 ③ Type A Hepatitis is not infectious within a week or so after the onset of jaundice, and the child can return to school. Options #1 and #2 are not necessary. Option #4 depends on the child's energy level.

6.55 ① Type A Hepatitis is spread by oral-fecal route, so it is important to teach effective hand washing every time the client uses the bathroom, or has genital-rectal contact. Options #2, #3, and #4 are not true for Hepatitis A. **I CAN HINT:** Notice that options #2 and #3 both address blood/needles. Since this is not a *Select all that apply* question, you can cluster the similar options together. This will provide you with a 50% chance of getting the right answer even if you have no idea what the correct answer is!

6.56 ① This is a priority to prevent accidental countershock. Option #2 is incorrect because the equipment should be checked every 8 hours. Option #3 is incorrect because the equipment should remain plugged in at all times. Option #4 is correct information, but is not a priority.

6.57 ④ Protecting the client's safety is a priority for the nursing care plan. Options #1, #2, and #3 are not necessary for this client and do not address safety. The BUN and creatine levels are elevated. The contrast could result in further renal compromise.

6.58 ④ The foundation of aseptic technique is meticulous hand washing prior to a procedure. Options #1 and #3 are inappropriate. Option #2 is incomplete.

6.59 ③ The total cholesterol level for an adult male should be under 200 mg/dL (5.17 mmol/L). Higher levels require a low-fat diet. Levels higher than 250 mg/dL (6.47 mmol/L) may require medication, if diet therapy is not effective. Option #1 is not necessary prior to working on diet. Option #2 is incorrect. Option #4 is incorrect because blood levels should be checked sooner than 2 years.

6.60 ① Option #1 is the only answer that does respect the client's right to refuse. Options #2, #3, and #4 may be considered malpractice.

6.61 ② Option #2 is correct. If faulty equipment, client's treatment is interrupted, and for safety it is imperative for the PCA pump to be replaced. Option #1 is incorrect; the settings will have been checked by 2 RN's prior to initiating PCA. Option #3 is incorrect, reporting does not address the issue of client not receiving medication. Option #4 is incorrect, replacing is correct; however, the faulty one must be investigated for safety.

6.62 ①②③⑤ Options #1, #2, #3, and #5 are ways to keep the waiting clients from becoming belligerent. Hopefully we will never get to option #4 as being the only answer.

6.63 ② Option #2 is the priority instruction. Option #4 may be necessary if the client is having trouble with balance. Options #1 and #3 should not be necessary at this time.

6.64 ① Option #1 is the only safe answer. The device must be removed by special handling materials, so that the person touching the radiation will not be exposed. Options #2 and #4 are secondary. Option #3 is an incorrect statement and a safety hazard to other clients, employees, family members, etc. that may come in contact with the radiation.

6.65 ① Option #1 should be priority. The rest is as easy as "RACE":

Rescue client

Activate the alarm

Contain fire, and

Extinguish

This is a strategy to assist in remembering the sequence of events for fire safety.

CHAPTER 7
Health Promotion and Maintenance

Just when the caterpillar thought the
world was over, it became a butterfly.
— ENGLISH PROVERB

✔ Clarification of this test …

There have been no changes in percentages. This chapter still represents 6–12% of exam items. The minimum standards include performing and directing activities that promote and maintain the health of client/family. This includes performing a comprehensive health assessment, provide care and education throughout the growth and development stages and through the aging process, disease prevention, health promotion programs, ante/intra/postpartum/newborn care and immunizations, plan and/or participate in community health education programs. Activities in this chapter are not as heavily weighted as many of the activities in pharmacology and management.

- Provide care and education for the adult client ages 18 through 64 years.
- Perform comprehensive health assessments.
- Provide care and education for the adult client ages 65 years and over.
- Assess client's readiness to learn, learning preferences, and barriers to learning.
- Educate client about preventative care and health maintenance recommendations.
- Perform targeted screening assessments (e.g., vision, nutrition, depression).
- Educate client about prevention and treatment of high risk health behaviors.
- Assess client ability to manage care in home environment and plan care accordingly.
- Assess and educate clients about health risks based on family, population, and community.
- Provide care and education for the newborn, infant, and toddler client from birth through 2 years.
- Plan and/or participate in community health education.
- Provide care and education for the preschool, school age and adolescent client ages 2 through 17 years.
- Provide prenatal care and education.
- Provide postpartum care and education.
- Provide care and education to an antepartum client or a client in labor.

Adapted from: © National Council of State Boards of Nursing, Inc. (NCSBN). (2022). 2021 *RN Practice Analysis: Linking the NCLEX-RN® Examination to Practice*. Chicago: Author.

Adapted from: © National Council of State Boards of Nursing, Inc. (NCSBN). (2023) *Next Generation NCLEX® NCLEX-RN® Test Plan. Chicago*: Author.

Chapter 7: HEALTH PROMOTION AND MAINTENANCE

7.1 Which of these clinical assessment findings for a maternity client should the nurse report to the health care provider? **Select all that apply.**
① Blurred vision
② Board like abdomen
③ Breast tenderness
④ Edema in the lower extremities
⑤ Heartburn
⑥ Periorbital edema

7.2 Which of these clinical assessment findings would be important for the nurse to monitor and report for a maternity client in hypovolemic shock? **Select all that apply.**
① BP 150/80
② HR—120 bpm weak
③ FHR—98/min
④ HR—decrease in variability
⑤ Respiratory Rate—36/min

7.3 Which system-specific assessment findings for a maternity client diagnosed with hyperemesis gravidarum indicate a need for further intervention? **Select all that apply.**
① BP increase from 110/70 to 136/80
② Urine output decrease from 95 mL/hour to 75 mL/hour
③ Pulse increase from 68 bpm to 118 bpm
④ Weight change from 148 lbs to 143 lbs. in 48 hours
⑤ Dry lips and mucous membranes with increase in thirst

7.4 What plan of care is important for a Hispanic maternity client during delivery?
① Encourage the partner to be involved in the labor and delivery suite.
② Encourage family to be involved in birth and allow the use of herbs during labor.
③ Encourage and support the mother of the client to be present during labor versus the client's partner.
④ Maintain a silent labor and do not include partner as an active participant.

7.5 What is appropriate for the nurse to include in the plan of care for a maternity client who is presenting with early decelerations?
① Stop oxytocin immediately.
② Initiate new order for magnesium sulfate.
③ Evaluate for a prolapsed cord.
④ Continue to monitor since this is from head compression.

7.6 Which of these clinical assessment findings for a 2-hour postpartum client requires further intervention?
① Uncontrollable shaking
② Complaints of chilling
③ Saturated perineal pad in 12 minutes
④ Fundus is firm, midline with and at level of umbilicus

7.7 Which of these nursing actions by the LPN/VN for postpartum clients require immediate intervention by the charge nurse? **Select all that apply.**
① Massages the leg that is swollen and tender.
② Measures leg circumferences for a client that the health care provider suspects a DVT.
③ Positions the client with a pulmonary embolus in the supine position to assess the fundus and lochia.
④ Massages the fundus for the client who is bleeding.
⑤ Encourages client with thrombophlebitis to rest in bed.

7.8 Which of these plans will the nurse include in the care for the newborn and new parents? **Select all that apply.**
① Administer phytonadione IM into the gluteus maximus.
② Review with parents that stools of a breastfed newborn will be yellow and seedy and will occur 3 to 4 times daily.
③ Administer phytonadione and hepatitis B in the same thigh.
④ Explain to parents that phytonadione assists with clotting.
⑤ Explain to the new mother that the newborn should pass the meconium within the first 72 hours.
⑥ Explain to the new mother the cord clamp stays in place for 1 week.

7.9 Which of these nursing actions indicate an understanding of how to safely provide care to the neonate?
① When handling the newborn, gloves should be worn by providers until after the first bath.
② When handling the newborn, gown, mask, and gloves should be worn throughout hospitalization.
③ When handling the newborn, wash hands thoroughly with antibacterial foam to minimize the risk of transmission of organisms.
④ When handling the newborn, use air-borne precautions.

7.10 What is priority of care for a newborn who chokes, coughs, and becomes cyanotic with the first feeding?
① Position newborn at a 45-angle.
② Provide nothing by mouth.
③ Only provide clear liquids.
④ Position newborn on left lateral side.

7.11 Which clinical assessment findings for a newborn with a cleft lip require further intervention? **Select all that apply.**
① Heart Rate—138 bpm
② Respiratory Rate—38/min
③ Sunken anterior fontanel
④ Dry lips and mucous membranes
⑤ Weight loss
⑥ One wet diaper in 6 hours

7.12 Which activity would be a priority in planning the use of resources for secondary prevention in a community clinic that serves a population of predominantly migrant families?
① Skin testing from tuberculosis.
② Review of food pyramid to prevent altered nutrition.
③ Information pamphlets about diabetes mellitus.
④ Ongoing eye exams to follow up clients with glaucoma.

7.13 What assessment finding is priority to report to the health care provider for a neonate who is being treated with phototherapy for hyperbilirubinemia?
① Decrease in the number of wet diapers.
② Bronze discoloration of the skin.
③ Yellowish tent to skin.
④ Stool containing some bile that is loose and green.

7.14 Which of these clinical observations would be appropriate and a priority for the UAP to report to the L&D nurse for clients in the birthing units?
① Contractions occurring 4 minutes apart and lasting 45 seconds.
② FHR—140, with good variability for a client with a small amount of bright-red bleeding.
③ Presentation consistent with spontaneous rupture of the membranes.
④ Patellar reflex decreased with a client who has Magnesium Sulfate infusing as prescribed for a diagnosis of pre-eclampsia.

7.15 Which of these nursing actions would be priority for a preschool age child newly admitted to the pediatric unit presenting with constant scratching of the head?
① Recommend parents to notify an exterminator.
② Evaluate the scalp for small white specks.
③ Advise the parents to wash out comb and brush each time after using.
④ Discuss the importance of not sleeping with pets.

7.16 What would be the priority to include in the health promotion plan for an older adult client with a diagnosis of multiple sclerosis?
① Discuss the importance of decreasing antioxidants (vitamins C and E, beta-carotene) due to the risk of losing the myelin sheath.
② Educate client to consume a low-fat, high-fiber diet, with a calcium supplement, and daily cranberry juice.
③ Review importance of keeping warm due to improving the neurologic function.
④ Teach about the importance of avoiding aerobic exercise due to muscle weakness.

7.17 What plan would be most appropriate for the common complaint in pregnancy during the third trimester with the problem with leg cramps? **Select all that apply.**
① Discuss the importance of doing Kegel exercises.
② Demonstrate the pelvic rocking exercises.
③ Increase broccoli in diet.
④ Increase dairy products in diet.
⑤ Increase raisins in diet.

7.18 In preparation for discharge of a client with arterial insufficiency and Raynaud's phenomenon, what is the priority to include in the teaching plan?
① Walk several times each day as a part of an exercise routine.
② Keep the heat up, so that the environment is warm.
③ Wear thromboembolic disease (TED) hose during the day.
④ Use hydrotherapy for increasing oxygenation.

7.19 What would be the priority of care for a client with Stage 2 Alzheimer's Disease who becomes agitated and refuses to answer further questions during an interview?
① Ask client if questions are upsetting in any way.
② Discontinue the interview.
③ Explain that the questions are necessary to complete plan of care.
④ Give client a small break and reconvene in five minutes.

7.20 Which of these plans would be most appropriate to incorporate while educating the family members of an older Asian American client regarding the discharge teaching?
① Avoid making eye contact with authority figures during the teaching.
② Touch client on the head to demonstrate respect.
③ Hug family after the teaching session is complete to demonstrate caring and acceptance.
④ Direct most of teaching plan at the women in the family and the grandparents.

7.21 A female client is diagnosed with human papilloma virus (HPV). Which client statement illustrates an understanding of the possible sequelae of this illness?
① "I will take all of the antibiotics until they are finished."
② "I will use only prescribed douches to avoid a recurrence."
③ "I will return for a pap smear in 6 months."
④ "I will avoid using tampons for 8 weeks."

7.22 Which of these questions is the highest priority for the nurse when discussing safety for a preschool child with the parents?
① "Do you have all of your kitchen cabinets locked?"
② "Do the parents in your neighborhood feel comfortable reporting strangers?"
③ "Are you able to discuss your child's disagreements while playing with his friends to other parents?"
④ "Does your child have appropriate safety equipment for the games he plays?"

7.23 Which intervention would be most important to implement during a teaching session for an elderly client who has bilateral hearing loss and macular degeneration?
① Frequently touch client when speaking.
② Maintain a dimly lit environment.
③ Remain on the side of the client.
④ Use a lower tone of voice when speaking.

7.24 When performing nursing care for a newborn after delivery, which of the following nursing interventions would be the highest priority?
① Adhere to Droplet Isolation precautions.
② Conduct a full physical assessment.
③ Suction the nose prior to the mouth.
④ Cover the newborn's head with a cap.

7.25 A hypertensive client returns to the clinic for reevaluation of his medication. His blood pressure is 180/100. The nurse questions the client regarding how he is taking his medication. What response by the client indicates that he understands and has been taking the medication as prescribed?
① "I take my medication every morning. If my blood pressure is high, I take another dose in the evening."
② "I take my medication every day at the same time regardless of how I feel. I have not missed any doses."
③ "I take my medication every day and make sure that I drink a large amount of liquid each time I take it."
④ "If I have a headache, I don't take my medication. If I miss the morning dose, then I take two pills in the evening."

7.26 Which statement made by the parents of an infant with hydrocephalus indicates they understand how to care for a child with a new ventriculoperitoneal shunt?
① "We will position our child on the operative side to facilitate draining."
② "We will report if our child starts vomiting."
③ "We understand the home health nurse should pump the shunt daily."
④ "We will position our child in the semi-Fowler's position after surgery."

7.27 What question is most important to ask a male client who is being evaluated for a digital rectal examination?
① "Have you noticed a change in the force of the urinary stream?"
② "Have you noticed a change in tolerance of certain foods in your diet?"
③ "Do you notice polyuria in the AM?"
④ "Do you notice any burning with urination or any odor to the urine?"

7.28 A young female client has just been told by the health care provider that her biopsy results indicate breast cancer. What is the next appropriate action for the nurse to take?
① Ask the client if she has any questions.
② Encourage client to talk about her feelings.
③ Leave client alone for awhile.
④ Call the chaplain for the client.

7.29 A female client reports that for the last 4 months a lump in her right breast has been growing larger. The nurse would recommend the client take which action?
① Notify her physician to schedule a mammogram.
② Begin taking large doses of vitamins.
③ Limit sodium intake.
④ Immediately stop any hormone treatment.

7.30 The nurse is preparing a middle-aged client for diagnostic tests to determine if she has a malignancy in her reproductive system. The client is having difficulty concentrating, appears tense, and is wringing her hands constantly. Which response would the nurse make?
① "You seem to be anxious about the tests. Tell me what you are thinking about."
② "You need to pay more attention to what I'm saying. You'll be less anxious if you understand these tests."
③ "Why are you so restless? Your physician is very good."
④ "I know you're worried about these tests, but I'm sure everything will be fine."

7.31 The nurse assesses a prolonged late deceleration of the fetal heart rate while the client is receiving oxytocin to stimulate labor. What is the priority nursing intervention?
① Turn off the infusion.
② Turn client to left side.
③ Change the fluids to Ringer's Lactate.
④ Increase mainline IV rate.

7.32 What clinical finding would cause the nurse to be concerned with the quality of home care for the toddler?
① Has a bruise on the knee.
② Cries and is fearful when parents leave.
③ Is lacking required immunizations.
④ Throws a temper tantrum during an injection.

7.33 Which assessment is a priority in documenting the nursing history of a toddler upon admission to the hospital?
① The child's rituals and routines at home.
② The child's understanding of hospitalization.
③ The child's ability to be separated from parents.
④ The parent's methods for dealing with temper tantrums.

7.34 Which nursing approach would be most appropriate to use while administering an oral medication to an infant?

① Place medication in 45 mL of formula.
② Place medication in an empty nipple.
③ Place medication in a full bottle of formula.
④ Place in supine position. Administer medication using a plastic syringe.

7.35 What is the priority of care for an infant in this type of traction?

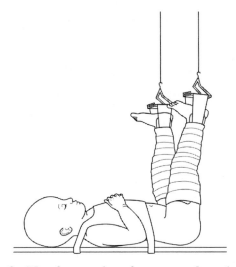

① Notify provider of care regarding the traction set up.
② Assess the infant for signs of infection under the ace wraps.
③ Evaluate brachial pulses and document in the chart.
④ Encourage the mom to assist with care and stroke and talk with infant during care.

7.36 Which statement made by the new mother indicates an understanding of screening for PKU for her newborn son who she is breastfeeding?

① "I will have him tested 24 hours after birth."
② "I will return to the clinic in 48 hours for the screening."
③ "I will return in 1 week to obtain blood samples."
④ "I will return in 1 month for the screening."

7.37 While performing a physical examination on a newborn, which assessment would be reported to the physician?

① Head circumference of 40 cm.
② Chest circumference of 32 cm.
③ Acrocyanosis and edema of the scalp.
④ Heart rate of 160 and respirations of 40.

7.38 To assist the mother in providing appropriate foods for her toddler, the nurse would identify which priority as being the highest?

① Provide the child with finger foods.
② Allow the child to eat favorite foods.
③ Encourage a diet higher in protein than other nutrients.
④ Limit the number of snacks during the day.

7.39 Which action by the mother of a preschooler indicates a disturbed family interaction?

① Tells her child that if he does not sit down and shut up she will leave him there.
② Explains that the injection will burn like a bee sting.
③ Tells her child that the injection can be given while he's in her lap.
④ Reassures child that it is acceptable to cry.

7.40 Planning anticipatory guidance for parents of a beginning school-aged child, what is most important for the nurse to include in the teaching plan?

① Teaching the child to read and write.
② Teaching the child sex education at home.
③ Giving the child responsibility around the house.
④ Expecting stormy behavior.

7.41 Which statement by the parent of a toddler indicates a lack of understanding of this child's nutritional needs?

① "I spend a lot of time planning and preparing my family's meals."
② "I realize she eats more at some meals than at others."
③ "She is a picky eater so I give her one of my vitamins every day."
④ "She likes starchy foods so I decorate them with vegetables."

7.42 What is the priority plan for preventing falls in the older adult?
① Recommend removing all the rugs in the home.
② Encourage installation of appropriate lighting in the home.
③ Review the normal aging changes that place one at risk.
④ Complete a comprehensive risk assessment.

7.43 What would the nurse emphasize when guiding parents teaching their children about human sexuality?
① Parents should determine exactly what the child knows and wants to know before answering questions.
② Parents' words will have more influence than their actions.
③ Anatomic terms should be avoided because they are difficult for the child to understand and learn.
④ Children should be allowed to play "physician" as it will satisfy their sexual curiosity.

7.44 What is most important to teach a child's parents about the treatment of pediculosis capitis (head lice) with Kwell shampoo?
① Treatment should be continued every other day for 1 week with a follow-up treatment in 14 days.
② Clothing and personal belongings require only normal cleansing with soap and water.
③ Application of the shampoo may be repeated at a later date to destroy any surviving live lice.
④ Never repeat the shampoo application as it is readily absorbed through the scalp.

7.45 During the nursing history interview, a preschool client's mother reports frequent hospitalizations for gastroenteritis. Which question reveals the most information regarding the cause of these frequent readmissions?
① "Are there other children in the family?"
② "Does the child attend a day care center?"
③ "Does your child play with neighborhood children?"
④ "Is the child current with his immunizations?"

7.46 Which assessment indicates a need to order a magnesium sulfate blood level?
① Urine output decreased from 80 mL/hour to 45 mL/hour.
② Respiratory rate increased from 14/min to 18/min.
③ Hypertonic patellar reflexes.
④ Blood pressure 150/90 increased to 170/100.

7.47 Which client would be the most appropriate for the nurse to administer Rh immune globulin?
① A client with a husband who is Rh positive.
② A client with a positive indirect antiglobulin (indirect Coomb's) test.
③ A client who is sensitized to the Rh antigen.
④ A client who is Rh negative and has an Rh-positive infant.

7.48 Which of these schedules is most appropriate to recommend to a pre-menopausal woman regarding her self breast exam?
① One week prior to the monthly period
② One week after the menstrual period
③ During every shower
④ The same day monthly

7.49 Which fetal monitor pattern indicates a problem with a cord compression?
① Early decelerations
② Late decelerations
③ Variable decelerations
④ Loss of variability

7.50 After the termination of pre-term labor, what action by a client indicates her ability to monitor herself at home for fetal well-being?
① Counts uterine contractions
② Measures her urine output
③ Counts fetal kicks
④ Weighs herself daily

7.51 Which of these nursing actions would be initiated when the nurse is evaluating the Rinne test?
① The nurse occludes one of the client's ears while the nurse whispers in the other ear from 30 cm away.
② The nurse places a vibrating tuning fork midline on top of the head and the client is asked when the sound is heard best.
③ The nurse places a vibrating tuning fork on the mastoid process and then placed near the ear until the sound is no longer heard.
④ The nurse evaluates the eyes for equality of pupil constriction.

7.52 After the anesthesiologist administers an epidural, which nursing action has the highest priority?
① Decrease IV fluid to prevent fluid overload.
② Assess fetal heart monitor for variable decelerations.
③ Place the client on their right side.
④ Evaluate the blood pressure.

7.53 A multigravida client presents to the labor and delivery area and has a precipitous birth with labor lasting only 45 minutes. Which would be the first nursing action for this client who now has a change in blood pressure from 120/70 to 94/50?
① Prepare client for surgery for retained placental fragments.
② Place the client in Trendelenburg position.
③ Massage uterus.
④ Apply oxygen.

7.54 During a health fair, which of these clients would be highest priority for receiving the seasonal influenza vaccination?
① A young adult client who is the mother of two young children.
② A young adult post-op client following an appendectomy.
③ A premenopausal female client with osteoporosis.
④ A middle-aged adult providing care for a spouse following a renal transplant.

7.55 Which of these pediatric clinical assessment findings would be referred to a specialist for further assessment?
① A 6-month-old infant who can only sit with support.
② A 12-month-old infant who is not walking.
③ A 2-year-old who has a vocabulary of 300 words, but only combines two or three words.
④ A 3-year-old who has a vocabulary of 400 words and can correlate these with objects.

7.56 What action would the nurse implement immediately for an OB client when at the peak of a contraction fluid gushes from a client's vagina?
① Evaluate for a prolapsed cord.
② Evaluate fetal monitor for early decelerations.
③ Perform a pH on the fluid to determine it is amniotic fluid.
④ Evaluate fetal monitor for an increase in the variability.

7.57 The mother of a 2-year-old reports that her son is becoming a very picky eater. What is the best response from the nurse?
① "This is a common behavior since he is becoming more autonomous. Try giving him some finger foods."
② "You may try setting better limits between meals regarding snacks."
③ "Try mixing his food together so there is not so much to select from."
④ "I will report this to the nurse practitioner. He may have a virus."

7.58 Which statement made by a mother who is breast feeding most indicates a need for further teaching about birth control?
① "I will go to my health care provider and get fitted for a diaphragm."
② "I will have my husband use a condom."
③ "I will get a prescription from my health care provider for the pill."
④ "I will practice abstinence during my fertile time."

7.59 Which statement by the parents of a newborn indicates a need for further teaching about newborn care?
① "We will notify the physician for absence of breathing for 10 seconds."
② "We will notify the physician for more than one episode of projectile vomiting."
③ "We will notify the physician if the infant's temperature is greater than 101°F (38.3°C)."
④ "We will rock and cuddle our infant to promote trust."

7.60 What would be a plan for a tertiary prevention activity for an older female client who had a cerebrovascular accident (CVA)?
① An annual mammogram
② An annual influenza vaccine
③ An annual ophthalmologic examination to evaluate for macular degeneration
④ A physical therapy program

7.61 A 3-month-old is placed in Bryant's traction for congenital hip dysplasia. Which toy is appropriate to offer the infant during hospitalization?
① Rattle
② Stuffed animal
③ Colorful blocks
④ Tape of nursery rhymes

7.62 While planning care for an elderly client with dementia, which plan is a priority?
① Encourage dependency with activities of daily living.
② Provide flexibility in schedules due to mental confusion.
③ Limit reminiscing due to poor memory.
④ Speak slowly and in a face-to-face position.

7.63 Which observation would most likely represent caregiver burnout in the daughter of an older adult client with Alzheimer's disease?
① Failure of daughter to get parent into wheelchair daily.
② Home environment extremely cluttered at each visit.
③ Daughter remains involved in family's activities.
④ Husband is seen assisting in mother-in-law care.

7.64 During the newborn assessment, the nurse is evaluating the rooting reflex. Locate where the nurse would stroke to elicit this response.

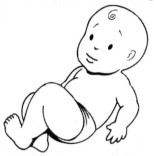

7.65 While assessing cranial nerve 11, which part of the body would the nurse ask the client to move?

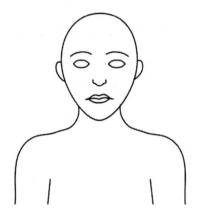

Answers & Rationales

7.1 ① Options #1, #2, and #6 are correct. The clinical
② decision-making strategy is to identify the
⑥ normal assessment findings that are expected during pregnancy. When you master this, then the other findings indicate a problem and need further assessment and intervention. Options #1 and #6 may indicate signs of preeclampsia. Option #2 may indicate a complication with abruptio placenta. Options #3, #4, and #5 are normal findings, and do not need to be reported.
I CAN HINT: Apply the clinical judgment/cognitive skill, analysis of cues (analysis), for a prenatal client who is experiencing complications.
NCLEX® Standard: Provide prenatal care and education.

7.2 ② Options #2, #3, #4, and #5 are correct. The
③ strategy is to organize the system-specific
④ assessments findings around altered
⑤ perfusion, an outcome from bleeding. When the heart does not have a lot of volume to pump, then it would make sense the blood pressure would decrease. This is the reason the HR and RR are elevated, so they can attempt to compensate for the blood loss. The only difference between assessments for a maternity and a medical surgical client is that the fetus must be evaluated. The alteration in perfusion can have negative effects on the fetus which can present with a fetal heart rate change out of the defined reference range, late decelerations, and a decrease in the variability.
I CAN HINT: Apply the clinical judgment/cognitive skill, analysis of cues (analysis), for a maternity client who is hypovolemic. You need to be competent in recognizing which cues (assessments) need to be reported for this maternity client who is hypovolemic.
NCLEX® Standard: Provide care and education to an antepartum client or a client in labor. Manage the care of a client with alteration in hemodynamics, tissue perfusion, and hemostasis.

7.3 ③ Options #3, #4, and #5 are correct. The
④ strategy is to understand the concept that
⑤ needs to be linked to hyperemesis gravidarum is fluid deficit. The assessments indicate a fluid volume deficit. Option #1 is incorrect because the increase in BP does not require further intervention, since the challenge would be a drop in the BP from the decrease in volume. Option #2 is incorrect because the decrease is not significant. Options #3, #4, and #5 are correct since they indicate a complication with fluid deficit. The concept of fluid deficit is the same for any pediatric or medical surgical client. The etiology will be different, but the outcomes will be the same for any client with fluid deficit. This is not new information; it is simply applying a concept you already know to a maternity client with a medical condition resulting in fluid deficit. You CAN do this! There are only so many concepts you need to master to be successful with the maternity client!
I CAN HINT: Apply the clinical judgment/cognitive skill, analysis of cues (analysis), for a prenatal client who is experiencing hyperemesis gravidarum resulting in fluid deficit.
NCLEX® Standard: Provide prenatal care and education. Manage the care of the client with a fluid and electrolyte imbalance.

7.4 ③ Options #3 is correct. The strategy is to understand the cultural differences and apply to maternity client. Hispanic client prefers mother as the supportive person versus the partner. Culturally Sensitive Care section in the book, *Maternal Newborn Nursing Made Insanely Easy* by Manning, L. (I CAN Publishing, Inc., pp. 142-143) will assist you in organizing the priority care for different cultures. Option #1 is consistent with the care for European American client and family. Option #2 is consistent with Native American clients and family members. Option #4 would be practiced with an Asian American client and family.
I CAN HINT: Apply the clinical judgment/cognitive skill, generate solutions (first-do priority plan), to incorporate cultural practices for a maternity client.
NCLEX® Standard: Incorporate client cultural practices and beliefs when planning and providing care.

7.5 ④ Options #4 is correct. Review the priority care for a maternity client presenting with early decelerations. "VEAL CHOP" in the book, *Nursing Made Insanely Easy*, can assist you in organizing this information. Option #4 is correct. Option #1 would be correct if client was presenting with late decelerations. Option #2 would be correct if client was presenting with preterm labor or preeclampsia. Option #3 would be correct if client was presenting with variable decelerations.
I CAN HINT: Apply the clinical judgment/cognitive skill, generate solutions (first-do priority plan), for the maternity client in labor.
NCLEX® Standard: Provide care and education to an antepartum client or a client in labor.

7.6 ③ Options #3 is correct. The strategy is to remember that excessive bleeding is considered to be one pad saturated in 15 min. or less or pooling of blood under buttocks (Option #3). This does need further intervention. Options #1 and #2 are incorrect, since postpartum chills that occur in first 2 hours and are related to a nervous system response, vasomotor changes, a shift in fluids, and/or work during labor. This is an expected finding for the first 2 hours in the postpartum client and does not require further intervention. Option #4 is incorrect since it is an expected finding and does not require further intervention.
I CAN HINT: Apply the clinical judgment/cognitive skill, analysis of cues (analysis), for a postpartum client.
NCLEX® Standard: Provide postpartum care and education.

7.7 ① ③ Options #1, #3 are correct. The strategy for answering this question is to recognize unsafe care for the postpartum client. Options #1 and #3 both would be unsafe care and require immediate intervention by the charge nurse. Option #1 may be a deep vein thrombosis and massaging could result in dislodging the thrombosis. The position in option #3 is incorrect. This client with a pulmonary embolus should be positioned in the semi-Fowler's position. Options #2, #4 and #5 include safe nursing practice for the postpartum client and do not require further intervention.
I CAN HINT: Apply the clinical judgment/cognitive skill, take-action (first-do priority interventions), for the postpartum client. .
NCLEX® Standard: Provide postpartum care and education. Manage the care of a client with alteration in hemodynamics, tissue perfusion, and hemostasis. Report, intervene, and/or escalate unsafe practice of health care personnel (e.g., improper care).

7.8 ② ④ Options #2 and #4 are correct. Option #1 is incorrect. Should be administered in the vastus lateralis where there is adequate muscle development. Option #3 is incorrect. These should not be given in same thighs. Sites should be alternated. Option #5 is incorrect. Meconium should be passed within 24 to 48 hours. Option #6, the cord clamp should only stay in place for 24 to 48 hours.
I CAN HINT: Apply the clinical judgment/cognitive skill, generate solutions (first-do priority plans), for the parents of a newborn.
NCLEX® Standard: Provide care and education for the newborn, infant, and toddler client from birth through 2 years.

7.9 ① Options #1 is correct. The clinical decision-making strategy requires an understanding of infection prevention. Options #2, #3, and #4 are not infection prevention protocols for newborn care. Option #1 is a correct nursing action to promote infection prevention.
I CAN HINT: Apply the clinical judgment/cognitive skill, take-action (first-do priority interventions), for newborn infection prevention.
NCLEX® Standard: Provide care and education for the newborn, infant, and toddler client from birth through 2 years. Apply principles of infection prevention.

7.10 ② Options #2 is correct. The clinical decision-making strategy for this client is to prevent aspiration. Esophageal Atresia should be suspected with these findings: coughing, choking, and cyanosis. Until this has been repaired, the newborn should be NPO to prevent aspiration. The options that do not address NPO are incorrect. Option #1 should read upright for this condition, but priority still is to provide nothing by mouth. Option #3 should read NPO, and option #4 should read upright with these assessment findings.
I CAN HINT: Apply the clinical judgment/cognitive skill, take-action (first-do priority interventions) for the newborn who is

presenting with coughing, choking, and cyanosis.
NCLEX® Standard: Provide care and education for the newborn, infant, and toddler client from birth through 2 years.

7.11 ③ ④ ⑤ ⑥ Options #3, #4, #5, and #6 are correct. The strategy is to connect the concept of fluid deficit to the congenital anomaly of clept lip. Compare and contrast each of the assessment findings and determine which are normal findings for a newborn. Options #1 and #2 are within the defined limits for a newborn and do not require further intervention. Options #3, #4, #5, and #6 all indicate fluid deficit that can be a complication from a cleft lip due to a decrease in fluid intake. The great news is when you master the concept of fluid deficit, you can apply this to appropriate medical surgical, pediatric conditions, etc.
I CAN HINT: Apply the clinical judgment/cognitive skill, analysis of cues (analysis), for a newborn who is experiencing fluid deficit.
NCLEX® Standard: Provide care and education for the newborn, infant, and toddler client from birth through 2 years. Manage the care of the client with a fluid and electrolyte imbalance.

7.12 ① Option #1 is correct. Secondary prevention focuses on health promotion, which includes screening, early detection and diagnosis of disease. Among migrant families, tuberculosis rates are typically high and should be a priority focus for secondary prevention. Options #2 and #3 are important, but are primary prevention. Option #4 is tertiary prevention.

7.13 ① Option #1 needs to be reported due to the risk of fluid volume deficit from the fluid loss that can occur from the frequent stools. Options #2 and #3 are the clinical findings that occur with hyperbilirubinemia. Option #4 does not need to be reported.

7.14 ③ Option #3 is correct. The L&D nurse would need to know if a client had clinical findings consistent with rupture of the membranes, since this could result in danger to the fetus if a prolapsed cord occurred. This would lead to an emergency situation mandating a cesarean delivery. This report is within the scope of practice for the UAP. Even a mother, can tell by the leaking membranes that there is a risk of rupture of the membranes. Option #1 is normal findings. Option #2 would be important for the RN to further evaluate, but is not a priority over option #3 that could lead to an emergency. Option #2 is presenting with a normal FHR, and the variability does indicate good oxygenation. The other focus of this question is that the UAP does not assess, and to make a decision that the variability is good is not within the scope of practice for the UAP. Option #4 is incorrect for several reasons. First, this is an expected outcome for a client receiving Magnesium Sulfate, so it would not be a priority over option #3 due to the safety. Second, this is an assessment, so it is not within the scope of practice for the UAP to report this.

7.15 ② Option #2 is correct. Constant scratching may indicate pediculosis (lice). Assessment of the scalp is priority for white eggs (nits) on hair shafts, itchy; on the body inspect for papules and macules; in pubic area inspect for red macules. Option #1 is incorrect; there is not enough information to make this conclusion. Option #3 is incorrect because it is ignoring identifying the etiology of the clinical finding. Option #4 is incorrect because as stated in option #3's rationale, further assessments need to be made to determine the etiology of this finding of constant scratching.

7.16 ② Option #2 is correct. It is important to maintain an ideal body weight, have rest, and become informed about the need to supplement calcium and daily intake of cranberry juice. Option #1 is incorrect because a daily intake of multiple vitamins, antioxidants, and low-dose aspirin (81 mg) are recommended. Option #3 is incorrect. Keeping cool, not warm, is associated with improvement of the neurologic function. Option #4 is incorrect since clients should exercise routinely.

7.17 ③ ④ Options #3 and #4 are correct. Leg cramps during the third trimester may occur due to the compression of lower extremity nerves and blood vessels by the enlarging uterus. This can result in poor peripheral circulation as well as an imbalance in the calcium/phosphorus ratio. In this situation, the options are focusing more to the cause being from hypocalcemia. Both broccoli and dairy products are high in calcium. Additional foods high in calcium include kale,

Chapter 7: ANSWERS & RATIONALES

grains, egg yolks. Foods high in phosphorus include dairy, peas, soft drinks, meat, eggs, and some grains. Option #1 is incorrect. Kegel exercises are done to strengthen the perineal muscles and have nothing to do with leg cramps. Option #2 is incorrect since the pelvic rocking exercises stretch out the muscles of the lower back and help relieve lower back pain. Option #5 is incorrect. Raisins are high in iron.

7.18 ② Option #2 is correct. Raynaud's phenomenon consists of intermittent episodic spasms of the arterioles, most frequently in the fingers and toes. Symptoms are precipitated by exposure to cold, emotional upset, or nicotine and caffeine intake. The client's instructions should include keeping the environment warm to prevent vasoconstriction. Wearing gloves, warm clothes, and socks will also be useful in preventing vasoconstriction (option #3), but TED hose would not be therapeutic. Option #1 is incorrect. Walking will most likely increase pain. Option #4 is incorrect. Spasms are not necessarily correlated with other peripheral vascular problems.

7.19 ② Option #2 would be the most appropriate response due to the agitation and refusal to answer questions. The client may be getting overwhelmed. Option #1 is incorrect. The behavior of the client demonstrates that these questions are upsetting the client. Option #3 does not answer the question. The question indicates the client is becoming agitated and refuses to answer further questions. The answer needs to address the problem the client is experiencing versus what the nurse needs to get accomplished. Option #4 is not correct since this time frame will not allow the client to regroup.

7.20 ① Option #1 would be important since this behavior is viewed as a sign of respect and trust for the Asian Americans. Option #2 may be considered to be disrespectful since the head may be considered sacred. Option #3 is not correct. Client and family members may be very modest and public display of affection are not typical. The African American, on the other hand, shows affection by touching, hugging, and being close. Option #4 is incorrect since this group is more patriarchal. In the African American culture, however, the women typically head the household.

7.21 ③ Several strains of the human papillomavirus (HPV) are associated with cervical cancer. Option #1 is incorrect because antibiotics are not used for viral infections. Option #2 is incorrect because douches will not prevent recurrence. Option #4 is incorrect because tampons do not contribute to the problem as in toxic shock syndrome.

7.22 ④ Option #4 is a priority due to the developmental stage of the preschoolers. They are into initiative vs. guilt. The preschooler is very active and safety is most important. Option #1 would be priority for the toddler. Options #2 and #3 are important but not a priority.

7.23 ④ Option #4 is correct. As the older clients age, they lose the ability to hear high tones. It is difficult for an older client to understand the voices of both children and women due to the high tones. Option #1 is incorrect since the touch may offend the client and actually be a distractor to the client. Options #2 and #3 are incorrect since the client may not be able to see.

7.24 ④ Option #4 is correct. The priorities immediately following delivery include: I CAN HINT: The 4 H's: hypoxia, hypothermia, hypoglycemia, and heart rate. One of the greatest risks to the newborn is cold stress. Due to the risk of developing hypothermia from the loss of heat from the head due to excessive evaporation, a priority in this question would be to cover the newborn's head with a cap. Option #1 is not required for the newborn unless the clinical situation indicates the growth of an organism that requires droplet isolation precautions such as: pertussis, streptococcal (group A) pharyngitis, pneumonia or scarlet fevers in infants, etc. Of course, standard precautions are practiced for all clients. Option #2 is not the highest priority following delivery. Yes, it is important to perform a full physical assessment, but the priority is safety during this time which would be the possible issue with hypothermia. Option #3 is incorrect since the mouth should be suctioned prior to the nose.

7.25 ② This option best describes how the client should take the medication for hypertension. It is important that he take it every day. However, it may be a problem if he is consuming a large amount of water during the day. If he is taking the medication correctly, he needs to have the medication reevaluated since his blood pressure remained high.

7.26 ② Option #2 is correct. Parents that understand how to provide care for their child with a ventriculoperitoneal shunt would need to know the signs and symptoms of increasing ICP. Refer to I CAN HINT below. Option #1 is incorrect. If the child had surgery, then infant would be positioned in the supine position with head turned operative side up to prevent pressure on the shunt valve and to prevent too rapid depletion of CSF. Option #3 is incorrect. The parents will learn how to provide care to the shunt. Option #4 is incorrect. This position would result in a rapid depletion of CSF.

I CAN HINT: An easy way to remember symptoms of increased intracranial pressure for the infant is "PIES." The book *Nursing Made Insanely Easy*, has a fun image to assist you with this, but for now I will share with you the mnemonic memory tool "PIES":

Projecile vomiting, posturing

Irritability (early symptoms); high-pitched cry (headache)

Enlarged head (bulging fontanels, ↑ head circumference), eye changes (pupillary changes)

Suture separation (cranial), seizures

7.27 ① Option #1 is correct. This change would be most indicative of a potential complication with (BPH) benign prostate hypertrophy. Options #2, #3, and #4 are incorrect. Option #4 would be indicative of an infection.

7.28 ② Encouraging the client to talk about feelings allows the client to cry or express her reaction. Options #1, #3, and #4 do not allow for immediate expression of reaction to this crisis.

7.29 ① A mammogram is an x-ray of the breast. It usually shows the presence of a lesion if one is present. Positive zero radiography (type of mammogram) has the ability to detect carcinomas 1 to 2 years prior to formation of a palpable 1 cm. lesion. Option #2 is incorrect because specific vitamin therapy may be useful in some cases. It is not curative alone. Option #3 is incorrect because sodium has not been associated with breast cancer. Option #4 is incorrect because hormones have not been known to cause breast cancer.

7.30 ① This response acknowledges the client's concerns and allows exploration of her fears. Options #2, #3, and #4 provide false reassurance and do not allow the client an opportunity to express and deal with her feelings.

7.31 ① Stopping the infusion will decrease contractions and possibly remove uterine pressure off the fetus, which is a possible cause of the late deceleration. Option #2 may help the deceleration by removing the placenta off of the inferior vena cava and increasing blood flow to the fetus; however, the initial action should be to stop the infusion which is causing ongoing stimulation of the uterus. Option #3 would be appropriate if the nurse was going to bolus the client with isotonic fluid due to the epidural, but this is not addressed in the question. Option #4 would be appropriate if the late deceleration was from the decrease in blood pressure from the epidural, but NEVER read into the questions. There is NO indication that this is the clinical situation.

I CAN HINT: *Nursing Made Insanely Easy*, by Manning & Rayfield has a great acronym to assist in recalling how to answer this type of question in chronological order. There is an image of a fire truck uncoiling the hose to help put out "Fetal Distress." UN "COIL": #1 STOP OXYTOCIN, then, Change position to the left side, Oxygen, Increase IV fluids, then Lower the head of the bed.

7.32 ③ This may indicate a lack of concern for child's well-being and may be a sign of poor quality of home care. Option #1 is a common assessment during the toddler years. Options #2 and #4 are expected behaviors for a toddler.

7.33 ① During a crisis such as hospitalization, children are able to establish a sense of security through a consistency of the rituals and routines from home. Option #2 is inappropriate for this age. Option #3 is incorrect because separation anxiety is a major fear during this age. Option #4 is not as high a priority as Option #1 in decreasing psychological trauma from hospitalization.

7.34 ② This is a convenient method for administering medications to an infant. Options #1 and #3 are incorrect. Medication is not usually added to infant's formula feeding. Option #4 is partially correct. However, the infant is never placed in a reclining position during procedure due to potential aspiration.

7.35 ④ Option #4 is correct. This is Bryant's traction and the infant's buttocks are slightly off the bed with the legs suspended in the air bilaterally. This is typically used for infants with congenital hip dysplasia. This is an example of skin traction, so option #2 is incorrect. The correct answer would have been to assess for skin integrity. Option #1 is incorrect since it is set up appropriately. Option #3 is incorrect since the pulses should be distal to the traction to evaluate arterial perfusion. The pulses that should be evaluated would be the dorsalis pedis and/or posterior tibial. Option #4 is correct since tactile stimulation is imperative for an infant's normal emotional development to continue to grow. Deprivation can result in a complication with failure to thrive.

7.36 ③ Option #3 is correct since the newborn is only getting colostrum for the first few days. This screening may have a possible false negative result with the initial screening. Options #1, #2, and #4 are inaccurate and would not provide valid information.

7.37 ① Average circumference of the head for a neonate ranges between 32 to 36 cm. An increase in size may indicate hydrocephaly or increased intracranial pressure. Options #2, #3, and #4 are normal newborn assessments.

7.38 ① The child is going through the autonomy versus shame and doubt stage. Finger foods allow the child the necessary independence for this stage. Options #2 and #4 may or may not be correct because the child may eat food without appropriate nutrients. Option #3 does not represent accurate nutritional information.

7.39 ① Threatening a child with abandonment will destroy the child's trust in his family. Option #2 is not necessarily accurate, but does not indicate a disturbed family interaction. Option #3 is inappropriate but does not indicate a disturbance in family interaction. Option #4 indicates a healthy interaction.

7.40 ③ Giving children responsibilities allows them to develop feelings of competence and self-esteem through their industry. Option #1 may require some assistance from the parents, but children this age learn at their own rate. Option #2 may be premature. Option #4 usually does not occur until about age 11.

7.41 ③ Children should not be given adult doses of vitamins because a child's need for vitamins is different than adults. Toddlers are picky eaters, and children's daily vitamins are appropriate. Option #1 shows concern about family nutrition. Option #2 is accurate because toddlers usually eat only one or two adequate meals each day. Nutritious snacks are helpful in assuring adequate nutritional intake. Option #4 is true because toddlers do prefer a "white diet" of starchy foods.

7.42 ④ Option #4 is priority in preventing falls. Options #1, #2, and #3 would be a part of doing a complete assessment.

7.43 ① Children often have misinformation about human sexuality; and if not identified, the child will incorporate the misinformation into the parent's answer. To be able to answer a question adequately, it is important to determine what the child wants to know. Option #2 is contra to human behavior. Option #3 is incorrect because most experts believe correct anatomic names are appropriate. Option #4, "Oh, please …"

7.44 ③ Kwell shampoo should be used as directed as it is an organic solvent and can be toxic as well as absorbed through the skin of the scalp. It may be repeated, but usually at least 5–7 days after the first application. Option #1 is too often for applying the shampoo. Option #2 is incorrect because very hot water and a special detergent (Rid) need to be used for cleansing clothing and personal belongings. Option #4 is incorrect because the shampooing must be repeated after the eggs hatch.

7.45 ② Environments where there are increased numbers of children, such as day care centers, are more likely to have infections due to close living conditions facilitating the transmission of disease. Options #1 and #4 do not pose a problem or solution regarding gastroenteritis. Option #3 is a possible source of infection but not as likely as a day care center.

7.46 ① Magnesium sulfate is excreted by the kidneys. A decrease in the urine output can lead to toxicity. Option #2 indicates an improvement. Options #3 and #4 are incorrect because these assessments indicate a need to start magnesium sulfate.

7.47 ④ RhoGam is administered to this client to prevent sensitization to the Rh antigen. Option #1 is irrelevant because it is the mother and infant's Rh type that the decision is based on. Option #2 may or may not be correct depending on what specific antibody was detected. If the mother has anti-D and did not receive antenatal RhoGam, she is sensitized and not a candidate. Option #3 is incorrect because the client is sensitized and RhoGam is given to prevent sensitization from occurring.

7.48 ② Option #2 is correct because this is when the breasts are least congested. Option #1 is when the breasts are most congested. Option #3 is unnecessary. The recommended frequency is monthly. Option #4 is for post-menopausal women.

7.49 ③ Variable decelerations indicate a problem with cord compression. Option #1 indicates head compression. Option #2 indicates uteroplacental insufficiency. Option #4 could indicate fetal acidosis, fetal neurological immaturity, or maternal medication.

7.50 ③ Being able to count fetal kicks assures the fetus is moving and makes the mother aware of the importance of monitoring fetal movement daily. Option #1 might indicate the onset of premature labor. Options #2 and #4 relate to maternal, more than fetal well-being.

7.51 ③ Option #3 is correct. This accurately describes the Rinne test. Option #1 is incorrect. This is the description for the Whisper test. Option #2 is incorrect since this is the description for the Weber test. Option #4 is incorrect. This describes the evaluation of the 3rd cranial nerve which is the oculomotor cranial nerve.

7.52 ④ A side effect of an epidural is hypotension from the vasodilation which occurs. Option #1 is incorrect because the client must be well hydrated before and after the procedure. Option #2 may be done as ongoing management but is not a priority. Option #3 is incorrect because the client would be placed on her left side to promote uterine perfusion.

7.53 ③ Option #3 is correct. Massaging the uterus will make it less boggy and more firm, reducing the bleeding that may be causing the decrease in blood pressure. The three major causes of bleeding following delivery are boggy fundus, cervical lacerations, and retained placenta. The answers for this question could be what is currently written or other options may include starting oxytocin or placing the neonate to the breast for the natural release of oxytocin while the neonate is nursing. Option #1, a retained placenta is an emergency, but the way the question reads is "what would be the first nursing action," and it is unlikely that the nurse would begin by preparing for surgery prior to initiating the massaging of the uterus. This may correct the cause, since the most common cause of bleeding is insufficient uterine contractions. Option #2, Trendelenburg position may help increase blood pressure, but does not address the etiology for the lowered blood pressure in a mutigravida client following a precipitous deliver. Option #4, applying oxygen may be indicated if the bleeding did not stop; however, this would not be the first nursing action.

7.54 ④ Option #4 is correct. Individuals who provide care home care for a loved one who is immunosuppressed and are at high risk for the flu need the vaccination. Options #1, #2, and #3 are not a priority over option #4 due to the risk involved.

I CAN HINT: Due to the treatment being increased immunosuppressive therapy; usually high- doses of steroids, polyclonal or monoclonal antibody therapy, it is imperative to prevent infection. This would also include any family member, friend, relative, etc. that will be having ongoing contact with the client.

7.55 ④ Option #4 is correct. A 3-year-old should have a vocabulary of 900 words and should be able to use a complete sentence of three or four words. This child needs a referral due to the developmental delay. Option #1 does not need a referral since a 6-month-old infant is only able to sit with support. By the time the infant is 8 months of age, the infant should be able to sit without support. Option #2 does not need a referral since this is normal. Not all children walk at 12 months of age. Option #3 is an expected outcome for this age.

7.56 ① Option #1 is most important due to safety. Option #2 reflects head compression. This deceleration indicates a problem with cephalopelvic disproportion versus a prolapsed cord. Option #3 is not an immediate concern. The fetus is the priority! Option #4 is good; increase in oxygenation is not a problem. Variability = good oxygen!

I CAN HINT: Remember, the question reads "immediately." The question to ask yourself is *"Do I need to immediately perform a pH on the fluid, or do I need to immediately intervene if the fetus has a prolapsed cord?"*

7.57 ① Finger foods will assist the child in establishing his autonomy. Options #2 and #3 are inappropriate. This age of child does not like food mixed together. In Option #4, there are no other concerns stated by the mother to make the nurse even consider a virus.

7.58 ③ The pill (oral contraceptive) will suppress production of breast milk. During breast-feeding, another method of contraception should be used. Options #1, #2, and #4 could be used and do not indicate a need for further teaching.

7.59 ① This is normal for a neonate. Apnea lasting longer than 15 seconds should be reported. Options #2, #3, and #4 do not indicate a need for further teaching.

7.60 ④ Option #4 is the correct answer. The physical therapy will assist client in restoring optimum level of functioning after a CVA. Options #1 and #3 are examples of secondary prevention activities nonspecific to a CVA. Option #2 is a primary prevention activity nonspecific to a CVA. The test taking strategy here is that options #1, #2, and #3 are unrelated to the client with a CVA. Another approach is to use the **I CAN HINT:** Primary prevention has an "i" which can assist you in remembering immunizations. Secondary prevention has an "s" for screening. Tertiary prevention has an "r" for rehab or restore a function.

7.61 ① A 3-month-old can grasp a rattle. Options #2 and #4 are correct but not a priority to option #1. Option #3 is for an older child.

7.62 ④ This is most effective when communicating with an elderly client. Option #1 is incorrect because independence is encouraged. Option #2 is incorrect because schedules need to be routine, reinforced, and repeated. Flexibility leads to confusion. Option #3 is incorrect because reminiscing helps the client resume progression through the grief process associated with disappointing life event and increases self-esteem.

7.63 ② Cluttered environment may represent depression and burnout. Option #1 may be impossible for the daughter to do alone. Options #3 and #4 are very healthy and desirable.

7.64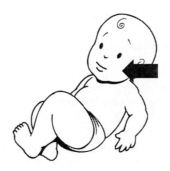

7.65 Cranial nerve 11 is the spinal accessory.

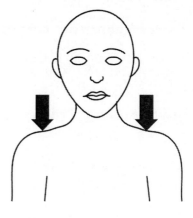

CHAPTER 8
Psychosocial Integrity

> Hope is being able to see
> that there is a light despite
> all of the darkness.
> — DESMOND TUTU

✔ Clarification of this test …

There have been no changes in percentages. This chapter still represents 6–12% of exam items. The minimum standards include performing and directing activities related to caring for client/family providing and directing care that promotes and supports mental, emotional, and social well-being of the client with an acute or chronic mental illness in addition to clients attempting to cope with stressful situations in life.

- Use therapeutic communication techniques.
- Promote a therapeutic environment.
- Recognize nonverbal cues to physical and/or psychological stressors.
- Assess client support system to aid in plan of care.
- Assess psychosocial factors influencing care and plan interventions (e.g., occupational, spiritual, environmental, financial).
- Provide appropriate care for a client experiencing visual, auditory, and/or cognitive alterations.
- Assess client's ability to cope with life changes and provide support.
- Assess client for substance abuse and/or toxicities and intervene as appropriate (e.g., dependency, withdrawal).
- Incorporate behavioral management techniques when caring for a client.
- Provide care and education for acute and chronic psychosocial health issues (e.g., addictions/dependencies, depression, dementia, eating disorders).
- Assess the potential for violence and use safety precautions.
- Incorporate client cultural practices and beliefs when planning and providing care.
- Assess client for abuse or neglect and report, intervene, and/or escalate.
- Provide care for a client experiencing grief or loss.
- Provide end-of-life care and education to clients.

Adapted from: © National Council of State Boards of Nursing, Inc. (NCSBN). (2022). 2021 *RN Practice Analysis: Linking the NCLEX-RN® Examination to Practice*. Chicago: Author.
Adapted from: © National Council of State Boards of Nursing, Inc. (NCSBN). (2023) *Next Generation NCLEX® NCLEX-RN® Test Plan. Chicago*: Author.

8.1 A middle-aged client is diagnosed with a chronic illness. Which of these would the nurse assess first?
① Support from spouse
② Previous coping skills of the client
③ Support from extended family
④ Client's understanding and thoughts of the diagnosis

8.2 A young adult client is presenting with anorexia nervosa. Which plans will the nurse include in the care for this client? **Select all that apply.**
① Include client in decision making.
② Encourage ongoing exercise throughout the day.
③ Assess for syncope.
④ Advise client to decrease fiber in diet.
⑤ Encourage client to journal.

8.3 A daughter is providing care for her elderly mother who has Alzheimer's disease. The daughter reports to the health care provider that she is struggling to manage her family, career, and her mother's care. What would be most appropriate to include in the plan of care for this daughter and her mother?
① Review resources for respite care with the daughter.
② Discuss time management with the daughter.
③ Encourage other family members to support daughter with the care.
④ Encourage daughter to seek legal counsel regarding advanced directives.

8.4 When providing care for a client with a personality disorder, which nursing action indicates an understanding of how to safely manage this client?
① The nurse establishes consistent limit-setting with this client.
② The nurse provides a plan for the client to provide a structure.
③ The nurse should discuss assertiveness training for a client who is flirtatious.
④ The nurse should provide a schedule of daily events.

8.5 Which plans of care indicate the nurse understands how to manage the client who is taking amitriptyline? **Select all that apply.**
① "I need eat fiber when taking this medication."
② "I can expect to experience insomnia when taking this medication."
③ "I may experience some drowsiness for several days after taking this medication."
④ "I should drink fluids when taking this medication."
⑤ "I should take St. John's Wort with this medication."

8.6 Which plans will the nurse include in the nursing care for a client who is presenting with mild anxiety? **Select all that apply.**
① Encourage client to discuss feelings.
② Ask client what the cause is for the anxiety.
③ Remain calm when interacting with client.
④ Discuss the importance of exercise.
⑤ Explain to client that anxiety will subside.

8.7 Which newly admitted client on the psychiatric unit will need to be assessed immediately following shift report?
① A client who is depressed and crying after experiencing the loss of a child.
② A client who has Alzheimer's disease and is sitting in the chair unable to remember the names of her grandchildren.
③ A client who has been depressed but is presenting with more energy and is giving away favorite possessions to another client on the unit.
④ A depressed client sitting on the floor rocking back and forth.

8.8 A client has a new prescription for bupropion for an anxiety disorder. Which plans are important for the nurse in include in the nursing care for this client? **Select all that apply.**
① Review importance for client to report complications with diarrhea.
② Encourage to drink fluids and practice meticulous oral hygiene.
③ Recommend only drinking one glass of wine daily.
④ Review importance of eating fiber when taking this medication.
⑤ Monitor weight and food intake.

8.9 Which of these dietary selections are priority for the nurse to instruct the client to avoid when taking buspirone for an anxiety disorder?
① Chicken salad sandwich
② Grapefruit juice
③ Yeast rolls
④ Grilled cheese sandwich

8.10 What is the priority plan of care for a client with severe Alzheimer's Disease who has a new prescription for memantine?
① Identify wrist bracelet for correct client identity prior to administering.
② Hold the medication and report a Blood urea nitrogen (BUN): 38 mg/dL and creatinine level: 3.5 mg/dL.
③ Educate family that medication can cure the Alzheimer's Disease.
④ Initiate fall and safety precautions.

8.11 Which plan of care should the nurse include when teaching a client about a new prescription for lithium carbonate?
① Limit playing tennis in the hot weather.
② Limit the use of acetaminophen for headaches.
③ Limit fluid intake to less than 1,500 mL daily.
④ Review with client that the effects will begin within 2-3 days.

8.12 During the assessment, the RN evaluates the client experiencing difficulty talking and swallowing, and complaining of muscle tightness in the throat. What would be the most appropriate nursing action for this client who is taking haloperidol?
① Explain that this is expected when taking this medication.
② Discuss the importance of decreasing the dose with these symptoms.
③ Notify the health care provider regarding findings and obtain a prescription for diphenhydramine.
④ Review the importance of increasing fluids to 1 liter per day.

8.13 Which of these statements made by the adolescent client with anorexia nervosa would require immediate intervention by the nurse?
① "Today I am feeling faint and weak."
② "I am experiencing some tenderness with my mouth when I brush my teeth."
③ "I know that the reason I do not have any friends is because I am ugly and fat."
④ "I am not thin enough."

8.14 What would be the priority of care for a client who is experiencing a manic episode and starting to become combative?
① Assist the client to the recreation room for a game of pool.
② Escort client to a quiet room with no other people or activities.
③ Encourage client to verbalize thoughts and feelings.
④ Set firm limits on client's behavior and expectations.

8.15 Which of these clients when making out assignments would be highest risk for suicidal completion?
① A young adult client who has recently had a mastectomy.
② A middle-aged client who has been diagnosed with cancer.
③ An older adult client who has been diagnosed with diabetes mellitus.
④ An elderly male client who lives alone following the death of his wife.

8.16 What would be the best response from the nurse for a client with diabetes mellitus who begins crying during a home health visit and says, "I cannot give myself this shot every day"?
① Report the statement to the health care provider.
② "What is your concern that bothers you to administer the insulin to yourself?"
③ "You can do this! You will get used to it once it becomes a habit."
④ "I will arrange for the home health nurse to visit you routinely and assist with the shots."

8.17 While the nurse is taking a history for an older client diagnosed with depression, what is the most important question for the nurse to ask?
① "Have you ever attempted suicide or thought about suicide?"
② "Do you take antidepressant medications or any other medications?"
③ "Have any of your family ever had a psychiatric disorder?"
④ "Are you currently experiencing delusions, illusions, or hallucinations?"

8.18 Which of these clinical findings would alert the nurse to suspect abuse for an elderly client who is admitted to the emergency department with injuries of unknown etiology?
① A diagnosis of a midshaft fracture of the femur.
② A daughter with the client who fills in the information that the client (her mother) is unable to recall.
③ Bruises and lesions on the inner aspects of the extremities.
④ Bruises on the extensor surfaces of the arms.

8.19 An elderly client is admitted to the emergency department (ED) with several bruises and cuts on body in various ages of healing. What is the nursing priority action after documenting these findings?
① Follow the agency policy for reporting elder abuse.
② Ask the client how the cuts and bruises occurred.
③ Notify the provider that abuse is suspected.
④ Immediately report to social worker.

8.20 A client rings the call bell requesting assistance to ambulate to the bathroom. The RN delegates this to the UAP. The UAP states, "I am so glad that I am the only one that is qualified to take someone to the bathroom. I guess they don't teach that in nursing school." How should the RN respond?
① "That was rude."
② "You sound like you are upset about something."
③ "Ambulating clients to the bathroom is within your scope of practice."
④ "We all have things about our job we do not like."

8.21 Which of these symptoms may be assessed for a client experiencing alcohol withdrawal? **Select all that apply.**
① HR—56 beats per minute
② BP—102/68
③ Fine tremor of both hands
④ Vomiting
⑤ Inability to sleep

8.22 A client with a severe thought disturbance has not been taking medication and appears to be more actively hallucinating. The client claims that the medicine makes him too drowsy during the day. Which action by the nurse is most likely to increase medication compliance?
① Ask the physician to schedule the client's entire dose at bedtime.
② Tell the client he is getting sicker and must take his medicine.
③ Teach the client about the side effects of the medication.
④ Ask the family to talk to the client about this problem.

8.23 A client, admitted for treatment of alcohol dependence, displays the following symptoms: slurred speech, ataxia, uncoordinated movements, and headache. Which nursing action would be taken first?
① Observe the client for 8 hours to collect additional data.
② Perform a complete physical assessment.
③ Collect a urine specimen for a drug screen.
④ Encourage the client to talk about whatever is bothering him.

8.24 What would be the most effective plan to assist with communication for a client who is being admitted to the medical unit, but only speaks Spanish?
① Notify the nursing assistant on another unit to come and interpret the questions for the client.
② Attempt to have the family interpret for the client to assist in understanding the questions the nurse is asking about client's history.
③ Notify the hospital's interpreter to assist client to understand the questions being asked in Spanish.
④ Since one of the client's friends speaks English, communicate with him.

8.25 What would be the priority plan of care following the death of a female client who is Muslim?
① Private room to gather the family for grieving
② A muslin wrap, preferably white, for the body
③ Post-mortem care of the body by a female nurse
④ Immediate referral to a crematory

8.26 An elderly man diagnosed with major depression is demonstrating decreased problem-solving ability, psychomotor retardation, and social isolation. In planning activities for this client during the early phase of hospitalization, which nursing action is appropriate?
① Prepare and give client a schedule of activities to follow and monitor participation.
② Encourage client to choose own activities.
③ Allow client some time to get acclimated to the milieu before scheduling activities.
④ Allow client to rest quietly to restore energy and fatigue level.

8.27 Which of these psychiatric clients would be evaluated first?
① Depressed client sitting on the floor rocking back and forth.
② Bipolar client pacing and clenching fist.
③ Psychotic client who is having a delusion that she is the Queen of England.
④ Schizophrenic client laughing and waving hands up in the air.

8.28 Which of these nursing interventions are appropriate for a client experiencing alcohol withdrawal? **Select all that apply.**
① Offer extra fluids and a nutritious diet.
② Place suction at bedside.
③ Place an airway at bedside.
④ Encourage to go to group therapy.
⑤ Place an ambu bag at bedside.

8.29 Which of these assessments is most important to report to provider of care for the wife of a spinal cord injury client with a C4 fracture?
① The wife indicates to the nurse that there may be a need for counseling to help cope with this current situation.
② The wife has elicited the support of family and friends in helping to provide care for the husband after discharge.
③ The wife has lost 10 lbs. (4.5 kg) since the accident, and shares with the nurse feelings of hopelessness about the future have resulted in an inability to sleep at night.
④ The wife reports going to bed one hour earlier to get the needed rest to assist in handling the current situation of with the husband.

8.30 What is the priority for an elderly client who has Alzheimer's disease and wanders the halls of the nursing unit during the day?
① Encourage client to watch television in room.
② Administer prn lorazepam as prescribed to calm client.
③ Assess client's gait to determine balance and steadiness.
④ Only allow client to wander in the unit with the assistance from a UAP.

8.31 Which plan is most appropriate for meeting the needs for a Hindu family after the loved one has died?
① Allow the family to wash the body.
② Allow the priest to touch the body.
③ Allow chanting to be done during the "last rites."
④ Do not consult with family about organ donations since it is considered a sin.

8.32 A client was minimally injured in a motor vehicle crash six months ago though client's friend was killed. The client comes to Student Health Services with complaints of not being able to study, not sleeping, and thinks "I'm going crazy." What is the most important information for the nurse to obtain?
① Complete physical and social history.
② Complete drug and alcohol history including reports from a drug screen.
③ Review of significant events in the last year.
④ Coping behaviors concerning the motor vehicle crash and friend's death.

8.33 What alternative plan of care would be most effective for clients with cancer who experience ongoing fatigue?
① Discuss the power of prayer and/or meditation as a regular part of plan of care.
② Drink several glasses of hot tea prior to lying down to go to sleep.
③ Encourage client to watch a favorite comedy on television.
④ Review the importance of taking an aspirin daily.

8.34 Which nursing action is of primary importance during the implementation of a behavior modification treatment program?
① Confirm that all staff members understand and comply with the treatment plan.
② Establish mutually-agreed-upon, realistic goals.
③ Ensure that the potent reinforcers (rewards) are important to the client.
④ Establish a fixed interval schedule for reinforcement.

8.35 Which of these statements made by a female client who has been abused by her spouse indicates the counseling has been effective?
① "I know my husband will never hurt me again."
② "I know it is my fault that he hits me."
③ "I promise I will get him to promise that he will not do it again."
④ "I have made arrangements to go to the battered women's shelter the next time he hits me."

8.36 An elderly client is frantically yelling for the nurse. The nurse enters the room as the client states, "See it? It's the devil!" What is the most therapeutic response?
① "The devil is here?"
② "Show me where the devil appeared to you."
③ "I don't see the devil, but I understand that it is real to you."
④ "The devil is not here. Your mind is playing tricks on you."

8.37 Which of these clinical findings is the first sign of opioid withdrawal?
① abdominal cramping
② diaphoresis
③ fever
④ nausea

8.38 An alcoholic client who occasionally uses marijuana and cocaine is attending his second group therapy meeting. The client comments, "I am having difficulty sitting still. Am I bothering some of the group members? Maybe I should stop coming to these group meetings." Which nursing action is most appropriate?
① Encourage client to share problem with the group.
② Remove client from the group and further assess needs.
③ Recognize that this is manipulative behavior and encourage client to remain in the group.
④ Tell client not to be concerned about the group members and to continue in the group.

8.39 Family members of clients with eating disorders would be instructed to watch for which of these possible problems?
① Aggressive behavior and feeling angry
② Self-identity and self-esteem
③ Focusing on reality
④ Family boundary intrusions

8.40 Which evaluation indicates a disoriented client with poor nutrition has made a positive response to the plan of care?
① Reports relationship of weight loss to change in mental status.
② Identifies basic four food groups.
③ States he needs to drink more water.
④ Feeds self when the nurse stays with and cues him.

8.41 Policemen bring a client to the emergency room after standing barefoot in the rain for more than 2 hours. The policemen report that the client had to be restrained after resisting and becoming agitated. What is the first nursing action?
① Do a preliminary physical exam.
② Reassure and help maintain client safety.
③ Ascertain the client's mental status.
④ Orient the client to place and time.

8.42 An infant is scheduled for open-heart surgery. The mother begins to cry and says, "I'm a terrible mother!" What is the best nursing response?
① "Do you want to talk about the surgery?"
② To place a comforting arm around the mother.
③ "Is your family here to be with you?"
④ "You have done everything that you can, and the baby is in the best of hands."

8.43 An adolescent client is being discharged after an attempted suicide. What is the priority of care for this client?
① Schedule the follow-up visit for the family and client.
② Review the side effects of the prescribed anti-depressant medication.
③ Obtain the client's signature on the behavior contract.
④ Encourage client to attend group therapy every Wednesday evening.

8.44 A client admitted to the mental health unit experiencing hallucinations is not wearing an identification band. What is the best action before giving the client a scheduled medication?
① Compare the picture and the hospital identification number on the medication administration record (MAR) to the information in the client's chart.
② Ask the client to verify name and date of birth before giving the medication.
③ Ask another staff member who knows the client to give the medication for you.
④ Use the client's photograph and the hospital identification number on the client's chart and compare this to the client's physical appearance.

8.45 A psychiatric client with the diagnosis of schizophrenia tells the nurse that he is the President of the United States. What is the priority action for the nurse?
① Confront the client regarding this delusion and bring him back to reality.
② Reflect this statement back to the client to encourage therapeutic communication.
③ Respond with an open-ended response to get client to further discuss his thoughts.
④ Verify the identity of the client prior to administering his medications.

8.46 Before undergoing an electroconvulsive therapy (ECT), the client reports being very anxious. Which action by the nurse would be the most therapeutic?
① Allow the client to have a cup of coffee to calm down.
② Encourage the client to sit quietly in her room and listen to a relaxation tape.
③ Administer lorazepan 1 mg IM to the client.
④ Ask if you can remain with client and discuss any fears.

8.47 Which assessment data would indicate a severely paranoid client is likely to need nursing interventions to promote self-care abilities?
① Speaks in a low, monotone voice.
② Has had suicidal ideation on 2 previous admissions.
③ Is very fearful that people are putting poison in his food.
④ Is unable to make eye contact with the nurse.

8.48 Which nursing action is most appropriate in helping an elderly depressed client complete activities of daily living?
① Medicate the client before the activities are begun.
② Develop a written schedule of activities, allowing extra time.
③ Assist the client with grooming activities for her so it doesn't take so long.
④ Provide frequent forceful direction to keep the client focused.

8.49 Which plan would be most likely to help the family of an emotionally disturbed client in managing behavior at home after discharge from inpatient treatment?
① Refer the family to Alliance for the Mentally Ill meetings for educational programs and support groups.
② Provide the family with pamphlets that describe the desired action and side effects of medications the client is taking.
③ Tell the family that it is not their fault that the client behaves inappropriately.
④ Involve the family in the assessment of the client when he is first admitted to the hospital.

8.50 Which approach should be included in the nursing care plan for a client who displays the following: restless and tense behavior, complaints of feeling empty, history of several threats of self-mutilation?
① Monitor weight and dietary intake.
② Medicate with chlordiazepoxide for tremors.
③ Provide foods in client's own containers to decrease suspiciousness.
④ Take inventory of unit and remove hazardous or sharp objects.

8.51 What would be the nurse's initial priority when managing a physically assaultive client?
① Restrict client to room.
② Place client on a 1-1 supervision.
③ Restore the client's self-control and help prevent further loss of control.
④ Clear the immediate area of other clients to prevent harm.

8.52 Before giving medication to a client who identifies himself as Jesus Christ, which action by the nurse is necessary?
① Ask several UAPs to be available for safety.
② Ask the priest to come and speak with the client.
③ Check the client's name band to make sure of the client's identity.
④ Make sure the client has eaten a full meal.

8.53 A client on lithium therapy should be on which dietary plan to receive increased nutritional requirements?
① Restricted sodium diet with increased fluid intake.
② High calorie diet with sodium and potassium restriction and adequate fluid intake.
③ Regular diet with normal sodium and increased fluid intake.
④ Reduced calorie diet with a reduced sodium and reduced fluid intake.

8.54 What is the priority nursing action when coordinating a community placement for an alcoholic schizophrenic client who has been homeless?
① Collaborate with members of the client's family to explore placement options.
② Collaborate with health care team and the client to schedule a pre-discharge visit to residential placement facility.
③ Visit the placement facility alone to make an independent decision about the facility and report to the client and family.
④ Review with the client specific rules of the facility.

8.55 Which behavior indicates a client is beginning to develop a trusting relationship with the nurse?
① The client describes delusions to the nurse.
② The client can describe his feelings to the nurse.
③ The nurse feels more comfortable with the client.
④ The client states feeling less anxious.

8.56 Which post electroconvulsive therapy (ECT) treatment observations would the nurse report to the physician?
① Headache
② Disruption in short and long-term memory
③ Transient confusional state
④ Backache

8.57 Which information would indicate that the therapeutic interaction is in the working stage with a client who has an addiction problem? **Select all that apply.**
① The client reluctantly discusses the family history of addiction.
② The client addresses how the addiction has resulted in family distress.
③ The client experiences difficulty with identifying personal strengths.
④ The client discusses the financial burden related to the addiction.
⑤ The client is uncomfortable in meeting with the nurse.
⑥ The client discusses the addiction's effects on the children.

8.58 What would be the priority nursing action when dealing with a client who is a victim of interpersonal violence?
① Encourage the client to verbalize feelings.
② Assess for physical trauma.
③ Provide privacy for the client during the interview.
④ Help the client identify and mobilize resources and support systems.

8.59 What would be a positive outcome of treatment with a victim of paternal sexual abuse?
① Acknowledges willing participation in an incestuous relationship.
② Reestablishes a trusting relationship with mother.
③ Verbalizes that she is not responsible for the sexual abuse.
④ Describes feelings of anxiety when speaking about father and the sexual abuse.

8.60 Which nursing intervention is the highest priority for a client receiving aripiprazole for a diagnosis of schizophrenia?
① Recommend that the client reduces his alcohol intake to one drink per day.
② Instruct client to take the medication only before meals.
③ Review the importance of taking aripiprazole at bedtime since it causes sedation.
④ Advise to increase his exercising in order to optimize the drug action.

8.61 Which plan indicates the nurse understands the characteristics of a therapeutic nurse-client relationship?
① Establishing priorities and goals for the client.
② Utilizing the nursing process to establish client goals.
③ Collaborating to establish mutually agreed upon goals and priorities.
④ Directing interactions to assist the client to meet needs.

8.62 A client with terminal cancer is nearing the end of life. Which plan best meets the client's emotional needs?
① Provide the client with a room where family can be present.
② Make sure that the client has an advanced directive on the chart.
③ Consult the hospital chaplain or client's personal spiritual advisor.
④ Provide the client with a journal to record final thoughts for family and friends.

8.63 Which is a positive response to fluoxetine HCL?
① Hand tremors and leg twitching
② Increased ability to sleep
③ Increased energy level and participation in unit activities
④ Hypervigilance and scanning of the environment

8.64 Which nursing intervention is most important when working with clients with a diagnosis of dementia?
① Reinforce the client's thought patterns.
② When speaking with the client, use simple, short sentences.
③ Administer anti-anxiety medications.
④ Facilitate an exercise program with the client's physical limitations.

8.65 Which assessment would have priority in an initial assessment of an alcoholic client?
① Has the client been taking over-the-counter medication?
② What has been the client's usual daily intake of alcohol?
③ When did the client have his last drink?
④ Has the client ever had a withdrawal seizure?

Answers & Rationales

8.1 ④ Option #4 is correct. Prior to the development of a plan of care, it is most important to assess the client's understanding and thoughts of the diagnosis. Options #1, #2, and #3 are not priority.
I CAN HINT: Apply the clinical judgment/cognitive skill, analysis of cues (analysis), for a client with a chronic illness. The key to success is an understanding of the importance to "Assess client" prior to the spouse, extended family, etc.
NCLEX® Standard: Assess client's ability to cope with life changes and provide support.

8.2 ① ③ ⑤ Option #1, #3, and #5 are correct. The client should be included in the initial plan of care to assist in determining client's food preferences. The client with anorexia nervosa may experience hypotension and bradycardia which can present a risk for injury to the client due to potential falls. Option #5 is correct. Journal writing is encouraged to assist client to document thoughts and feelings regarding self, food, coping, etc. Option #2 should not be included in the plan. Option #4 is incorrect. A diet high in fiber is advised to minimize risks of alteration in elimination (constipation).
I CAN HINT: Apply the clinical judgment/cognitive skill, generate solutions (first-do priority plans), for a client with anorexia nervosa. An understanding of anorexia nervosa is important for answering this question.
NCLEX® Standard: Provide care and education for acute and chronic psychosocial health issues (e.g., depression, dementia, eating disorders).

8.3 ① Option #1 is correct. Reviewing resources for respite care with the daughter will provide the daughter with some support with the caregiving responsibilities of her mother. Option #2 is incorrect. There is no indication of any time management issues. Option #3 is incorrect. There is no indication that other family members are not supporting the daughter with the mother's care. Option #4 is incorrect. It does not answer the question. The question focuses on how the daughter is struggling to manage her mother's care, manage her family, and career.
I CAN HINT: Apply the clinical judgment/cognitive skill, generate solutions (first-do priority plans). Focus on the question. It is about the struggle for the daughter to manage her responsibilities.
NCLEX® Standard: Provide care and education for acute and chronic psychosocial health issues (e.g., depression, dementia, eating disorders).

8.4 ① Option #1 is correct. This will decrease the client being able to manipulate. Options #2 and #4 are not priority over option #1 for a client with a personality disorder. These would be important for a depressed client. Option #3 is incorrect. There is no need for assertiveness training for this client.
I CAN HINT: Apply the clinical judgment/cognitive skill, take-action (first-do priority interventions).
NCLEX® Standard: Provide care and education for acute and chronic psychosocial health issues (e.g., depression, dementia, eating disorders, personality disorders).

8.5 ① ③ ④ Options #1, #3, and #4 are correct. Anticholinergic effects can occur when taking amitriptyline. Fluids and fiber will assist in decreasing the risk of constipation (anticholinergic effect) from this medication. Drowsiness can initially occur when taking this medication. Option #2 is incorrect since it can result in drowsiness. Option #5 is incorrect. St. John's Wort may alter the serum concentration of the medication.
I CAN HINT: Apply the clinical judgment/cognitive skill, generate solutions (first-do priority plans).
NCLEX® Standard: Evaluate client's understanding of safe medication management.

8.6 ① ③ ④ Option #1, #3, and #4 are correct. Therapeutic communication is crucial in letting clients know you care and are willing to listen (i.e., examples incude open-ended statements, exploring, and assessing client for further clarification, etc.). Option #3 is important for the interaction and environmental management in assisting to decrease client's anxiety. Option #4 is correct for a client with

anxiety. This activity will provide an outlet for anxiety and promote endorphin release. This will result in an improvement in the client's mental health. Option #2 is unrealistic. This will not assist in decreasing anxiety. Option #5 is not therapeutic. It is providing false assurance and may even result in an increase in anxiety.
I CAN HINT: Apply the clinical judgment/ cognitive skill, generate solutions (first-do priority plans).
NCLEX® Standard: Provide a therapeutic environment for an anxious client.

8.7 ③ Option #3 is correct. These assessments indicate a high risk for suicide. Option #1 is an expected assessment. Option #2 is an expected finding with a client with Alzheimer's disease. Option #4 is not priority due to the fact the client has no energy to hurt self. The suicidal risk is when client begins presenting with more energy, has a plan to hurt self, and is giving away favorite possession to other people.
I CAN HINT: Apply the clinical judgment/ cognitive skill, analysis of cues (analysis).
NCLEX® Standard: Assess the potential for violence and use safety precautions.

8.8 ② ④ ⑤ Options #2, #4, and #5 are correct. This atypical antidepressant can cause anticholinergic side effects which may include a dry mouth and constipation. Fluids, oral hygiene, and fiber are important to include in the plan to prevent the anticholinergic effects from occurring. Options #4 and #5 are correct due to the GI effects such as nausea and vomiting and weight loss that can also occur. Option #1 is incorrect. The complication would be constipation versus diarrhea. Option #3 is incorrect. Alcohol and/or other CNS depressants should be avoided.
I CAN HINT: Apply the clinical judgment/ cognitive skill, generate solutions (first-do priority plans). An understanding of bupropion, an atypical antidepressant, is important for answering this question. Options #2 and #4 are secondary to anticholinergic effects which is a good clinical decision-making strategy, since many mental health drugs do have these effects. Diarrhea would be more of a concern with antibiotics!
NCLEX® Standard: Educate client about medications.

8.9 ② Option #2 is correct. Grapefruit can increase effects of buspirone. Options #1, #3, and #4 are incorrect.
I CAN HINT: Apply the clinical judgment/ cognitive skill, generate solutions (first-do priority plans). The nonbarbiturate, buspirone, is reviewed in the book, *Pharmacology Made Insanely Easy* by Manning and Rayfield, with the image of a buspirone bus indicating there should be no sudden stops. This medication is used to decrease anxiety
NCLEX® Standard: Review pertinent data prior to medication administration (e.g., contraindications, potential interactions such as fluid/food-drug interactions).

8.10 ② Option #2 is correct. Use cautiously in moderate renal impairment. Drugs or diets that cause alkaline urine should be avoided. Condition that increases urine pH, including urinary tract infections or renal tubular acidosis may lead to a decrease in excretion and increase levels. This increase in the BUN and creatinine indicates an alteration in renal function. Options #1 and #4 would be included in the plan of care for the client but are not priority over option #2. Option #3 is an incorrect statement. It is not a cure, but the client should experience an improvement in cognitive function (i.e., memory, attention, language, ability to perform activities of daily living).
I CAN HINT: Apply the clinical judgment/ cognitive skill, generate solutions (first-do priority plans).
NCLEX® Standard: Review pertinent data prior to medication administration (e.g., lab results, contraindications, and potential interactions).

8.11 ① Option #1 is correct. Lithium is a salt and with any sodium loss from hot weather, fever, etc., there is a risk for fluid deficit resulting in hypernatremia and lithium toxicity. Clients should notify health care provider if they experience fever, vomiting, diarrhea, and/or sweating. These assessment findings may result in lithium toxicity. Options #2, #3, and #4 are incorrect. Option #2 is an incorrect statement. Option #3 should be between 1,500 mL to 3,000 mL daily. Option #4 is incorrect because the effects begin within 5-7 days.
I CAN HINT: Apply the clinical judgment/ cognitive skill, generate solutions (first-do priority plans).

Chapter 8: ANSWERS & RATIONALES

NCLEX® Standard: Manage the care of the client with a fluid and electrolyte imbalance. Educate client about medications.

8.12 ③ Option #3 is correct. The key to answering this question appropriately is to recognize these clinical findings to be tardive dyskinesia which can become irreversible and result in airway obstruction as well. The treatment for these clinical findings are diphenhydramine (Benadryl) or benztropine (Cogentin). Option #1 is not correct information. This should not occur and is an undesirable effect if it does occur. Option #2 is incorrect. This is not the role of the nurse or client. The health care provider is the only professional who should be adjusting the medication. Option #4 is incorrect because it does not address the severity of the clinical findings.

8.13 ① Option #1 is correct. The client may be experiencing some alteration in fluid and electrolytes leading to cardiovascular complications. These may result in a fall. Option #2 is not correct. It would not be a priority. Requiring immediate intervention. Options #3 and #4 are not correct. Both of these statements are symptoms of a low self-esteem, but are not priority to option #1.
I CAN HINT: The key to answering this correctly is to focus on the anorexia nervosa and the "immediate intervention". This indicates there is a complication that is an immediate threat to the client's safety. After clustering options #3 and #4, this would leave options #1 and #2 for the selection. While we are concerned with option #2, the question for you to ask is, *"Would mouth tenderness cause an immediate threat to the client?"* versus *"Would a feeling of being faint and weak cause an immediate threat to the client?"*

8.14 ② Option #2 is correct. This will assist client with establishing some control over behavior with no outside stimuli and activities for distraction. Option #1 would only contribute to the manic episode and would not be therapeutic. The last thing the nurse would want the client to engage in would be a competitive activity. Option #3 is not correct. During the manic episode, the client is out of control and needs time to regroup. Option #4 is not correct for the manic client. This would be appropriate if client was demonstrating manipulative behavior.

8.15 ④ Option #4 is correct. The high-risk factors for suicide include Caucasian males, advanced age, hopeless, living alone, family history of suicide, substance abuse. Males 65 and older are high risk, especially males 85 and older. Diagnosis (psychiatric) are some of the most reliable factors for suicide such as substance disorders, schizophrenia, and depression. The client alone following the death of his wife is a high risk for suicide. Options #1, #2, and #3 are not within this category. They will have concerns, but will not consider suicide.

8.16 ② Option #2 is correct. The best response is to encourage client to ventilate thoughts, feelings, and concerns regarding giving the insulin shot. This is the most therapeutic response that will assist the nurse in identifying the reason the client has so much fear. Option #1 may need to be implemented in the future. Option #3 is non-therapeutic! It is ignoring the feelings behind the statement. Option #4 is not correct. First of all, the client needs to learn how to perform the injection and be held accountable. Second, home health will most likely not continue to pay for this service, since there is no reason for the client not to administer insulin to self.
I CAN HINT: The key to success on this question is to understand "Therapeutic Communication."

8.17 ① Option #1 is correct. While the other options are important to assess during this initial history, it would be most important to assess if the client is at risk for injury related to suicide. Safety is a priority concern for depressed clients. Some assessments that are very valuable to determine if the client has a plan are giving away valuable possessions and if there has been an increase in the client's level of energy. Option #2 is not a priority over #1. It is important to assess the medications, but not more important than assessing for risk for suicide. Options #3 and #4 are not a priority over option #1.
I CAN HINT: Testing strategy would be that Options #3 and #4 include general psychiatric disorders. The question is asking *"What would be the most important question to ask?"*

8.18 ③ Option #3 is correct. Research has concluded that bruising on the inner surfaces of the extremities and areas with different stages of resolution are often found in the elderly client who has been abused. Option #1 is not conclusive of abuse. This could have resulted from a fall or an injury due to the complication from osteoporosis. Option #2 is not a finding for abuse. This is a finding of a caring daughter. Option #4 may be common findings for the elderly client, and does not indicate a complication with abuse.

8.19 ② Option #2 is correct. This question is evaluating the ability to "*Identify clients at risk for abuse.*" The priority nursing action is to assess how the client perceives the cuts and bruises occurred. Option #1 is an important intervention, but would not come before assessment. Option #3 is also important, but not a priority over option #2. Option #4 would not be a priority over option #2 since the nurse should start with the client, and then evaluate if the stories are the same from both the client and family member accompanying client.

8.20 ② Option #2 is the correct answer. This is an example of how to incorporate "therapeutic communication" with staff. This statement allows the UAP to know that the nurse is paying attention to the statement that was made. This will allow the UAP to ventilate the concerns to the RN and facilitate clarification as to the request. Option #1 is nontherapeutic. It is a statement, and does nothing to assist in understanding the reason the statement was made, even if in reality it was a rude statement. A strategy for "*therapeutic communication*" is to assist the client, staff member (or anyone who is making the statement) to further discuss statement, know they are being heard, and take time to listen to their concerns. While option #3 may be a true and valid statement, it does not address the feelings behind the statement. Option #4 is not therapeutic and also does not address the feelings behind the question.

8.21 ③ ④ ⑤ Options #3, #4, and #5 are correct. This question is evaluating the NCLEX® activity: "*Assess client for drug/alcohol withdrawal.*" These options include clinical findings for clients experiencing alcohol withdrawal. Additional clinical findings for client may include restlessness, depressed mood, irritability, vital signs are elevated, so the HR would be elevated and the BP would be increased (Options #1 and #2). A late symptom is tactile hallucinations of "bugs crawling" on the skin.

8.22 ① Medication dose non-compliance is often associated with negative side effects and a multiple dosing daily schedule. When the client has only one daily dose at bedtime, it is easier for him to remember to take the medication. The other advantage is that the sedative effects of the drug peak while the client is sleeping. Options #2 and #4 do not offer concrete solutions and may foster dependent behaviors. Option #3 may help to some degree, but a more concrete solution is possible.

8.23 ② The best way to identify possible physical complications of alcohol dependence is through a complete physical assessment. Option #1 is important but will not provide the data that a physical assessment would. This may be a medical emergency requiring an immediate intervention. Option #3 is also a helpful source of data but can be done after the physical assessment is finished. Option #4 is inaccurate since the symptoms are most likely caused by physical and not psychological stressors.

8.24 ③ Option #3 is correct. This will be more professional, more accurate, and will not violate any client confidentiality. The interpreter has a sense of accountability; whereas, the other options do not have this responsibility. Options #1, #2, and #4 are inaccurate due to confidentiality and accountability.

8.25 ③ Option #3 is correct. The Muslim culture believes that the same gender should provide care after death. Option #1 is incorrect because the Muslim culture grieves at home. Option #2 is secondary to option #3. Option #4 is incorrect because cremation is not typically practiced in the Muslim culture.

8.26 ① A regular daily routine of scheduled activities provides structure and decreases the degree of problem-solving. Depressed clients need to have structure provided because of impairment in decision-making and problem-solving. Options #2, #3, and #4 may promote further social isolation and increase the client's impairments. This may further decrease the client's self-esteem.

8.27 ② Option #2 needs to be evaluated first due to safety issues. Options #1, #3, and #4 are not going to hurt anyone.

8.28 ② ③ ⑤ Options #2, #3, and #5 are correct. This question is evaluating "*Safe use of equipment*" for a client who is experiencing alcohol withdrawal.
I CAN HINT: Always think about equipment for airway due to the risk of airway obstruction during the withdrawal activities such as delirious tremors. Think of equipment the nurse should have at the bedside for a client with seizure activity. This will assist in answering this question. Option #1 is incorrect for this question. The priority is safety for the client "experiencing alcohol withdrawal". Option #4 is incorrect for this question. This is the last thing the nurse will consider during this behavior with alcohol withdrawal.

8.29 ③ Option #3 is correct. This question is evaluating the NCLEX® activity, "*Recognize impact of illness on individual/family.*" This assessment would be most important due to the feelings of hopelessness, insomnia, and significant weight loss. This assessment indicates a need for additional support.
Option #1 is a healthy statement, indicating self-awareness with the need to seek additional support. Option #2 is also a healthy statement, indicating an awareness of not attempting to cope with this situation alone. Option #4 is also a healthy behavior.

8.30 ③ Due to medications, changes in eye sight, hearing, balance, etc., this client is at risk for falls. Option #1 is incorrect, since this does not allow client to ambulate and be independent. Option #2 is incorrect, since this may actually contribute to falls. Option #4 is unrealistic and unnecessary.

8.31 ① Option #1 is correct for the Hindu family. For an Islamic family member's death, only relatives or a priest may touch the body. The family washes the body and then turns it to face Mecca. Option #3 is appropriate for a Buddhist family. Option #4 is not true. Donation of organs may be done.

8.32 ④ All of these options are important and relevant to a thorough physio-psychosocial evaluation. However, initially ascertaining focused information about a very traumatic event, is helpful and provides the nurse with an opportunity to understand how this client has coped up to this point with a tragedy that has made client vulnerable.

8.33 ① Option #1 is correct. Studies show that cancer clients who practice meditation and/or pray experience a decrease in fatigue levels. These have been scientifically measured to be less than those clients who do not use these types of practice. Option #2 is incorrect due to the caffeine. This will not facilitate rest. Option #3 is going to result in laughing which can result in an increase in the endorphins that create more energy. Option #4 does not address the issue of fatigue.

8.34 ① To successfully implement a behavior modification plan, all staff members need to be included in the program development and to allow time for discussion of concerns from each nursing staff member. Consistency and follow-through are of utmost importance to prevent or diminish the level of staff manipulation by the client during the implementation of this program. Options #2, #3, and #4 are important in designing an effective behavior modification program. However, option #1 is a priority.

8.35 ④ Option #4 is correct. Most abused women eventually leave the situation. Interventions may not produce quick outcomes, but they can begin to facilitate the process of healing. Options #1, #2, and #3 are incorrect. Option #1—the husband will not change without identifying cause of anxiety and altering the manner he deals with it. Options #2 and #3 do not indicate counseling was effective.

8.36 ③ The nurse does not want to reinforce the client's hallucinatory experiences. Option #1 is incorrect because reflection techniques usually do not work in this situation. Option #2 is incorrect because attempts to reason or argue with the client may entrench him more firmly into this distortion. Option #4 is a direct challenge to the client's belief about sensory-perceptual intake and may increase mistrust and conflict between the nurse and client.

8.37 ② Option #2 is correct. Diaphoresis can occur between 6–12 hours. Abdominal cramping, fever and nausea may occur later between 48 to 72 hours.

8.38 ① The client is probably experiencing some mild level of anxiety related to detoxification as well as his participation in the group process. He needs reinforcement and encouragement to continue attending the group meetings and to share his feelings. Options #2, #3, and #4 would not be therapeutic.

8.39 ② Clients with eating disorders experience difficulty with self-identity and self-esteem which inhibits their ability to be a self-advocate and act assertively. Some assertiveness techniques that are taught include: giving and receiving criticism, giving and accepting compliments, accepting apologies, being able to say no and set limits on what they can realistically do, rather than just doing what others want them to do. Options #1 and #4 are secondary because these clients may have problems with family boundary intrusion and having difficulty with feelings of anger. Family therapy sessions can be helpful in identifying some of these feelings and difficulties with family boundaries. Option #3 is usually not an issue.

8.40 ④ A disoriented client who is not able to be an independent self-care agent will need prompting from the nurse to accomplish self-feeding. Options #1, #2, and #3 are not usually indicative of a client who is disoriented. They are more characteristic of a client with a higher level of cognitive functioning.

8.41 ② The major priority of the nurse is to provide and maintain safety for the client who is unable to provide this for him/herself. A safe environment will generate trust and rapport. This will decrease resistance to the next critical steps. Options #1, #3, and #4 are important, but cannot be done effectively until option #2 is accomplished.

8.42 ④ Option #4 is the priority answer. It is important to promote a sense of hope. Option #1 would provide for listening to client/family concerns, and options #2 and #3 may provide comfort.

8.43 ③ Option #3 is a priority due to safety and placing some accountability with the client. Options #1, #2, and #4 are an important part of the plan but are not a priority to option #3.

8.44 ④ Option #4 is correct. Using a client photograph for identification is acceptable in behavioral and long-term care areas. Option #1 compares one chart item to another. It does not identify the client. Option #2 is incorrect because a client experiencing hallucinations may not be able to respond reliably. Option #3 is inappropriate.

8.45 ④ Option #4 is a priority due to safety. Option #1 is partially correct, but nurses do not confront this client. Options #2 and #3 are part of therapeutic communication and are not answering the question.

8.46 ④ This allows the client some control over how to mutually deal with the anxiety related to ECT. The interpersonal contact provided by remaining with the client and discussing any fears will assist in anxiety reduction. Option #1 is inappropriate because the client must remain NPO before the ECT treatment, and coffee (especially caffeinated) is a CNS stimulant which could escalate her anxiety. Option #2 represents nurse avoidance but could be a beneficial strategy if the exercise had been instructed and practiced with the nurse. Option #3 is incorrect because medicating anxiety does not encourage the development of any additional coping strategies. Only if the level of anxiety were severe would psychopharmacologic intervention be necessary.

8.47 ③ When the client is fearful of being poisoned, he will not eat willingly and may suffer from problems with nutrition. Options #1 and #4 will have little bearing on his self-care abilities. Option #2 warrants further observation for depressive symptoms which might impair self-care, but at this point, there is no evidence to support this.

8.48 ② A written schedule with built-in extra time will allow the client to understand what is expected and will allow her to participate at a slower pace. Options #1, #3, and #4 will not increase the client's independence and may interfere with the client's self-esteem.

8.49 ① This group provides ongoing support and educational information. People who attend have common needs and goals focused on managing the client's behavior at home. Options #2, #3, and #4 may be helpful, but will not have the ongoing impact that option #1 would have.

8.50 ④ Option #4 is the correct answer. Protecting the client's safety is a priority for the nursing care plan. Options #1, #2, and #3 are not a priority for this client. Safety is the priority due to threats of self-mutilation.
I CAN HINT: The key to answering this question appropriately is to have an understanding of risk for suicide.

8.51 ④ Option #4 is correct. The most important priority in the nursing management of an assaultive client is to maintain safety of the client and others. A quick assessment of the situation, psychological intervention, chemical intervention and possible physical control are important when managing the physically-assaultive client. Option #1 may be a useful strategy before the client becomes assaultive. However, once the client is assaultive, this behavior may continue in room without any redirection and support. Option #2 may be unsafe to the other person. Option #3 is helpful, but not a priority.

8.52 ③ It is always necessary for the nurse to verify the client's identity before administering medications, particularly when the client cannot verbalize his identity. Options #1, #2, and #4 will be unnecessary.

8.53 ③ The client receiving Lithium needs to maintain a regular diet with a normal sodium intake and increased fluid intake (approximately 2–3 liters per day). Lithium is a salt preparation, and its retention within the body is directly related to the body's sodium and fluid salience. Option #1 is incorrect because a depletion of sodium is to be avoided because Lithium replaces sodium in the cells, therefore precipitating Lithium toxicity. Options #2 and #4 are incorrect because diets that are low in sodium, regardless of caloric intake, do not provide adequate nutritional balance for Lithium regulation.

8.54 ② Option #2 is correct. It is important that the multidisciplinary team discuss and collaborate with the client regarding discharge placements. The client will need support and assistance in making decisions about discharge and residential living arrangements. Option #1 may not be optimum because of possible codependence. Option #3 is incorrect because if the nurse visits independent of the client, that can diminish the sense of self-worth and decision-making. Option #4 is incorrect because reviewing rules with the client prematurely can inhibit the opportunity to explore feelings about this decision.

8.55 ② The client who is suspicious and delusional begins to demonstrate trusting behaviors when he/she shares their feelings with the nurse. Option #1 is incorrect because their delusional system is an indication of anxiety and delusions will increase with greater anxiety. Trust with the nurse is not related to an explanation of the client's delusions. Option #3 is incorrect because the nurse's response can be an indication of transference counter-transference issues and is not indicative of the client beginning to enter a trusting relationship. Option #4 may be secondary to option #2. It is very beneficial that the client's anxiety level is becoming less intense, and this will facilitate the development of a trusting relationship.

8.56 ④ A client undergoing ECT needs to be instructed by the nurse concerning symptoms that could be experienced during and post ECT. A backache is not a usual effect. A thorough description of the pain in relation to severity, duration, location and what makes the pain better, needs to be assessed and reported to the physician. Options #1, #2, and #3 are expected effects of the procedure.

8.57 ②④⑥ Options #2, #4, and #6 are correct. In option #1 the client is reluctant and still not confident with self. In option #3 the client is not comfortable enough to be self-aware of positive attributes. In option #5 the client is not comfortable with nurse which means there is still not a degree of comfort with interaction.

8.58 ② The victim of interpersonal violence may have physical trauma and concealed injuries. This assessment is of utmost importance, so that the client's physiologic integrity is maintained. Options #1, #3, and #4 are done concurrently as the nurse is assessing for physical injury. Privacy and encouraging the client to verbalize feelings are important. Facilitating the client to identify and rally their family or significant others to assist them during the crisis are important in the care of the victim of interpersonal violence.

8.59 ③ A positive outcome of treatment of a sexually abused client is the verbalization that they are not responsible for the sexual abuse. The victim needs assistance to challenge the "belief of victims" which includes, "I am bad and deserve the abuse." Option #1 continues the myth of badness and that they deserved the abuse and actively consented to it. Option #2 is an outcome that would be positive, but usually is not an initial result of treatment. Option #4 is an expected outcome—though not a positive one.

8.60 ③ Option #3 is correct. Aripiprazole (Abilify) is an antipsychotic agent referred to as a dopamine system stabilizer. Since these antipsychotic agents cause sedation, sleeping during the night and decreasing daytime drowsiness can be done by administering the agent at bedtime. Option #1 is incorrect because it should be avoided, not limited. Option #2 is incorrect because Abilify may be administered with or without food since it is well absorbed either way. Option #4 is an incorrect statement.

8.61 ③ The therapeutic nurse-client relationship is a mutual learning and corrective emotional experience. The nurse utilizes self and specified clinical techniques in working with the client to facilitate insight and behavioral change. Options #1, #2, and #4 are incorrect because in a nurse-client relationship, the client's needs are of primary concern.

8.62 ① Option #1 is correct. Providing a room for the client's family would be the best plan to meet the client's emotional needs. Option #2 does not meet the client's emotional needs. Option #3 and option #4 are secondary.

8.63 ③ Fluoxetine HCL (Prozac) is an "energizing" antidepressant, and as clients begin to demonstrate a positive response. They have an increased energy level and would be able to become more participative in the milieu. Options #1 and #4 can be side effects of the medication. Option #2 is not indicative of Prozac which can actually inhibit sleep and is useful with clients who experience increase in sleeping and psychomotor retardation and lethargy.

8.64 ② The client with dementia has significant difficulty with communication. Therefore, simple and short sentences can enhance the client's ability to process the information. Option #1 is incorrect because reality orientation, not reinforcement of the client's altered thought process, is an important goal. Option #3 is incorrect because anti-anxiety (anxiolytic) agents are not appropriate in the care of a dementia client and can worsen their confusional state. Option #4 is important but secondary to option #2.

8.65 ③ It is imperative that the nurse obtain the time of the client's last drink so that anticipation of when the client would most likely experience withdrawal symptoms will be known (usually occurring within 48-72 hours after the last drink). Options #1, #2, and #4 are important to note but do not take priority over option #3.

Notes

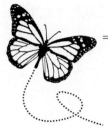

CHAPTER 9
Physiological Adaptation

*What we think determines what happens to us,
so if we want to change our lives, we need to
stretch our minds.*

— WAYNE DYER

✔ **Clarification of this test ...**

There are no changes in percentages, still representing 11–17% of exam items. The minimum standards include providing direct care for clients with acute, chronic, or life-threatening conditions: including fluid and electrolyte imbalances, alteration in hemodynamics, illness management, and emergencies.

- ☛ Educate client regarding an acute or chronic condition.
- ☛ Manage the care of a client on telemetry.
- ☛ Evaluate the effectiveness of the treatment plan for a client with an acute or chronic diagnosis.
- ☛ Manage the care of the client with a fluid and electrolyte imbalance.
- ☛ Maintain optimal temperature of client.
- ☛ Recognize signs and symptoms of client complications and intervene.
- ☛ Identify pathophysiology related to an acute or chronic condition.
- ☛ Manage the care of a client with impaired ventilation/oxygenation.
- ☛ Manage the care of a client with alteration in hemodynamics, tissue perfusion, and hemostasis.
- ☛ Perform wound care and dressing change.
- ☛ Provide post-operative care.
- ☛ Perform suctioning.
- ☛ Monitor and maintain devices and equipment used for drainage (e.g., surgical wound drains, chest tube suction, negative pressure wound therapy).
- ☛ Provide pulmonary hygiene (e.g., chest physiotherapy, incentive spirometry).
- ☛ Manage the care of a client receiving hemodialysis or continuous renal replacement therapy.
- ☛ Manage the care of a client with a pacing device.
- ☛ Monitor and care for clients on a ventilator.
- ☛ Monitor and maintain arterial lines.
- ☛ Perform emergency care procedures.
- ☛ Provide ostomy care and education (e.g., tracheal, enteral).
- ☛ Assist with invasive procedures (e.g., central line, thoracentesis, bronchoscopy).
- ☛ Perform and manage care of client receiving peritoneal dialysis.
- ☛ Implement and monitor phototherapy.

Adapted from: © National Council of State Boards of Nursing, Inc. (NCSBN). (2022). 2021 *RN Practice Analysis: Linking the NCLEX-RN® Examination to Practice*. Chicago: Author.

Adapted from: © National Council of State Boards of Nursing, Inc. (NCSBN). (2023) *Next Generation NCLEX® NCLEX-RN® Test Plan*. Chicago: Author.

Chapter 9: PHYSIOLOGICAL ADAPTATION

9.1 Which clinical findings require further follow-up for an elderly client experiencing diarrhea? **Select all that apply.**
 ① Serum sodium 135 mEq/L
 ② Specific gravity > 1.030
 ③ Poor skin turgor
 ④ Unable to identify son
 ⑤ BP from 145/90 to 102/58 mm Hg
 ⑥ Weight loss of 2 pounds in 24 hours

9.2 What is the immediate nursing action for a client who is presenting with poor skin turgor with tenting present and presenting with a BP change from 140/80 to 86/62 and pale in color after vomiting and experiencing diarrhea for 48 hours?
 ① Position client in supine position with legs elevated.
 ② Notify health care provider.
 ③ Position client in Fowler's position.
 ④ Evaluate characteristics of mucous membranes.

9.3 What is the priority plan of care for a client who is experiencing neck distention, crackles in the lungs, and peripheral edema?
 ① Position client in the supine position.
 ② Elevate legs to promote venous return.
 ③ Decrease the IV fluids and notify the health care provider.
 ④ Orient client to time, place, and situation.

9.4 Which of these nursing actions is priority for a client who was admitted for vomiting 24 hours and presenting with the ABG results: pH - 7.55; $PaCO_2$ - 43 mm Hg; HCO_3 – 30 mEq/L?
 ① The unlicensed assistive personnel weighs the client daily.
 ② The LPN irrigates the NG tube with tap water.
 ③ The RN administers sodium bicarbonate per protocol.
 ④ The RN administers oxygen via a rebreathing device per protocol.

9.5 Which nursing actions and teaching will the nurse include in the plan of care for a client requiring deep vein thrombosis (DVT) management, including anticoagulant therapy, and prevention of a new DVT? **Select all that apply.**
 ① Monitor blood pressure and heart rate per protocol.
 ② Elevate the legs for 15 minutes, two to three times daily when wearing sequential compression device.
 ③ Explain the importance of wearing sequential compression device while in bed on unaffected leg.
 ④ Report a sudden onset of chest pain, rapid heart rate and respiratory rate.
 ⑤ Review the importance of using an electric razor and soft toothbrush.
 ⑥ Discuss the importance of taking an aspirin with the intravenous heparin therapy.
 ⑦ Review the rationale for frequent ambulation.
 ⑧ Review the importance of drinking fluids.

9.6 What is the priority clinical finding that the nurse needs to report to the health care provider for a client with WBC - 3,000 mm³ (3×10^9/L), platelets 400,000 mm³ (400×10^9/L), and RBC - 5 million /uL (5×10^{12}/L) who is receiving chemotherapy?
 ① Bruising easily
 ② Fatigue
 ③ Oozing of blood at IV site
 ④ Sore throat

9.7 Which client would be the priority to assess on a Neurological Intensive Care Unit?
 ① The client with a closed head injury and increased intracranial pressure with a Glasgow Coma Scale that changed from 7 to 14.
 ② The client with meningitis who is presenting with a stiff neck and irritability with stimulation.
 ③ The client with a C-6 spinal cord injury who has a HR that went from 90 bpm to 46 bpm, BP from 140/80 to 96/48, and hyperreflexia.
 ④ The client with a cerebrovascular accident who presents with large toe moving toward the top surface of the foot with other toes fanning out after the sole of the foot has been stroked firmly.

9.8 Which client would be appropriate to assign to the RN with two years of experience?
① The client with Parkinson's disease who presents with a tremor and pill rolling.
② The client with amyotrophic lateral scleroscosis (ALS) presenting with dysarthria, dysphagia, and crackles in the bilateral breath sounds.
③ The client with Alzheimer's disease and wanders during the evening hours.
④ The client who is lethargic following a seizure.

9.9 Which of these clinical findings for a client with Addison's disease needs to be reported to the health care provider?
① Serum sodium level of 145 mEq/L (145 mmol/L)
② Serum glucose 48 mg/dL (2.7 mmol/L)
③ Blood pressure 174/90
④ Serum potassium level of 2.8 mEq/L (2.8 mmol/L)

9.10 Which of these clinical assessment findings would indicate a therapeutic response with the cardiac output from a bolus of isotonic fluids for a client who is in hypovolemic shock? **Select all that apply.**
① Pulmonary artery wedge pressure from 14 to 5 mm Hg.
② Urine output increased from 45 mL/hour to 60 mL/hour.
③ BP went from 140/90 to 98/64 in 2 hours.
④ CVP went from 2 mm Hg to 8 mm Hg.
⑤ Client alert and answering questions.

9.11 Which of these clinical assessment findings would be important to monitor and report for a client who experienced blood loss secondary to surgery? **Select all that apply.**
① BP 150/88
② Heart Rate from 78 bpm to 130 bpm (weak) in 1 hour
③ CVP 7 mm Hg
④ Respiratory Rate: 40/minute
⑤ Urine output from 80 mL/hour to 38 mL/hour in 1 hour

9.12 An older client was admitted to the emergency department presenting with atrial fibrillation. Three hours following the initiation of telemetry monitoring per health care provider's order, the central alarm sounds at the monitoring station, and the dysrhythmia has now changed to ventricular tachycardia. What is the first nursing action?
① Assess the client and check placement of leads.
② Call a Code Blue.
③ Notify the health care provider regarding the rhythm change.
④ Immediately administer lidocaine.

9.13 Which of these clients would be the priority to be assessed immediately following report?
① A client with a spinal cord injury who has a $PaCO_2$—36 mm Hg; ICP—15 mm Hg; and systolic arterial pressure (SAP)—120 mm Hg and is unable to move extremities.
② A client with a head injury with a MAP—90 mm Hg and ICP—8 mm Hg.
③ A client with a brain tumor who is complaining of a headache, with BP—170/58 mm Hg; HR—50 BPM; and motor, verbal, and eye opening responses to deep pain only.
④ A client who is 1 hour post-seizure and is resting on side with SaO_2—95%, but is lethargic.

9.14 Which clinical assessment findings would alert the nurse that an elderly client may be developing the complication of pneumonia?
① Change in functional and mental status
② Congestive and frequent cough
③ Temperature—102.4° F (39.1° C)
④ WBC—18,000 mm^3

9.15 A client presents with the following ABG report: pH—7.47; pCO_2—34 mm Hg; HCO_3—24 mEq/L (24 mmol/L). What is the priority of care for this client?
① Assist client to slow down breathing and assist with rebreathing device.
② Call the provider of care and report the arterial blood gas report of respiratory acidosis.
③ Place in the high-Fowler's and encourage breathing and coughing.
④ Place in prone position to prepare for respiratory therapy.

9.16 The UAP screams that the client with a diagnosis of atrial fibrillation who is being ambulated is suddenly feeling very dizzy. What action would the RN immediately assist the UAP to do with this client?

① Assess the client's blood pressure.
② Assess the client's apical pulse.
③ Encourage client to take deep breaths.
④ Help client to sit down.

9.17 Which of these plans are important for the nurse to implement when performing tracheostomy care? **Select all that apply.**

① Suction the tracheostomy tube every hour to maintain patency.
② Use cotton-tipped applicators and gauze pads to clean exposed outer cannula surfaces. Begin with hydrogen peroxide to clean the cannula and sterile saline to rinse it.
③ Use standard precautions when removing and cleaning the inner cannula.
④ Change and secure new tracheostomy ties after removing soiled ones.
⑤ If a knot is needed for the ties, tie a square knot that is visible on the side of the neck. One or two fingers should be able to be placed between the tie tape and the neck.

9.18 An older adult is admitted with a new onset of heart failure. A graduate nurse in orientation receives report for this client at 0700, including these lab reports. What is the priority of care for this client?

Serum Potassium—3.0 mEq/L (3.0 mmol/L)
Serum Glucose—110 mg/dL (6.11 mmol/L)
Creatinine—1.2 mg/dL (106 µmol/L)

① Consult with the preceptor regarding the care of a client with an elevated creatinine.
② Consult with the pharmacist to determine the procedure for administering glucagon.
③ Call the health care provider and question the prescription for furosemide.
④ When the health care provider (HCP) makes rounds, determine if there will be any revisions in the client's care due to these abnormal findings.

9.19 Which of these symptoms should be reported to the health care provider with these hemodynamic readings? Central Venous Pressure (CVP)—20 mm Hg; Pulmonary Artery Wedge Pressure (PAWP)—10 mm Hg; Cardiac Output (CO)—4-6 L/min. **Select all that apply.**

① Peripheral edema
② Hepatomegalyy
③ Poor skin turgor
④ Dry mucous membranes
⑤ Jugular vein distention

9.20 A nurse is providing care for an older client when the client becomes unresponsive and has the following cardiac dysrhythmia. After the nurse activates the emergency response system and determines there is no pulse, what would be the next action?

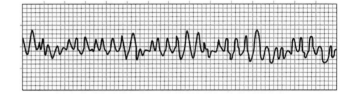

① Assess for response to noxious stimuli.
② Apply the defibrillator pads and administer a shock.
③ Begin giving 20 chest compressions.
④ Give two rescue breaths, and then start chest compressions.

9.21 Which one of these nursing actions indicates an understanding of how to successfully perform an IV access?

① Cleanse area at the site using friction in a circular motion from outward to middle with alcohol, iodine preparation or chlorhexidine. Allow to air dry for 1 to 5 min.
② Insert the catheter with bevel up at an angle of 15 to 20 degrees using steady motion (or as recommended by catheter manufacturer).
③ Advance the catheter through skin and into vein, but if flashback of blood is seen remove catheter from the site.
④ When using clean tourniquet, apply 8 to 10 inches above proposed insertion site to compress only venous blood.

9.22 A client is 3 days post-operative mitral valve replacement. Which recommendation would the nurse include in the nursing care plan to prevent post-operative complications?
① Maintain in supine position to prevent tension on the mediastinal suture line.
② Encourage deep breathing, but discourage coughing because of increased central venous pressure.
③ Decrease fluids to prevent fluid retention and development of heart failure.
④ Encourage early activity to promote ventilation and improve quality of circulation.

9.23 Which of these clients would be assessed immediately after shift report?
① A client who is presenting with the tracheal deviating to the unaffected side several hours after having chest tube inserted.
② A client who is 1 hour post bronchoscopy and is presenting with a depressed gag reflex.
③ A client post thoracentesis after having 1000 mL of fluid aspirated and is now complaining of syncope 2 hours later when getting up too quickly.
④ A client with SARS who is presenting with sneezing and coughing.

9.24 Which finding would the nurse identify as interfering with the effective functioning of chest tubes?
① 15 cm. water suction on chest tube system
② An air leak in water seal chamber
③ Leaking blood around chest tube site
④ Clots of blood in the chest tube

9.25 A permanent demand pacemaker set at a rate of 72 is implanted in a client for persistent third degree block. Which nursing assessment indicates a pacemaker dysfunction?
① Pulse rate of 88 and irregular
② Apical pulse rate regular at 68
③ Blood pressure of 110/88, pulse at 78
④ Tenderness at site of pacemaker implant

9.26 Which assignment is most appropriate for a new RN of 8 months who is pulled from the surgical unit to the medical unit?
① A middle-aged client with SARS and is on airborne precautions.
② A middle-aged client following thoracic surgery and is on a ventilator.
③ An older adult client who just returned from a bronchoscopy.
④ An elderly client who needs teaching regarding the use of an incentive spirometer.

9.27 A client is 2 days post-operative aortic aneurysm resection. A complete blood count reveals a decreased red blood cell count. Which symptoms is the nursing assessment most likely to reveal?
① Fatigue, pallor, and exertional dyspnea
② Nausea, vomiting, and diarrhea
③ Vertigo, dizziness, and shortness of breath
④ Malaise, flushing, and tachycardia

9.28 A client has tested positive for tuberculosis and is started on isoniazid for 6 months. What information would the nurse plan to include in the client's teaching plan?
① The color of the urine will change.
② Subsequent TB tests will be negative after drug administration.
③ Other medications should be withheld during therapy.
④ Alcohol consumption is contraindicated.

9.29 A client is scheduled for a left lower lobe lobectomy. Which nursing observation most indicates the need for an anti-anxiety agent?
① Agitation and decreased level of consciousness
② Lethargy and decreased respiratory rate
③ Restlessness and increased heart rate
④ Hostility and increased blood pressure

9.30 Organize the following steps to suctioning in chronological order (with 1 being the first step in this procedure).

| ① Put on sterile glove. |
| ② Lubricate catheter with normal saline. |
| ③ Apply suction for 5-10 seconds. |
| ④ Explain procedure to client. |
| ⑤ Wash hands thoroughly. |

| |
| |
| |
| |
| |

9.31 A client is admitted with dehydration secondary to diarrhea. A nursing history reveals the client has been on daily medications of digoxin 0.25 mg and furosemide 40 mg, which are to be continued according to admission orders. Which symptom is most important for the nurse to report to the next shift?

① Confusion and reports of yellow lights.
② Character and time of daily stools.
③ Intake and output for the last 24 hours.
④ Irritability toward friends and family.

9.32 A non-ventilated client with an ineffective breathing pattern related to severe dyspnea presents with cyanosis, tachycardia and hypotension. Which intervention has the highest priority?

① Encourage rest to conserve energy.
② Explain emergency procedures as they are happening.
③ Assess vital signs and respiratory status every 15 minutes.
④ Assess for bleeding tendencies and the potential for disseminated intravascular coagulation.

9.33 When changing the tubing on central lines, what is most important for the nurse to instruct the client to do?

① Sit in semi-Fowler's position, and take a deep breath prior to the procedure.
② Lie down, hold breath, and bear down when the line is opened.
③ Lie in the left lateral position, and hold breath during the procedure.
④ Sit in the Fowler's position, and exhale during the procedure.

9.34 Which nursing action is appropriate for a client with orthopnea, dyspnea, and bibasilar crackles?

① Elevate legs to promote venous return.
② Decrease the IV fluids, and notify the physician.
③ Orient the client to time, place, and situation.
④ Prevent complications of immobility.

9.35 A client is 3 hours post-operative thoracotomy. For the past 2 hours, there has been 200 mL per hour of bloody chest drainage. Which action would the nurse take?

① Increase the IV fluid rate.
② Administer oxygen at 5 liters/min. per face mask.
③ Elevate the head of the bed.
④ Advise the physician of the amount of drainage.

9.36 Which of these clients would the nurse intervene with immediately after shift report?

① A client with a newly implanted demand ventricular pacemaker, who has occasional periods of sinus rhythm, heart rate of 88-98 BPM.
② A client who has an order for verapamil with a history of atrial fibrillation.
③ A client diagnosed with atrial fibrillation and has a heart rate of 88 BPM at rest.
④ A client with an acute myocardial infarction (MI) and has a sinus rhythm, rate 74 BPM, with frequent premature ventricular contractions.

Chapter 9: PHYSIOLOGICAL ADAPTATION

9.37 A client awakens during the night with dyspnea, severe anxiety, jugular vein distension (JVD), and frothy pink sputum. After the nurse begins oxygen at 4 liters per nasal cannula, which action would be done next?
① Place 2 pillows behind head, and elevate the legs.
② Notify physician about change in client's condition.
③ Increases IV fluids to liquefy the secretions.
④ Dim lights and provide privacy.

9.38 It is 0600 and a client is scheduled for a cardiac catheterization at 0800. Laboratory work completed 5 days ago showed: K⁺—3.0 mEq/L (3.0 mmol/L), Na⁺—148 mEq/L (148 mmol/L), glucose—178 mg/dL (9.88 mmol/L). Client complains of muscle weakness and cramps. Which nursing action would be implemented at this time?
① Hold 0700 dose of spironolactone.
② Encourage eating bananas for breakfast.
③ Call the physician to suggest a stat K⁺ level.
④ Call for a twelve lead ECG.

9.39 A client is being treated for hypovolemia. Which observation would the nurse identify as the desired response to fluid replacement?
① Urine output 160 mL/8 hours
② Hgb—13g/dL; Hct— 49%
③ Arterial pH—7.34
④ CVP reading—8 mm Hg

9.40 The nurse is caring for an intubated, mechanically ventilated client. The nurse notes a "high pressure alarm" and finds the client coughing with secretions visible in the endotracheal tube. What are the priority nursing interventions?
① Silence the alarm and sedate the client for anxiety.
② Ambu the client and notify respiratory therapy.
③ Suction the client and monitor pulse oximetry.
④ Disable the alarm and order an arterial blood gas.

9.41 A client is admitted with arterial blood gasses of pH—7.57; pCO₂—29 mm Hg; HCO₃—22 mm Hg (22mmol/L). In response, the provider of care's orders: O₂ via nasal cannula at 5L/min. What is the priority nursing action?
① Begin O₂ immediately.
② Determine the accuracy of the order.
③ Assess for pain.
④ Notify the laboratory to repeat the test prior to any action.

9.42 A nurse caring for a client with a complete heart block would contact the physician regarding which order?
① Administer Lidocaine 50 mg IV push for PVCs in excess of 6 per minute.
② Administer atropine sulfate 0.05 mg IV for symptomatic bradycardia.
③ Anticipate scheduling client for a temporary pacemaker if pulse continues to decrease.
④ Mix 10 mL of 1:5000 solution of Isoproterenol in 500 mL D₅W for sustained bradycardia below 30.

9.43 A client arrives at the emergency department with a penetrating chest wound and a rush of air through the trauma site. Organize the following interventions in chronological order (with 1 being the highest priority).

① Administer oxygen and begin set up for tube insertions.
② Place air-occlusive dressing over chest wound.
③ Monitor blood gases.
④ Medicate for pain.

9.44 A client develops severe crushing chest pain radiating to the left shoulder and arm. Which PRN medication would the nurse administer?
① Diazepam PO
② Meperidine IM
③ Morphine sulfate IV
④ Nitroglycerine SL

9.45 A client presents with peripheral venous disease. The nurse will make which assessments with this client?
① Hair loss distal to the occlusion and a cool limb.
② Brawny color of extremity and sudden pain with exercise.
③ Peripheral edema from foot to calf and no pain.
④ Pale extremity when elevated and red when dependent.

9.46 Which assessment data indicates a client with a chest injury has sustained severe thoracic damage?
① Irregular S_1 and S_2
② Symmetrical respiratory excursion
③ Respiratory rate 30
④ Paradoxical chest movement

9.47 Which of these medications would be questioned for the client with this dysrhythmia?

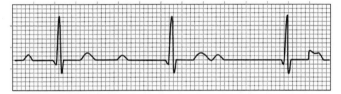

① Atropine
② Isoproterenol
③ Dopamine
④ Digoxin

9.48 A client receiving a continuous IV heparin infusion has a partial thromboplastin time (PTT) 1-1/2 times greater than normal. What would the nurse do next?
① Discontinue the heparin infusion.
② Slow down the heparin infusion.
③ Check the prothrombin time (PT) results.
④ Continue to monitor the client.

9.49 A nurse is the first on the scene of a motor vehicle accident. The victim has sucking sounds with respirations at a chest wound site and tracheal deviation toward the uninjured side. What is the priority nursing action prior to the emergency personnel arriving?
① Loosely cover the wound, preferably with a sterile dressing.
② Place sand bag over the wound.
③ Sit the client up.
④ Place a firm, airtight, sterile dressing over the wound.

9.50 The nurse is caring for a client who is immediate post-operative for an abdominal aortic aneurysm repair. Vital signs include: blood pressure—100/70, pulse—120, respirations—24, urine output—75 mL over the past 3 hours. Which nursing action is a priority for this client?
① Weigh the client to determine post-operative fluid loss.
② Obtain an ECG to evaluate the cause of the tachycardia.
③ Decrease the rate of the IV fluids and start nasal oxygen.
④ Maintain on bed rest; evaluate for decrease in CVP readings.

9.51 What action would a nurse take if a pleur-evac attached to a chest tube breaks?
① Immediately clamp the chest tube.
② Notify the physician.
③ Place the end of the tube in sterile water.
④ Reposition the client in the Fowler's position.

9.52 The nurse is caring for a client who has been immobilized for 3 days following a perineal prostatectomy. The client begins to experience sudden shortness of breath, chest pain, and coughing with blood-tinged sputum. What would be immediate nursing actions?
① Elevate the head of the bed, begin oxygen, assess respiratory status.
② Assist the client to cough. If unsuccessful, then perform nasotracheal suctioning.
③ Position in supine position with legs elevated. Monitor CVP closely.
④ Administer morphine for chest pain. Obtain a 12 lead ECG to evaluate cardiac status.

9.53 Which of these interventions is most appropriate for the LPN to initiate for safe and effective suctioning for a client?
① The LPN hyper-oxygenates client only after suctioning.
② The LPN positions client in the prone position for the procedure.
③ The LPN uses clean technique during the procedure.
④ The LPN tests the equipment for proper functioning prior to the procedure.

9.54 The nurse would identify which client as being at highest risk for development of a pulmonary emboli?
① A young-adult client four days postpartum with obstetrical history of a placenta previa.
② An obese middle-aged client with multiple pelvic fractures from an auto accident two days ago.
③ An older-adult client who is ten days post fractured hip repair and who is in physical therapy daily.
④ A young-adult client with leukemia who has a platelet count of 120,000/mm³ and hemoglobin of 9.0 g/dL.

9.55 Which of these nursing actions is a priority for a client with this ECG strip on the monitor?

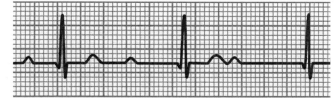

① Immediately begin CPR after establishing breathlessness.
② Administer amiodarone.
③ Prepare to cardiovert the client.
④ Have transcutaneous pacing ready at the bedside.

9.56 Two hours after a cardiac catheterization, the client begins to bleed from the femoral artery insertion site. Which nursing intervention is most appropriate?
① Assess pedal pulses and apply a sandbag.
② Apply manual pressure and notify the physician.
③ Place the client in Trendelenburg immediately.
④ Elevate the head of the bed 40 degrees and apply an ice pack.

9.57 When obtaining a specimen from a client for sputum culture and sensitivity (C&S), which instruction is best?
① After pursed lip breathing, cough into container.
② Upon awakening, cough deeply and expectorate into container.
③ Save all sputum for 3 days in covered container.
④ After respiratory treatment, expectorate into container.

9.58 Which assessment best indicates proper rehydration in a burn client with an IV order for 200 mL/hr?
① 400 mL of po intake over 3 hrs.
② Urine output of 100 mL per hr.
③ Heart rate of 105 per min.
④ Respiratory rate of 32 per min.

9.59 Which method is the most appropriate to assess or measure a client's jugular venous distension?
① Inspect the external jugular vein for distention with the client in the supine position.
② Observe for pulsations of the jugular vein that fluctuate with client's inspiration/exhalation.
③ Place the client in a Trendelenburg position for 5 minutes prior to assessment.
④ Recognize that a visible pulse at 2 cm above the sternal angle is recorded as distended.

9.60 While the nurse is providing care for a client who is on a volume cycled positive pressure ventilator, the low volume alarm sounds. What assessment would the nurse make?
① Client is biting on the tubing.
② Excessive fluid is in the ventilator tubing.
③ A leak in the client's endotracheal tube cuff.
④ Client is lying on the tubing.

9.61 To assess the right middle lobe (RML) of the lung, the nurse would auscultate at which location?

① Posterior and anterior base of right side.
② Right anterior chest between the fourth and sixth intercostals.
③ Left of the sternum, midclavicular at the fifth intercostal.
④ Posterior chest wall, midaxillary right side.

9.62 During a cardiac assessment, the nurse assesses an S_4. What additional assessments indicate an understanding of the implications of this assessment?

① Occipital headache
② Jugular vein distention
③ Weight loss
④ Hepatosplenomegaly

9.63 A client becomes extubated while being turned, and becomes cyanotic with bradycardia and dysrhythmias. Which action would be the highest priority while waiting for a physician to arrive?

① Immediately begin CPR.
② Increase the IV fluids.
③ Provide oxygen by ambuing and maintaining the airway.
④ Prepare the medications for resuscitation.

9.64 Place an X over the chamber that would be most important to assess for a client who has a chest tube connected to a water-seal chest tube drainage system and begins to present with the system below after the lung had expanded.

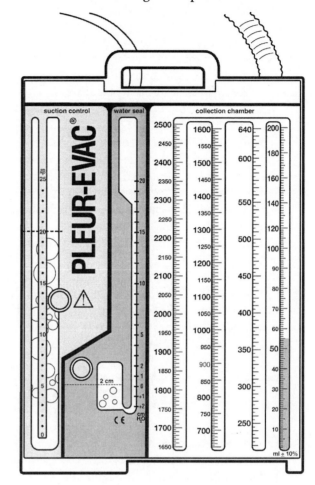

9.65 Identify the area where the nurse would place the stethoscope to auscultate the PMI during the physical assessment.

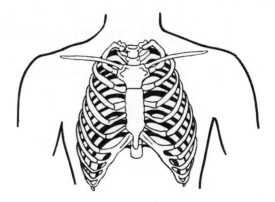

Answers & Rationales

9.1 ② Option #2 is correct. This value indicates
④ the urine is concentrated due to fluid deficit.
⑤ The normal reference range is 1.015 – 1.025.
⑥ Option #4 is correct. One of the first clinical assessment findings for elderly clients with fluid deficit is acute confusion. Option #5 is correct. This is indicative of a decrease in volume. Option #6 is correct. A weight gain or loss of 2 pounds or greater should be reported. Option #1 is incorrect. This is within the normal reference range which is 135-145 mEq/L (135-145 mmol/L). Option #3 is an invalid assessment for the elderly client because with aging the elasticity decreases which does not provide a reliable skin turgor.
I CAN HINT: Apply the clinical judgment/cognitive skill, analysis of cues, to the concept of fluid deficit. Remember, assessment findings all decrease (i.e., weight, BP, skin turgor [if not an older client], UO & peripheral pulses), HR is exception but the ↑ is due to ↓ volume, etc.) Lab values increase.
NCLEX® Standard: Manage the care of the client with a fluid and electrolyte imbalance.

9.2 ① Option #1 is correct. The client is experiencing fluid deficit with a drop in the blood pressure. Option #3 would result in a further drop in the blood pressure. Option #2 is important, but an intervention needs to be implemented prior to notifying the health care provider. Option #4 is not the immediate action with the clinical presentation; perfusion is priority.
I CAN HINT: Apply the clinical judgment/cognitive skill, take-action, to the concept fluid deficit.
NCLEX® Standard: Manage the care of the client with a fluid and electrolyte imbalance.

9.3 ③ The client is presenting in fluid overload and needs the IV rate decreased and health care provider notified in case the client needs an order for a diuretic. Options #1 and #2 are correct if client was experiencing hypovolemia (fluid deficit). Option #4 is not priority for this client who has fluid overload.
I CAN HINT: Apply the clinical judgment/cognitive skill, generate solutions, to the concept fluid imbalance. "RESTRICT" will assist you in organizing interventions for fluid overload. Reduce IV flow rate; reposition; Evaluate breath sounds, SaO_2, edema; Semi-Fowler's/high-Fowler's position; support extremities to decrease dependent edema as approved; Treat with oxygen and diuretics as prescribed; Reduce fluid and sodium intake; rest encouraged; I & O and daily weight, implement prescriptions for flid and sodium restrictions and intake; Circulation, color, and presence of edema, Turn and position at least every 2 hours.
NCLEX® Standard: Manage the care of the client with a fluid and electrolyte imbalance.

9.4 ① Options #1 is correct. Any client with alteration in fluid volume needs to have weight monitored daily to evaluate trend and the need to intervene appropriately. Option #2 is incorrect. The NG tube should be irrigated with Normal Saline solution instead of tap water. Client may need to have electrolyte replacement. Option #3 is incorrect. There is no need for sodium bicarbonate. Client is experiencing metabolic alkalosis from vomiting. Option #4 is incorrect. There is no need for a rebreathing device. This would be appropriate for respiratory alkalosis, but client is experiencing metabolic alkalosis. $PaCO_2$ is within the normal reference range (35-45 mm Hg), but HCO_3 is elevated (normal reference range is 22-26 mEq/L).
I CAN HINT: Apply the clinical judgment/cognitive skill, take-action, to the concept fluid deficit.
NCLEX® Standard: Manage the care of the client with a fluid and electrolyte imbalance.

9.5 ① Option #1, these vital signs can indicate
③ bleeding. Option #3 is correct. DVT
④ management should include teaching the client
⑤ to keep legs elevated when in bed and up in the
⑧ chair, and the importance of wearing sequential compression device on unaffected leg while in bed for the purpose of preventing additional DVT's. Option #4 is correct. A sudden onset of chest pain, tachycardia, and tachypnea may indicate the development of a pulmonary embolism, a potential complication. This must be reported. It is an emergency. Option #5 is correct. Since anticoagulation therapy has been

started, these bleeding precautions should be included in the plan.
Option #8 is correct. Fluids will keep blood moving! Option #2 is incorrect. Rationale explained with option #3. Option #6 is incorrect. Aspirin can contribute to bleeding. Option #7 is incorrect. If client ambulates with a DVT, the clot in the calf muscle may dislodge and result in a pulmonary embolus. The client diagnosed with a DVT should be on bedrest.
I CAN HINT: Apply the clinical judgment/cognitive skill, generate solutions, to the disease process of a DVT.
NCLEX® Standard: Manage the care of a client with alteration in tissue perfusion.

9.6 ④ Options #4 is correct. The low WBC count supports the risk of infection as evidenced by a sore throat. Other findings may include temperature, adventitious breath sounds, yellow drainage/secretions, etc. Options #1 and #3 are not supported with the platelet count that is within the normal reference range. Option #2 is not supported with the normal reference range for the RBC count.
I CAN HINT: Apply the clinical judgment/cognitive skill, recognize cues, for a client with neutropenia secondary to chemotherapy.
NCLEX® Standard: Recognize signs and symptoms of client complications and intervene.

9.7 ③ Option #3 is correct. These clinical assessments indicate spinal shock and need to be assessed initially. Option #1 is not correct. This is a good change from 7 to 14 and does not warrant an immediate assessment. Option #2 is not correct, since these are expected findings for clients with meningitis. Option #4 is not correct, since it is a positive Babinski which can occur with a cerebrovascular accident or with a brain stem herniation, so this would not indicate a need for immediate assessment.

9.8 ② Option #2 is correct. The nurse with several years of experience should be assigned to this client with alteration in the breath sounds. Progressive paralysis and wasting of the muscles with ALS can eventually result in respiratory paralysis and death. Option #1 is not correct because these symptoms are expected for this client. Option #3 is not a priority, since this is also expected for this client. Option #4 is not a priority; this describes what can occur following a seizure and does not mandate care by an RN with two years of experience.

9.9 ② Option #2 is correct. The key to making this decision is to master the labs that change with this medical condition that results in adrenocortical insufficiency. The sodium level is low, potassium is elevated, glucose is low, and calcium is high. Option #1 is not correct, since this value does not need to be reported because it is within the reference range. Option #3 is not correct. The concern would not be with hypertension. It would be with a low blood pressure. Option #4 is not correct, since the concern with Addison's disease would be with hyperkalemia.

9.10 ②④⑤ Options #2, #4, and #5 are correct. Option #2, the trend of the urine output increasing is a sign the bolus of IV fluids was effective. Option #4, CVP is within the reference range which does indicate a therapeutic response from the IV bolus. Option #5, client being alert and answering questions indicates a therapeutic response as well from the IV bolus. Option #1 does not indicate a therapeutic response. This drop would not be decreasing if the bolus was effective. Option #3, the BP would not be decreasing if bolus was effective.

9.11 ②④⑤ Options #2, #4, and #5 are correct. Option #2, heart rate increase is a sign of bleeding. Option #4, respiratory rate of 40/min is a sign of hypoxia from bleeding. Option #5, the trend of the urine output going down is a sign of blood loss as well. Option #1, the BP would not be high if client was bleeding. It would be low. Option #3, CVP is within the reference range which does not indicate a complication of blood loss.
I CAN HINT: The strategy is to identify that the client is experiencing blood loss secondary to surgery. This may result in hypovolemic shock.

9.12 ① Option #1 is correct. First assess the client and then the equipment for proper placement and connections. Lead placement needs to be assessed for accuracy of telemetry reading. If the dysrhythmia is truly a ventricular tachycardia, then follow the advanced directives outlined by client, including pulse assessment, medication administration, and/or initiating a code. Option #2 is incorrect since the accuracy of the dysrhythmia must be determined initially. Option #3 is incorrect. The assessment must be conducted first to determine if the information is accurate prior to notifying the health care provider. Option #4 is not the first nursing action until option #1 has been implemented.

9.13 ③ Option #3 is the correct answer. This client needs to be assessed initially due to the headache, high systolic pressure and low diastolic with a widening in the pulse pressure, low heart rate and motor, verbal and eye opening only to deep pain which indicates there is some increase in the intracranial pressure. The client may need immediate intervention in comparison to the other clients. Option #1 is not a priority. The $PaCO_2$ should be maintained around 35 mm Hg and a normal oxygen level by adjusting the rate of the mechanical ventilation if client is being maintained on a ventilator. The bottom line for this question is that this client does not have hypercarbia. This client is not able to move extremities due to the spinal cord injury. This does not mandate immediate intervention. Option #2 is incorrect. The cerebral perfusion pressure (CPP) is calculated by subtracting ICP from the MAP which would be 82 mm Hg. This is right where the range begins. The CPP should be maintained above 70 to 80 mm Hg. Option #4 is not a priority over option #3. This client is in the postictal phase which is expected during this time.

9.14 ① Option #1 is correct. The elderly client presents often times with symptoms that are atypical and subacute. There is often alteration in the functional and mental status when developing an infection such as pneumonia. Option #2 is incorrect; the cough may be absent or weak. In elderly clients with underlying congestive heart failure or emphysema, the auscultatory signs of pneumonia may be absent or masked. Option #3 is incorrect since the fever response may be blunted and pleurisy may be absent. Option #4 is incorrect since the WBC count may not be elevated initially when the client may just be starting to develop the complication of pneumonia.

9.15 ① Option #1 is correct since the client is experiencing respiratory alkalosis.
I CAN HINT: Always begin with the normal pH which is 7.35 to 7.45; then drop the 7 and decimal point to get the value range for the pCO_2 which is 35 to 45 mm Hg, and then the HCO_3 is 22 to 26 mEq/L (22 to 26 mmol/L). In the question, the pH is high and the pCO_2 is low, which means the client is breathing off too much CO_2. The goal for this client is to slow down the breathing and assist with rebreathing in order to hold on to more CO_2. Option #2 is incorrect. The client is not experiencing respiratory acidosis. If this were true, the pH would be < 7.35 and pCO_2 > 45 mm Hg. Option #3 does not address the concern with the respiratory alkalosis from hyperventilating. These nursing actions would be appropriate for a client in respiratory acidosis. Option #4 is incorrect, and does not address the clinical lab data outlined in the stem of the question.

9.16 ④ Option #4 is correct. The client may be experiencing a potential alteration in perfusion from the dysrhythmia. Safety is of paramount importance. While it is important to initiate an assessment, the immediate concern is fall prevention. Options #1, #2, and #3 are incorrect for this clinical situation.

I CAN HINT: Options #1 and #2 are both clinical assessments which is a hint they may not be the answer since the question requires immediate action. The keys are that the client *"is suddenly feeling very dizzy"* and *"what action should the RN immediately assist the UAP with?"*

9.17 ② Options #2 and #5 are correct. These ⑤ are included in the standard of care for tracheostomy care. Option #1 is incorrect. The tracheostomy tube should not be suctioned routinely, as this may cause mucosal damage, bleeding, and bronchospasm. The tracheostomy should be suctioned as necessary. Option #3 is incorrect. Surgical aseptic technique should be used when removing and cleaning the inner cannula. Option #4 is incorrect. The new ties should be secured before removing the soiled ones to prevent accidental decannulation.

9.18 ③ Option #3 is correct since the serum potassium is low (normal range is 3.5 to 5.0 mEq/L or 3.5 to 5.0 mmol/L). Furosemide (Lasix) should not be administered with this low potassium level. The provider of care must be notified since the level is low. This low serum potassium may result in cardiac dysrhythmis, such as atrial fibrillation. Option #1 is incorrect since the creatinine level is within a normal range, and there is no need for additional management. Option #2 is incorrect since the serum glucose is within the normal range. (normal range is 70 to 110 mg/dL or 3.89 to 6 .11 mmol/L). There is no need to administer glucagon (Glucogen) since the client is not hypoglycemic. Option #4 is incorrect since the potassium level is the only one that is low. The other values are normal.

9.19 ①
② Options #1, #2, and #5 are correct. The first
⑤ part for successfully answering this question is to understand the normal hemodynamic values and to understand what the measurements indicate. The CVP reading evaluates the right side of the heart and the PAWP evaluates the left side of the heart. The normal values are as follows: CVP: 1–8 mm Hg, PAWP: 4–12 mm Hg, CO: 4–6 L/min. As you can see by reviewing the stem of the question, the CVP is elevated. Note that the CVP reading indicates preload complications. As a result of this preload complication, the client would present with peripheral edema, hepatomegaly, and jugular vein distention. If the PAWP was elevated, then the client would present with crackles in the lungs. If the CVP was decreased, then the client would present with poor skin turgor and dry mucous membranes.

9.20 ② Option #2 is correct. Since the client is presenting with ventricular fibrillation, defibrillation should be initiated as soon as possible to convert the dysrhythmia to a normal rhythm. Option #1 is incorrect. The nurse is concerned with a cardiovascular assessment, and is not conducting a neuro exam. While these other options in #3 and #4 are components of CPR, these should never delay the use of a defibrillator, necessary for conversion of this dysrhythmia. Option #4 is incorrect.

9.21 ② Option #2 is correct. This is an appropriate action for the nurse when accessing the IV site. Option #1 is incorrect. The circular motion should be from middle to outward and the time from drying should be 1 to 2 min. versus 1 to 5 min. Option #3 is incorrect because the flashback of blood should be seen and the catheter should not be removed. Option #4 is incorrect. The tourniquet should be applied 4 to 6 inches above proposed insertion site.

9.22 ④ Post-operative open-heart clients should be encouraged to be out of bed and ambulate as soon as possible. Option #1 is incorrect because the client is maintained in semi-Fowler's position. Option #2 is incorrect because coughing and deep breathing should be encouraged. Option #3 is incorrect as fluids are encouraged unless there is evidence of cardiac failure.

9.23 ① Option #1 is correct. The client is experiencing a tension pneumothorax. The tracheal deviation is a definitive sign of tension pneumothorax. If not treated immediately, death can be a result. Option #2 is incorrect. A depressed gag reflex is an expected finding following this procedure due to the anesthesia received during the procedure. This is the reason the nurse must assess the gag reflex prior to administering any oral fluids. This return of the gag reflex usually takes approximately 2 hours. Option #3 is incorrect. This is not a priority over Option #1 which could lead to death. Option #3 is indeed a concern due to the risk for falls after having 1 L of fluid removed and attempting to get up quickly. This would be the second client to see if the nurse had to organize the order for seeing these clients. Option #4 is a concern, but these are expected findings for SARS and are not a priority over option #1.

I CAN HINT: The question you need to ask yourself is, *"Who would die first?"*

9.24 ② An air leak would not allow negative pressure to be reestablished and would hinder complete resolution of the pneumothorax. Therefore, partial atelectasis could be noted. Option #1 is an appropriate order for chest tubes. Option #3 does not hinder the chest tube functioning. Option #4 would be an expected finding. It would be important for the nurse to ensure tube patency.

9.25 ② Anytime the pulse rate drops below the preset rate on the pacemaker, then the pacer is malfunctioning. The pulse should be maintained at a minimal rate set on the pacemaker. Options #1 and #3 do not indicate malfunction of the pacemaker. Option #4 may be an early sign of infection at the site.

9.26 ④ Option #4 is correct. The new RN should be competent at teaching the appropriate use of an incentive spirometer since the nurse is from a surgical unit. Post-operative care which includes prevention of alteration in gas exchange from shallow breathing, immobility, etc., and should be a routine skill for this new nurse of only 8 months. The bottom line is that one of the decision making strategies for delegation is to always consider the nurse's level of expertise in addition to the Scope of Practice. Option #1 is incorrect since clients with SARS would not routinely be admitted to a surgical unit due to infection prevention which means the new RN may not have any experience with this type of infection prevention precaution. Option #2 is incorrect. While the new RN may provide care during the post-op period, the care of the client on the ventilator involves more clinical decision making skills and expertise than the new RN may have developed after this brief period of time. Option #3 is incorrect since it would not be a priority over option #4. If the new RN had not worked with a client immediately following a bronchoscopy, the nurse may not be knowledgeable about the Standard of Care which is to evaluate the gag reflex prior to administering any oral liquids.

9.27 ① These "constitutional symptoms" are characteristic of most types of anemia and are predominantly the result of tissue hypoxia secondary to inadequate red blood cells. Options #2, #3, and #4 are not as indicative of the loss of red blood cells.

9.28 ④ Alcohol consumption while on INH therapy has been reported to increase isoniazid-related hepatitis. Therefore, clients should be cautioned to restrict consumption of alcohol. Options #1, #2, and #3 are untrue.

9.29 ③ The most indicative observation for anti-anxiety drugs is restlessness and increase in heart rate due to circulating catecholamines (fight or flight syndrome). Options #1 and #2 are more indicative of preoperative complications and should be reported before medications are given. Option #4 may be best treated by ventilating feelings.

9.30

| ④ Explain procedure to client. |
| ⑤ Wash hands thoroughly. |
| ① Put on sterile glove. |
| ② Lubricate catheter with normal saline. |
| ③ Apply suction for 5-10 seconds. |

9.31 ① This describes characteristic signs and symptoms of digoxin toxicity. Digoxin toxicity is a great concern in the presence of diarrhea or any circumstance that leads to alteration in fluid and electrolyte balance. This is especially true with the young or elderly. Options #2, #3, and #4 are appropriate for this client, but are not as high a priority as option #1.

9.32 ③ Option #3: All are appropriate interventions to care for a client in acute respiratory distress. The priority of care for the non-ventilated client is to consistently assess airway and vital signs and to intervene if mechanical ventilatory support is needed.

9.33 ② This option is the safest procedure. Since the catheter goes into the thoracic cavity, it is subjected to changes in pressure which increase the risk of air emboli. Options #1, #3, and #4 are unsafe.

9.34 ② Orthopnea, dyspnea, and crackles are signs and symptoms of fluid excess. Decreasing the IV fluids is the priority. Option #1 would worsen the situation. Options #3 and #4 are not of priority to the situation.

9.35 ④ Chest drainage in excess of 100 mL/hr is not normal and the physician should be notified. Options #1 and #2 may be appropriate after the physician is notified. Option #3 may result in a decrease in blood pressure if client is bleeding.

9.36 ④ Option #4 is correct. Due to the frequent premature ventricular contractions, this client needs to be intervened with immediately after shift report due to the risk of progressing into a ventricular dysrhythmia which can be life threatening. Option #1 is not a priority to option #4. This client is stable with no life threatening dysrhythmia. Options #2 and #3 are not a priority over #4.

9.37 ② The next priority is to notify the physician since the signs indicate pulmonary edema. Options #1 and #3 would increase fluids to the lungs. Option #4 is incorrect because the nurse should stay with the client for reassurance.

9.38 ③ The signs and symptoms are indicative of hypokalemia. A stat serum K+ level is needed to confirm the K+ level prior to going for cardiac catheterization. Option #1 is incorrect because Spironolactone is potassium sparing and is an oral medication. Option #2 is not feasible prior to the cardiac catheterization since the client is NPO. Option #4 is unnecessary.

9.39 ④ The normal range for CVP is 1 to 8 mm Hg. A reading of 8 mm Hg would indicate a desired response from fluid replacement. Option #1 indicates a hypovolemic state. In Option #2, hematocrit is still high. Option #3 is acidosis which can result from various problems.

9.40 ③ Option #3 is correct. A high pressure alarm signals increased pressure in the airways. In the presence of visible secretions in the endotracheal tube, suctioning the client and monitoring pulse oximetry are priority to reducing airway pressure. Option #1 is never appropriate. Options #2 and #4 are inappropriate actions.

9.41 ② This blood gas indicates respiratory alkalosis and the intervention is to breathe into a paper bag or use a mask that causes the re-breathing of carbon dioxide. For this reason the accuracy of the order should be questioned. Option #1 is not indicated, option #3 is appropriate, but not the priority. Option #4 would be costly and unnecessary, since there is no reason to question the validity of the lab report outlined in the question.

9.42 ① In complete heart block, the AV node blocks all impulses from the SA node so the atria and ventricles beat independently. Because Lidocaine suppresses ventricular irritability, it may diminish the existing ventricular response. All cardiac depressants are contraindicated in presence of complete heart block. Options #2, #3, and #4 are appropriate treatments.

9.43

② Place air-occlusive dressing over chest wound to prevent further complications (pneumothorax, mediastinal shift).
① Administer oxygen and begin set up for tube insertions.
③ Monitor blood gases to determine early acid-base imbalances.
④ Medicate for pain with caution so as not to depress the respiratory center.

9.44 ③ Morphine sulfate is given to reduce pain, anxiety, and cardiac workload. Option #1 does not reduce this type of pain. Option #2 is less common because it may induce vomiting and initiate a vagal response. Option #4 is incorrect because the nurse would administer it by IV to reduce pain and decrease overload.

9.45 ③ Venous disease results from obstruction such as thrombus, thrombophlebitis, or incompetent valves. Signs and symptoms include: little or no pain, brawn (reddish-brown skin color), cyanotic if dependent, stasis dermatitis, limb warm to touch, statis ulcers, and peripheral edema present which may be from foot to calf. Options #1, #2, and #4 would be assessed with arterial insufficiency. While in option #2 part of it describes venous insufficiency, the sudden pain is a result of arterial complications.

9.46 ④ Paradoxical chest movement occurs with a flail chest. Immediate treatment of flail chest is directed toward improvement of ventilation and oxygenation as well as stabilization of the chest wall. Option #1 describes normal heart sounds. Option #2 is a normal finding. Option #3 occurs with increased anxiety.

9.47 ④ Option #4 is correct. The dysrhythmia is a third-degree or complete heart block. Notice the PR interval is getting longer. Digoxin is a cardiac glycoside that inhibits the sodium-potassium ATPase, resulting in an increase in cardiac contraction which may result in a decrease in the heart rate. If the client already has this potential complication occurring, then this would not be an appropriate drug for this client. Options #1, #2, and #3 may be included in the treatment plan for this dysrhythmia. Each of the actions of these drugs will actually cause the heart rate to increase.

I CAN HINT: Notice they spell "AID," Atropine, Isoproterenol, Dopamine. These will "AID" in increasing the HR for a client in a complete heart block.

9.48 ④ An expected result of Heparin therapy is prolonged PTT of 1.5 to 2.5 times the control, without signs of hemorrhage. Options #1 and #2 do not indicate a reason to discontinue or slow infusion since the PTT is appropriately prolonged. Option #3 is incorrect because the prothrombin time (PT) test is useful for assessing warfarin (Coumadin) therapy.

9.49 ① In an open pneumothorax, air enters pleural cavity through an open wound. Placing a sterile dressing loosely over the wound allows air to escape, but not re-enter the pleural space. Options #2 and #4 would prevent air from escaping. Option #3 is inappropriate since a chest tube has not yet been inserted.

9.50 ④ Client is at increased risk for development of hypovolemic shock. The vital signs and urine output correlate with the early signs of shock. CVP needs to be evaluated with previous readings. Option #1 is not a priority. Option #2 is incorrect because an ECG will not determine cause of tachycardia. Option #3 is incorrect because IV fluid may be be increased.

9.51 ③ Option #3 is the safest for the client and will allow the nurse time to set up another pleur-evac. Option #1 is unsafe and could result in a mediastinal shift. The majority of physicians will request the chest tubes not be clamped. Option #2 is not a priority. Option #4 is incorrect.

9.52 ① Based on the client's history, current immobility, and assessment factors, this client may be experiencing a pulmonary emboli. Priority nursing care is to prevent severe hypoxia and maintain ventilation. Option #2 is not appropriate. Option #3 is for hypotension. Option #4 is for a cardiac client who is experiencing severe chest pain.

9.53 ④ Option #4 is correct since it would be imperative for the LPN to test the equipment prior to using to verify the equipment is functioning properly. This is a standard of care that should be followed for all equipment. Option #1 is incorrect since the client should be hyper-oxygenated prior to being suctioned as well "versus only after suctioning." Option #2 is incorrect due to the incorrect position. Client should not be in the prone position, but in the Fowler's or semi-Fowler's position. Option #3 is incorrect. Surgical aseptic technique should be used when opening the suction catheter kits. Medical aseptic technique can be used to suction the mouth (oropharyngeal), whereas surgical aseptic technique must be used for all other types of suctioning.

9.54 ② Obesity, immobility, and pooling of blood in the pelvic cavity contribute to development of pulmonary emboli. Options #1 and #4 are high risk for shock and bleeding complications. Option #3 is incorrect because the client is not immobilized.

9.55 ④ Option #4 is correct. Transcutaneous pads should be placed on the client with this third degree heart block; this is the treatment of choice. Notice in the strip that the p wave has totally disappeared which is indicative of a third degree heart block. Option #1 is incorrect since the HR would need to be assessed prior to initiating CPR. Option #2 is incorrect. Amiodarone would be contraindicated for this dysrhythmia since it would further decrease the sinus rate. Option #3 would be for a client with atrial fibrillation who does not respond to medication.

I CAN HINT: The key to successful outcomes with this question is to understand that a third degree heart block was on the strip and then how to handle this dysrhythmia. "PACE" will assist you in organizing this information. Transcutaneous pacing is the treatment of choice. There is an A and E in "PACE" to assist you in remembering atropine or epinephrine can be administered for a block to help increase the heart rate. The LAST thing we want to administer is a drug that will SLOW the heart rate down.

9.56 ② Option #2 is correct. The client is bleeding and the intervention is to stop it. Option #1 is incorrect. The assessment of the pulses is not going to stop the bleeding. Option #3 is incorrect. Option #4 is not appropriate for this situation.

9.57 ② Specimens should be obtained in the early morning because secretions develop during the night. Option #1 is incorrect because coughing deeply is indicated but not pursed lip breathing. Option #3 is appropriate for Acid-Fast Stain. Option #4 is incorrect because the earliest specimen is most desirable.

9.58 ② This indicates appropriate renal function. Option #1 doesn't evaluate renal sufficiency. Options #3 and #4 are too rapid which may indicate a hypovolemic state.

9.59 ② In measuring JVD, pulsations that fluctuate upon respirations are observed. Options #1 and #3 are incorrect because the client is positioned at a 45-degree angle, and the nurse inspects the internal jugular vein. Option #4 is incorrect because 2 cm or less is considered normal.

9.60 ③ Option #3 is correct. When the low alarm sounds, this usually indicates a leak. Options #1, #2, and #4 would result in a high volume alarm.

9.61 ② The RML is found right anterior between the fourth and sixth intercostal spaces. Options #1 and #4 are incorrect because the RML cannot be auscultated from the posterior. Option #3 is the point of maximum impulse or apical pulse.

9.62 ① S_4 is indicative of problems with hypertension. A client may present with an occipital headache upon arising in the morning, blurred vision, and an elevated blood pressure. Options #2 and #4 are related to right-sided heart failure. Option #3 is incorrect.

9.63 ③ Airway is the priority. The client's clinical changes have occurred due to hypoxia. Providing oxygen will maintain the client until the physician can reintubate. Option #1 is inappropriate since the client still has a pulse. Option #2 is incorrect since the hypoxia is not secondary to hypovolemia. Option #4 is not a priority.

9.64 The answer is the underwater seal chamber which is bubbling after the lung has expanded indicating an air leak. The nurse would expect there to be some bubbling initially since the tube is draining air, but once the lung has reexpanded there should be no leaks in the system. The output in the drainage chamber is not an assessment that is a concern. If there had been more than 100 mL's in one hour, then further assessment would have been completed to determine if client was experiencing hypovolemia. The suction chamber should have continuous bubbling.

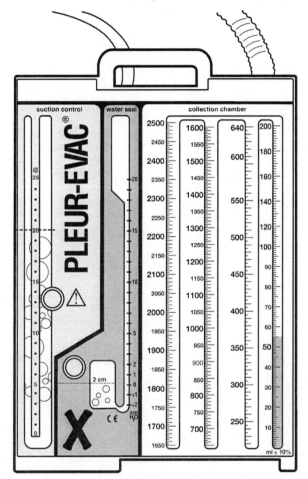

9.65

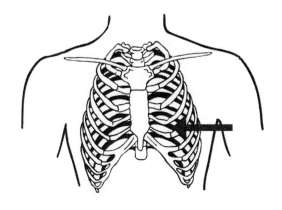

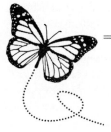

Notes

CHAPTER 10
Reduction of Risk Potential

Nothing is impossible, the word itself says 'I'm possible'!
— AUDREY HEPPBURN

✔ Clarification of this test ...

Note this percentage has remained 9–15% on the new NCLEX-RN®. These questions relate to focused assessments, care for the client undergoing treatments/procedures/surgery to reduce complications. These include diagnostic tests, lab values, therapeutic procedures, pre and post-operative care, monitor/maintain equipment used for drainage, and obtain blood specimens peripherally or through a central line.

- ☞ Perform focused assessments.
- ☞ Assess and respond to changes and trends in client vital signs.
- ☞ Evaluate responses to procedures and treatments.
- ☞ Recognize trends and changes in client condition and intervene as needed.
- ☞ Educate client about treatments and procedures.
- ☞ Perform testing within scope of practice (e.g., electrocardiogram, glucose monitoring).
- ☞ Use precautions to prevent injury and/or complications associated with a procedure or diagnosis.
- ☞ Monitor the results of diagnostic testing and intervene as needed.
- ☞ Insert, maintain, or remove a peripheral intravenous line.
- ☞ Apply and/or maintain devices used to promote venous return (e.g., anti-embolic stockings, sequential compression devices).
- ☞ Obtain blood specimens.
- ☞ Obtain specimens other than blood for diagnostic testing.
- ☞ Insert, maintain, or remove a urinary catheter.
- ☞ Manage client following a procedure with moderate sedation.
- ☞ Provide pre-operative or post-operative education.
- ☞ Maintain percutaneous feeding tube.
- ☞ Insert, maintain, or remove a nasal/oral gastrointestinal tube.
- ☞ Provide pre-operative care.
- ☞ Manage client during and/or following a procedure with moderate sedation.

Adapted from: © National Council of State Boards of Nursing, Inc. (NCSBN). (2022). 2021 *RN Practice Analysis: Linking the NCLEX-RN® Examination to Practice*. Chicago: Author.

Adapted from: © National Council of State Boards of Nursing, Inc. (NCSBN). (2023) *Next Generation NCLEX® NCLEX-RN® Test Plan. Chicago*: Author.

10.1 What is the priority intervention that the nurse will include in the plan of care to prevent complications from immobility in an elderly client with a fractured bone?
① Obtain an order for assistive devices to move the client.
② Turn, cough, and deep breathe every two hours.
③ Complete a comprehensive skin assessment every other week to check for breakdown.
④ Limit fluids to decrease risk of developing complications with fluid excess.

10.2 Which clinical findings indicate the client has improved following treatment for a deep vein thrombosis (DVT)?
① Denies pain in the calf of the leg
② Temperature is the same in bilateral lower extremities
③ SaO_2: 90%
④ RR: 32 breaths/min
⑤ HR: 120 bpm

10.3 A client's vital signs are being evaluated every 15 minutes during the post-operative period. What nursing action indicates the nurse understands how to safely use an electronic blood pressure device?
① Evaluates the skin integrity every 2-3 hours.
② Auscultates the blood pressure and compares with initial electronic reading.
③ Compares each reading with the arterial line pressure reading.
④ Ensures one finger fits between the cuff and skin.

10.4 The nurse is preparing to obtain a urinary specimen from an indwelling urinary catheter. Which action will the nurse implement prior to initiating this procedure?
① Advise client to void.
② Clean tubing port with an antiseptic solution.
③ Clamp tubing for 30 min. prior to obtaining specimen from the urinary bag.
④ Apply sterile gloves.

10.5 The nurse is preparing to apply a sequential compression device (SCD) to a client who is on bed rest. (Place the sequence of steps in chronological order for this task. All options must be included.)

①	Place SCD sleeve under leg.
②	Explain procedure to client.
③	Wrap and secure SCD sleeve around leg.
④	Assess a circulatory assessment baseline.
⑤	Evaluate functioning of SCD device for one total cycle.
⑥	Attach connector of SCD sleeve to device.
⑦	Place 2 fingers between sleeve and leg.

10.6 Which of these nursing interventions will the nurse implement prior to a client experiencing a paracentesis? **Select all that apply.**
① Place client in semi-Fowler's position.
② Explain importance of voiding prior to procedure.
③ Complete an abdominal assessment.
④ Explain that a decrease in blood pressure is expected.
⑤ Insert a Foley catheter.

10.7 Which client would require the nurse to intervene immediately following shift report?
① The client who received prednisone and is presenting with +1 edema in feet and ankles.
② The client who has been administered lisinopril and is presenting with a HR – 60 bpm.
③ The client with hypertension and has a BP of 149/90 mm Hg.
④ The client who is coughing up pink, frothy secretions with a diagnosis of congestive heart failure.

10.8 Which of these plans will the nurse include in the care for a client who has chronic kidney disease? **Select all that apply.**
① Discuss the importance of using salt substitutes.
② Assess for peaked T waves on the ECG monitor.
③ Encourage client to take an NSAID for discomfort.
④ Review the importance of monitoring and reporting trends in weight gain.
⑤ Review importance of taking the iron supplement with orange juice.

10.9 Which assessment finding is priority for the nurse to report for a client with an ileostomy?
① Urine specific gravity 1.003.
② Heart rate was 78 bpm and is now 86 bpm.
③ Urine output from 75 mL/hour to 43 mL/hour.
④ Weight from 150 lbs. to 144 lbs. in 4 weeks.

10.10 Which nursing action is appropriate for the nurse to delegate to the unlicensed assistive personnel (UAP) for a client who is one-day post-operative following a cholecystectomy?
① Empty the T-tube drainage bag and report the amount / characteristics of drainage noted.
② Instruct client to avoid broccoli, fried chicken, and cheese.
③ Obtain vital signs and monitor for changes.
④ Assist client to ambulate in the hall.

10.11 A client on the medical unit has this laboratory report.

Laboratory Report
Hemoglobin: 13 g.dL (130 g/L)
Hematocrit: 39%
Platelets: 36,000 mm^3 (36 x10^9/L)
White blood cell count: 6.10 (6.1 x10^9/L)

What nursing care is priority to include in the plan of care?
① Encourage frequent rest periods.
② Notify health care provider regarding an order for an IM medication.
③ Initiate protective isolation precautions.
④ Provide oxygen supplement during physical activity.

10.12 Which of these would be appropriate immediate nursing interventions for a client with Myasthenia Gravis and is presenting with a HR of 112 BPM, RR 24/min with accessory muscle use, anxiety, and restless? **Select all that apply.**
① Elevate head of bed.
② Administer furosemide 40 mg IV.
③ O$_2$ per health care provider's order.
④ Teach client importance of wearing a medical ID bracelet.
⑤ Apply a lubricating eye drop.

10.13 Which of these laboratory results require additional assessment by the nurse?
① BUN: 18 mg/dL (6.43 mmol/L); creatinine: 1.2 mg/dL (106.08 umol/L)
② Calcium level: 10 mg/dL (2.5 mmol/L)
③ pH: 7.38, pCO$_2$: 38 mm Hg, HCO$_3$: 23 mEq/L (23 μmol/L)
④ Hemoglobin: 8 g/dL (80 g/L) and hematocrit 24%

10.14 Which client would be the priority to assess following shift report?
① A post-operative client with a deep vein thrombosis who is requesting lorazepam.
② A client with cystic fibrosis who is expectorating small amounts of pale yellow secretions.
③ A one-day post-operative client with a hysterectomy.
④ A client with Hepatitis C.

10.15 Which interventions would be included in the plan of care for a client with a left-sided chest tube secondary to a pneumothorax? **Select all that apply.**
① Strip the chest tubes every shift.
② Maintain the tubing so there are no dependent loops.
③ Assess the chest tube drainage q 1-2 hours or per protocol.
④ Report serosanguinous drainage of 45 mL/hour.
⑤ Maintain bed rest with no bathroom privileges.

10.16 Which of these clients does the RN need to intervene with immediately due to the care the LPN is providing?
① The client is taken to the bathroom immediately following a lumbar puncture (spinal tap).
② The LPN encourages the client to wash hair prior to undergoing an electroencephalogram (EEG).
③ The LPN tries to keep client awake most of the night prior to undergoing an electroencephalogram (EEG).
④ The LPN inquires as to if the client has a history of claustrophobia and explains the tight space and noise that can be experienced with the scheduled Magnetic Resonance Imaging (MRI).

10.17 A client with a T6 spinal cord injury presents with a BP—170/72; HR—46 BPM; sudden severe headache and flushing on neck and face. What is the immediate nursing action for this client?
① Titrate the dopamine as prescribed.
② Elevate the legs if possible.
③ Apply compression stockings.
④ Position bed in reverse Trendelenburg.

10.18 What clinical finding would be most important to report for a client with a spinal cord injury who is receiving dexamethasone?
① Blood pressure—130/82; HR—72 BPM
② Daily weight has increased 1 kg
③ Pale yellow secretions suctioned from endotracheal tube
④ Serum glucose—128 mg/dL (7.10 mmol/L)

10.19 An older client has been admitted to the Medical Unit following a cerebrovascular accident (CVA). The client presents with left-sided paralysis and has been experiencing dysphagia. Which of these actions by the UAP requires intervention by the charge nurse?
① The UAP puts the food on the unaffected side in the back of the client's mouth.
② The UAP brings the tray in the room on the unaffected side and places within visual range.
③ The UAP starts the feeding with some chicken broth to assist with swallowing.
④ The UAP positions the head and neck slightly forward.

10.20 Which of these clinical findings would be reported for a client with a diagnosis of parathyroid disease and presenting with a calcium level of 6.0 mg/dL (1.5 mmol/L)?
① Depressed patellar reflex.
② Paresthesia in the hand is produced when tapping over the median nerve at the wrist crease.
③ Foot extension of the big toe while fanning the other toes when stimulating the outside of the sole of the foot.
④ Carpopedal spasm after BP cuff is inflated above systolic pressure.

10.21 What plan of care is the priority for a client who is presenting with nausea, diarrhea, muscle weakness, and an abnormal ECG and is taking spironolactone lisinopril and glipizide?
① Report a serum potassium level of 5.2 mEq/L (5.2 mmol/L).
② Report a serum sodium level 146 mEq/L (146 mmol/L).
③ Instruct client about the importance of eating bananas.
④ Assess characteristics of the lips and mucous membranes.

10.22 Which of these clinical findings would be reported to the health care provider immediately for a client who is being managed and treated for acute low back pain?
① Discomfort that has lasted approximately 3½ weeks.
② When the leg is elevated, there is pain in the lower back.
③ L4 to L5 has diffuse, aching sensation.
④ A new onset of urinary incontinence.

10.23 What is the first nursing action for a client who has returned from having a bowel resection, and as the nurse is making rounds at the beginning of shift notices that client is becoming restless?
① Administer pain medication as ordered.
② Order stat labs for electrolytes and blood gasses.
③ Ask client's family if the client has a history of drug or alcohol abuse.
④ Assess vital signs and urine output.

10.24 What clinical findings require immediate action for a client diagnosed with peptic ulcer disease?
  ① HR—80 BPM and increased to 90 BPM, BP—138/70 decreased from 150/88.
  ② HR—88 BPM and decreased to 78 BPM, R—18/min and increased to 22/min, and BP—120/80 and increased to 140/88.
  ③ Complaints of heartburn and bloating during the middle of the night.
  ④ Abdominal distention increased with increase in the pain and vomiting.

10.25 The nurse is observing a client for complications following a craniotomy. The client begins complaining of thirst and fatigue. Which nursing observation is most important to report to the physician?
  ① Specific gravity of urine is increased; urine is foul smelling.
  ② Fluid intake over past 24 hours has been 3000 mL.
  ③ Urine output in excess of 4000 mL in 24 hours.
  ④ Presence of diarrhea and excoriation of anal area.

10.26 Before teaching a CVA client about self-care, which plan would be a priority?
  ① Have the client identify perception of health status.
  ② Identify the client's strengths and weaknesses.
  ③ Encourage client to discuss concerns with another CVA client.
  ④ Provide client with a written plan of therapy.

10.27 Which of these procedures is correct for wrapping a stump after an amputation?
  ① Make three figure-eight turns to adequately cover the ends of the stump.
  ② Wrap the ace bandage in a circular motion around the stump.
  ③ Unroll the bandage upward over the stump and to the front of the leg.
  ④ Wrap the stump so that it narrows toward the proximal end.

10.28 A child weighing 80 pounds (36.3 kg) is sent home in a hip spica cast. Which instruction is most important to include in the teaching plan designed to promote bowel functioning?
  ① Give a soap suds enema every day.
  ② Perform range of motion exercises to the upper extremities four times a day.
  ③ Give at least six to eight 8-ounce (237 mL) glasses of fluid a day.
  ④ Give a strong laxative every day.

10.29 What is the highest priority for a client 72 hours after having second-degree burns to 20% of his body in the lower abdominal area, back, and both legs?
  ① Airway
  ② Body image
  ③ Fluid and electrolytes
  ④ Pain

10.30 Which is the most important post-operative nursing action for the client following a sceleral buckling procedure for detached retina?
  ① Remove reading material to decrease eye strain.
  ② Closely assess for presence of nausea and prevent vomiting.
  ③ Assess color of drainage from affected eye.
  ④ Maintain sterility for q 3 hr saline eye irrigations.

10.31 What would the nurse ask the client to do when evaluating the cranial nerve XI?
  ① Ask client to smell and identify different odors.
  ② Ask client to shrug the shoulders.
  ③ Ask client to read a Snellen chart.
  ④ Ask client to stick out tongue and move from side to side.

10.32 A client is admitted with a diagnosis of trigeminal neuralgia (Tic Douloureux) involving the maxillary branch of the affected nerve. The nurse would plan nursing care to assist the client with which problem?
  ① Intermittent blurred vision and tinnitus.
  ② Intense facial pain on affected side.
  ③ Attacks of severe dizziness and vertigo.
  ④ Impaired speech function due to muscle spasm.

10.33 The health care provider orders a wet-to-dry dressing for a client with a venous stasis ulcer. What is the correct method of implementing this order?

① Moisten the skin around the ulcer. Then apply a dry gauze dressing.
② Apply antibacterial ointment to the wound. Then apply a dry gauze dressing.
③ Apply a wet dressing and allow to dry. Then wet again to remove.
④ Apply a wet dressing. Allow to dry; then remove.

10.34 The nurse is caring for an elderly client with bilateral eye patches. Which nursing action would be most beneficial in preventing problems secondary to sensory deprivation?

① Maintain client sedation until eye patches are removed.
② Isolate client so others will not confuse him.
③ Maintain a calm, dark environment conducive to rest.
④ Speak to him frequently, and provide frequent touch.

10.35 Which statement made by the parents of a child with hydrocephalus indicates they understand how to care for a child with a ventriculoperitoneal shunt?

① "We will position our child on the operative side."
② "We will position our child in the semi-Fowler's position after surgery."
③ "We will report if our child starts vomiting."
④ "We will rely on the home health nurse to pump the shunt."

10.36 Which statement by the client best indicates an understanding of and preparedness for a scheduled magnetic resonance imaging (MRI)?

① "The dye used in the test will turn my urine green for about 24 hours."
② "I will be put to sleep for this procedure. I will return to my room in 2 hours."
③ "This procedure will take about 1-1/2 hours to complete. It will be noisy."
④ "The wires that will be attached to my head and chest will not cause me any pain."

10.37 When caring for a client with myasthenia gravis, what would be an important nursing consideration?

① Prevent accidents from falls as a result of vertigo.
② Maintain fluid and electrolyte replacement.
③ Control situations that could increase intracranial pressure and cerebral edema.
④ Assess muscle groups that are affected as they tend to be weaker toward the end of the day.

10.38 Which of these clients are a priority for the nurse to assess first after coming out of shift report?

① An infant with a tracheoesophageal fistula (TEF) who is presenting with substernal retractions, RR—60/min. at rest.
② An infant who is occasionally pulling at the right ear when awake.
③ A school-age child who is 2 hours post-operative for a tonsillectomy and adenoidectomy with HR—96 bpm and vomiting 30 mL of dark brown emesis.
④ A school-age child with cystic fibrosis (CF) who was admitted to the pediatric unit during the night shift and is presenting with large and foul-smelling stools.

10.39 What is the highest priority following a grand mal seizure?

① Remain with client and administer anticonvulsant medication.
② Document the events prior to the onset of the seizure.
③ Maintain a patent airway by turning client's head to the side and suctioning if necessary.
④ Protect client from injuring self by removing constricting clothes.

10.40 In planning the care of a client with an acute episode of Ménière's Syndrome, what would be included in the teaching plan?

① Adding salt to food.
② Avoiding sudden motion of the head.
③ Restricting fluids to 3–4 glasses daily.
④ Keeping cotton in affected ear.

10.41 Which instruction would the nurse include in a discharge teaching plan for the client with a diagnosis of glaucoma?

① Decrease intake of saturated fats and potassium.
② Eye pain and nausea should be reported to the physician.
③ Anticipate gradual increase in visual field.
④ Eye drops may be discontinued after two weeks.

10.42 Which clinical assessment finding would be documented in the nurses' notes indicating a complication of a deep vein thrombosis (DVT) for a client during the post-operative period?

① Client presents with a cool, painful, tingling pain.
② Client presents with weak peripheral pulses.
③ Client presents with pain in calf of leg when walking.
④ Client presents with a rapid onset of unilateral leg swelling with dependent edema.

10.43 Which statement made by a client with a left-sided hemiparesis from a CVA indicates an understanding of how to transfer out of the bed?

① "The wheel chair should be on the right side of the bed."
② "The wheel chair should be on the left side of the bed."
③ "I will use a cane."
④ "I will wait for the physical therapist to lift me out of the bed."

10.44 A client with a long leg cast on the right leg has a foot that is pale and cool to touch. An analgesic has offered no relief to severe leg pain after 45 minutes. What would be the first nursing action?

① Apply a heating pad to the right toes.
② Repeat the dose of analgesic stat.
③ Remove the cast immediately.
④ Notify the health care provider immediately.

10.45 Which of these clinical findings would the nurse monitor for with a client who has a nasogastric tube with suctioning? **Select all that apply.**

① Paresthesias
② Chvostek's sign
③ Flat T waves on ECG
④ Muscle cramps
⑤ Positive Trousseau sign

10.46 A client with a closed head injury has a nasogastric tube in place and begins to vomit. What is the highest priority?

① Check the nasogastric tube for appropriate placement.
② Reposition client in bed to the side lying position.
③ Notify physician.
④ Remove the tube immediately.

10.47 Which of these statements made by the client with Raynaud's phenomenon indicate a need for further teaching?

① "I will avoid all caffeine and nicotine."
② "I will take my calcium channel blocker to cure the Raynaud's phenomenon."
③ "I understand the symptoms can be precipitated by emotional upset."
④ "I will wear gloves when I go outside in the cold weather."

10.48 On the second day following a lumbar disc excision, the client complains of mild pain in both legs. The nurse's response is based on which understanding of leg pain in the early post-operative period?

① Should delay early ambulation.
② Can result from swelling which compresses the nerve.
③ Is common for months after surgery.
④ Indicates surgery was unsuccessful.

10.49 Which of these clients would be assessed immediately following shift report?

① A client with Trigeminal Neuralgia who is complaining of pain in the lips.
② A client with Bell's Palsy who is experiencing depression from a negative image.
③ A client with Guillain-Barré syndrome presenting with continuous drooling of saliva.
④ A client with dementia who is unable to remember the food that was served at dinner.

10.50 Which documentation indicates a clinical finding for a client exhibiting symptoms of myxedema?

① Increased pulse rate, from HR—68 bpm to HR—100 bpm
② Decreased temperature, from 98.9°F (37.2°C) to 97.2°F (36.2°C)
③ Fine tremors
④ Increased radioactive iodine uptake level

10.51 Which nursing assessment is the most important regarding proper fitting of crutches?
① With the client standing, the top of the crutch should be approximately 2 inches (5.08 cm) below the axillary area.
② The bottom of the crutches should be positioned next to the heel of the foot.
③ The arms should be fully extended to the crutch hand grips.
④ The crutches should fit snugly under the arm for weight-bearing.

10.52 Following a left above-the-knee amputation, the nurse is teaching a client regarding positioning. Which response by the client indicates an understanding of the importance of the prone position post-operatively?
① "I need to lie on my stomach to keep from getting a flexion contracture at my left hip."
② "Lying flat keeps my blood flowing and prevents my stump from swelling."
③ "I need to lie on my stomach to prevent a pressure sore on my hips."
④ "I will always elevate my stump when I am in a chair to keep it from swelling."

10.53 Which of these statements made by the client require immediate evaluation for a client who recently had a paracentesis?
① "I am feeling as if I may pass out."
② "My shirt feels tight."
③ "I feel some discomfort at the incision site."
④ "I need to go to the bathroom."

10.54 Which nursing measure would be the most appropriate in preventing complications of immobility with an elderly client?
① Consistent use of bedrails.
② Physical restraints.
③ Encourage isometric muscle contraction.
④ Encourage as much assistance from the caregiver with activities of daily living as needed.

10.55 Which statement made by a client with hypothyroidism started on levothyroxine sodium indicates a need for further teaching?
① "This medicine might affect my diabetes."
② "I'll take this little pill every day before I have breakfast."
③ "I'll be able to quit taking this pill when I start feeling better."
④ "This medicine may affect the action of my heart pill, digoxin."

10.56 What is the most important to monitor when evaluating the desired response of calcium gluconate in treating acute hypoparathyroidism?
① Intake and output
② Confusion
③ Tetany
④ Bone deformities

10.57 Which of these plans indicate an understanding of the priority care?
① The licensed practical nurse (LPN) positions a client following a thoracentesis on the unaffected side.
② The unlicensed assistive personnel (UAP) limits fluids for a client who experienced a myelogram in the AM.
③ The RN explains to the client who is going for a bronchoscopy to expect the voice to become hoarse.
④ The RN notifies the health care provider (HCP) that a client expectorated a small amount of blood tinged sputum 2 hours post-bronchoscopy.

10.58 What is most important for the nurse to caution client about during the discharge teaching for a client who is newly diagnosed with multiple sclerosis and is preparing to go home?
① Ambulating every day.
② Staying away from being over-exposed to heat or cold.
③ Participating in stretching and strengthen exercises.
④ Participating in social activities.

10.59 The nurse is preparing to administer a scheduled dose of insulin Lispro as prescribed by provider of care to a client with Type 2 Diabetes Mellitus. The AM glucose level is 175 mg/dL (9.71 mmol/L). What is the priority nursing action?

① Ensure that a meal is at the bedside.
② Hold the medication.
③ Administer the medication IM.
④ Verify the order.

10.60 Which statement made by the client indicates a correct understanding of steroid therapy for Addison's Disease?

① "I'll take the medicine in the morning because if I take it at night, it might keep me awake."
② "I'll take the same amount from now on."
③ "I'll increase my potassium by eating more bananas."
④ "This medicine probably won't affect my blood pressure."

10.61 Which statement made by the client with Cushing's syndrome indicates a need for further teaching?

① "I realize I'll have to begin an exercise program slowly and gradually."
② "I'm going to have to keep a close eye on my blood pressure."
③ "I'm not really worried about getting pneumonia this winter."
④ "I'll be eating foods low in carbohydrates and salt."

10.62 Which of these tests would be performed prior to initiating a radial arterial puncture to evaluate ABGs?

① Compress the ulnar and radial arteries simultaneously while instructing client to form a fist. Instruct client to relax hand while releasing pressure on radial artery.
② Tap over the median nerve at the wrist crease.
③ After BP cuff is inflated above systolic pressure, evaluate for color return.
④ Compress the top of the finger, and evaluate the time for color to return to the finger tips.

10.63 What is the priority clinical finding that the nurse must monitor for a client who has pheochromocytoma?

① Blood pressure
② Skin temperature
③ Urine for occult blood
④ Weight

10.64 What would be the priority nursing care specific for an adult in Buck's traction?

① Checking site of pins for bleeding or infection.
② Applying topical or antibiotic ointment as ordered.
③ Assessing that the elastic bandages are not too loose or too tight.
④ Removing the bandages daily to lubricate the skin.

10.65 For an elderly client who has just had a prosthetic hip implant, which post-operative position would be maintained?

① The affected hip should be internally rotated and flexed.
② The affected hip should be adducted when turning the client.
③ In the supine position, the knees should be elevated 90 degrees.
④ When side-lying, the affected hip should be in a position of abduction.

Answers & Rationales

10.1 ② Option #2 is priority due to the risk of developing pneumonia from immobility. Option #1 does not answer the question regarding complications from immobility. Option #3 needs to be completed more frequently to monitor for potential skin breakdown. Option #4 is incorrect. Fluids need to be **encouraged** to decrease risk of constipation, UTI, and decrease viscosity of potential pulmonary secretions, etc. There is no indication of complications with cardiac, neuro, and/or renal which would contraindicate encouraging fluids.
I CAN HINT: Apply the clinical judgment/cognitive skill, take-action (first-do priority interventions), to the concept of immobility. Master the concept of immobility. It can be "AWFUL": Atelectasis, Avoid venous thrombo-emboli (VTE); Wasting of bones; Functional loss of muscle; Urinary stasis; Last but not least, constipation.
NCLEX® Standard: Provide post-operative care.

10.2 ① ② Options #1 and #2 are correct. Clients with a DVT experience pain in the calf of the leg. This change with no pain indicates an improvement in the condition. Redness and warmth and induration along blood vessels on the affected leg ae clinical findings of a DVT. This change in temperature being the same in bilateral extremities indicates an improvement in the condition. This SaO_2 (option #3) may indicate a complication with a pulmonary embolism. This may result from the DVT dislodging and entering the venous circulation forming a blockage in the pulmonary vasculature. Due to hypoxia that may occur, the respiratory rate and heart rate may be elevated as they are in options #4 and #5. These client findings do not currently indicate an improvement following the treatment.
I CAN HINT: Apply the clinical judgment/cognitive skill, evaluate outcomes to deep vein thrombosis."DVT": Diameter of calf and thighs; compare bilaterally for swelling. Vein tenderness and redness, note; Temperature increase (also at site of clot, warm to touch)
NCLEX® Standard: Evaluate response to procedures and treatments.

10.3 ② The correct answer is option #2. The nurse should evaluate the accuracy of the electronic blood pressure device by comparing the auscultated blood pressure with the initial electronic reading. This is important since several medical conditions such as heart rate irregularity, tremors, etc. may affect the reliability of the electronic reading.
I CAN HINT: Apply the clinical judgment/cognitive skill, take-action (first-do priority interventions), when evaluating blood pressure.
NCLEX® Standard: Perform focused assessments.

10.4 ② Option #2 is correct. The port must be cleaned with an antiseptic such as povidone-iodine solution or alcohol. A 5 mL sterile syringe then should be used to aspirate the specimen from the port. Option #1 is incorrect. The client has a catheter in place. Option #3 is incorrect. This is not included in evidence-based practice. Option #4 is incorrect. This is not a part of the standard of care for this procedure.
I CAN HINT: Apply the clinical judgment/cognitive skill, take-action (first do priority interventions), when obtaining a urinary specimen from an indwelling catheter.
NCLEX® Standard: Obtain specimens for diagnostic testing (e.g., wound, stool, urine).

10.5

②	Explain procedure to client.
④	Assess a circulatory assessment baseline.
①	Place SCD sleeve under leg.
③	Wrap and secure SCD sleeve around leg.
⑦	Place 2 fingers between sleeve and leg.
⑥	Attach connector of SCD sleeve to device.
⑤	Evaluate functioning of SCD device for one total cycle.

I CAN HINT: Apply the clinical judgment cognitive skill, take-action (first-do priority interventions), when applying a sequential compression device (SCD) to a client who is on bed rest.

10.6 ① Options #1, #2, and #3 are correct. Option #1:
② The head of the bed should be elevated to a
③ minimum of 30 degrees to optimize lung expansion. Option #2 is important for client not to have a full bladder to prevent bladder perforations. Option #3 is correct since there is a risk of perforation of the bowel, so it is important for the nurse to evaluate vital signs for signs of bleeding, the abdomen for peritonitis; board like abdomen, decrease in bowel sounds, abdominal distention, and/or rigid abdomen. Option #4 is not expected. This would indicate a complication of hypovolemia secondary to bleeding. Option #5 is incorrect. It is not included in the standard of care for this procedure.
I CAN HINT: Apply the clinical judgment/cognitive skill, take-action (first-do priority interventions), when preparing a client for a paracentesis.
NCLEX® Standard: Use precautions to prevent injury and/or complications associated with a procedure.

10.7 ④ The assessment (option #4) supports the diagnosis of pulmonary edema. This is a complication of congestive heart failure and needs immediate care. Option #1 is not priority over #4. There is no immediate emergency with +1 edema. Option #2 is not a priority. Lisinopril is not going to affect the HR, since it works on suppressing the renin - angiotensin aldosterone system; blocks conversion of angiotensin I to angiotensin II (a potent vasoconstrictor). Option #3 is a concern but does not require immediate intervention.
I CAN HINT: Apply the clinical judgment/cognitive skill, take-action (first-do priority interventions), for a client experiencing pulmonary edema. The key is to focus on the word "immediately".
NCLEX® Standard: Recognize changes in client condition and intervene as needed.

10.8 ② Options #2 and #4 are correct for this client
④ These clients do not eliminate potassium due to the kidney disease, so this can result in peaked T waves (option #2). This dysrhythmia will alter the cardiac perfusion. Option #4 is correct due to fluid retention that occurs from the kidney disease. This will be monitored by trending the weight gain, HR and BP increase, changes in breath sounds, etc. Option #1 is incorrect because salt substitutes are high in potassium, and this is unsafe for renal clients. Options #3 is incorrect since these can result in nephrotoxicity. Option #5 is incorrect. The client will need an iron supplement, but it should not be taken with orange juice due to the high potassium in oranges.
I CAN HINT: Apply the clinical judgment/cognitive skill, generate solutions (first-do priority plans, when developing a plan of care for the client with alteration in elimination secondary to chronic kidney disease.
NCLEX® Standard: Use precautions to prevent injury and/or complications associated with a procedure or diagnosis.

10.9 ③ Option #3 is correct. Urine is trending down. Yes, it is not 30 mL/hour, but our goal as a nurse is to prevent complications from occurring. A complication from an ileostomy can be fluid deficit from diarrhea or in this case liquid stools, due to the location of the ileostomy. "Remember, Diarrhea = risk for fluid Deficit! You do NOT have to remember every GI disorder that has diarrhea or loose stools. As a nurse, you may not know the actual disease, but you will be able to recognize the trends in the changes in the vital signs, client's color, abdominal assessment (abdomen – soft, hard, distended, etc.) and the stools. Remember, HR ↑, RR ↑, ↑ color , later on BP ↓ , ↓ urine output = fluid deficit. The key is to assess the trends early, intervene, and not wait until client is in last signs of shock due to hypovolemia that had no early interventions. Option #1 is incorrect. This would indicate dilute urine which is not a complication from an ileostomy. Option #2 is not correct. This is not a significant change. Option #4 is incorrect due to the time frame.
I CAN HINT: Apply the clinical judgment/cognitive skill, recognize cues (system-specific assessments), for a client with an ileostomy. Fluid and electrolyte imbalance is a priority with clients with an ileostomy.
NCLEX® Standard: Assess and respond to changes and/or trends in client vital signs, urine output, etc.

10.10 ④ Option #4 is correct. Assist client to ambulate in within the scope of practice for the UAP and is an appropriate action during the post op period to promote deep breathing and prevent potential complications (i.e., deep vein thrombosis, atelectasis, etc.). The other options require decision making and is not within the scope of practice for the UAP. The strategy is to know post-op care. The priority post-operatively with many surgeries is to get the client moving! Moving is very important to prevent post-op complications such as atelectasis and DVTs. Clients with abdominal incisions do not like to take deep breaths because of the pain from the incision. This increases the risk for atelectasis and potential infections. Ambulation requires an upright position and helps ope up the airway. Prior to deep breathing and ambulation, remember to administer pain medication to help the client take deep breaths and move without pain.
I CAN HINT: Apply the clinical judgment/cognitive skill, take-action (first-do priority interventions), for a client experiencing post-operative care for a cholecystectomy. The link here is that even if you did not remember exactly what the nursing care is for this client, you understand POST-OP CARE and that it applies to any kind of GI surgery (i.e., cholecystectomy, thoracic, appendectomy, Biliroth I or II, etc.). You know it is important to promote perfusion, oxygenation, and help avoid any potential complications. You CAN do this! Congratulations on persevering! You are on your way to success!
NCLEX® Standard: Provide post-operative care.

10.11 ② Option #2 is correct. The platelets are decreased, so there is a risk client could bleed. Option #1 is not necessary. There is no indication of hypoxia. Hemoglobin and hematocrit are within the expected reference range. Option #3 is not correct. The WBC is normal with no indication of infection. Option #4 is not correct. There is no indication that this is necessary.

10.12 ① ③ Options #1 and #3 are correct. Elevating the HOB will assist with lung expansion. Option #3 addresses the clinical findings of hypoxia. Option #2 is not correct; there is no indication of fluid overload. Option #4 is important, but is not an immediate need. Option #5 is also not an immediate need. The strategy is to focus on the immediate concern with hypoxia and then to address these in the options. The strategy for answering this is using the guidelines for "ABC's".

10.13 ④ Option #4 is correct. These values are low and require further assessment to determine if client is symptomatic for this low level. Options #1, #2, and #3 are values within the expected reference range.

10.14 ① Option #1 is correct. This client may have a pulmonary embolism. Options #2, #3, #4 are not the priority over option #1 which can be an emergency.

10.15 ② ③ Options #2 and #3 are correct standards of care for clients with a chest tube. Looping the tubing prevents pressure on the tubing and maintains tubing from being on the floor. This focuses on infection prevention and safety. Option #1 is not correct. This is contraindicated for chest tubes due to the pressure. Option #4 is an expected finding and does not need to be reported. Option #5 is not correct. The client is able to go to the bathroom; ambulation will promote ventilation and lung expansion.

10.16 ① Option #1 is the correct answer. The LPN should not have the client up to the bathroom immediately following a lumbar puncture. The client should remain lying for several hours to ensure the site clots. The RN needs to intervene and assist client back to bed in addition to reviewing the Standard of Practice for clients following a lumbar puncture. Options #2 and #3 are the appropriate Standards of Practice for a client undergoing an EEG. Option #4 is incorrect. There is no need for intervention since the LPN is making the correct assessment for this procedure.

10.17 ④ Option #4 is correct. Clients who have lesions at the T6 or higher may experience the medical emergency of autonomic dysreflexia because the parasympathetic nervous system is unable to neutralize the sympathetic response. This condition may occur secondary to the stimulation of the sympathetic nervous system and inadequate compensatory response by the parasympathetic nervous system. Sympathetic stimulation is usually caused by a triggering stimulus in the lower part of the body. This stimulation may cause extreme hypertension, sudden severe headache, diaphoresis, restlessness, nausea, piloerection (goose bumps), and pallor below the level of the spinal cord's lesion dermatome. Stimulation of the parasympathetic nervous system causes bradycardia, flushing above the corresponding dermatome to the spinal cord lesion (flushed face and neck), and nasal stuffiness. The priority action is to sit the client up to decrease blood pressure secondary to postural hypotension. Notify the provider. Option #1 is incorrect. Dopamine will cause the blood pressure to increase further. Options #2 and #3 are incorrect for this client's clinical presentation.

10.18 ③ Option #3 is the correct answer. Dexamethasone (Decadron) may cause immunosuppression which places client at high risk for infection. The pale yellow secretions indicate an infection may be starting to occur. Option #1 is important to monitor the trends, but with only one BP report it is difficult to determine if this is a change in the blood pressure from the norm. This option as it reads would not be a priority to report. Option #2 must be continued to be monitored, but is currently not a priority over the symptoms of infection. Option #4 is slightly elevated, but is not a priority over option #3.

10.19 ③ Option #3 is correct answer. Dysphagia is difficulty swallowing. Clients usually handle soft or semi-soft foods better than liquids. Chicken broth does not have any thickening and may result in aspiration. The nurse does need to intervene due to this potential risk of aspiration. Option #1 is a correct nursing action. Feeding the client slowly in small amounts and on the unaffected side will reduce the risk of aspiration. Option #2 does not require intervention since this action will assist with the hemianopsia and assist with client's visual range. Option #4 is an appropriate action and does not require intervention. This will assist client with chewing and swallowing since the head and neck are positioned correctly.

10.20 ④ Option #4 is correct. The normal range for calcium is 9.0 to 10.5 mg/dL (2.25 to 2.62 mmol/L). This client indeed had hypocalcemia. This is how the nurse would check the Trousseau sign. The Trousseau's sign of latent tetany is more sensitive than Chvostek's sign in hypocalcemia. This Trousseau's sign may be positive prior to gross manifestations of hypocalcemia, specifically tetany and hyperreflexia. When the BP cuff is inflated and held in place for 3 minutes, this results in the occlusion of the brachial artery, and the hypocalcemia and subsequent neuromuscular irritability may induce a muscle spasm of the hand and forearm of the client's hand. Another test to check for hypocalcemia is the Chvostek's sign. This sign is initiated by tapping over the parotid gland and if the lip twitches this is a positive sign. Another assessment for hypocalcemia would be checking for tingling of toes and fingers and around the mouth. Option #1 is incorrect. This clinical finding would indicate too much of a CNS depressant such as Magnesium Sulfate or a sign of hypernatremia. Option #2 is incorrect. This is the tinel's sign which is least sensitive, but most specific for carpal tunnel syndrome. Another test to check for carpal tunnel syndrome is the Phalen's sign test. Option #3 is incorrect. This is the Babinski reflex which is used to assess adequacy of the higher (central) nervous system. Option #3, the examiner begins by stimulating the heel and going forward to the base of the toes. A Babinski reflex is positive when the big toe moves toward the top surface of the foot and the other toes fan out after the sole of the foot has been firmly stroked.

10.21 ① Spironolactone is a potassium-sparing diuretic, and when given with lisinopril, there is a potential problem with hyperkalemia. Option #1 is the answer due to the potassium level. (Normal: 3.5 to 5.0 mEq/L [3.5 to 5.0 mmol/L].) Option #2 is not the priority over option #1. In fact with the clinical presentation, the sodium would be low. (Normal: 135 to 145 mEq/L [135 to 145 mmol/L].) Option #3 is incorrect since these foods are high in potassium and could result in hyperkalemia. While option #4 is appropriate, it is not a priority to option #1.

10.22 ④ Option #4 is correct. This is a neurologic change and symptoms such as bladder or bowel changes or foot-drop should be reported to the health care provider immediately. Option #1 is incorrect, since when a client experiences acute low back pain, these symptoms may take 4 to 6 weeks to resolve. Options #2 and #3 are not findings that should be reported immediately. The client may present with both of these symptoms when there is a problem with acute low back pain.

I CAN HINT: The key to success with this question, as with many of the NCLEX® questions, it to remember that an "expected outcome" is most likely not going to be the priority to report or intervene with immediately! Options #2 and #3 are expected findings with acute low back pain.

10.23 ④ Post-operative restlessness should create a high degree of suspicion of hypoxemia (for instance—due to bleeding). Vital signs and urine output will give information regarding intravascular volume. Option #1 requires further assessment to rule out hypoxemia as the cause of the restlessness. Option #2 may be the second priority. Option #3 may indicate an erroneous assumption.

10.24 ④ Option #4 is correct. This may indicate a complication with perforation. This then is followed by increasing pain with fever and guarding of the abdomen. Peritonitis can occur rapidly, so these clinical findings are in need of immediate action. The nurse should maintain the client NPO, keep on bed rest, and notify the health care provider immediately. Option #1 is incorrect. The HR is not increased and BP not decreased enough to indicate a complication with bleeding. Option #2 is incorrect; there is no significant changes to make this a priority over this risk for perforation. Option #3 is a clinical presentation for a duodenal ulcer that is characteristic by high gastric acid secretion and rapid gastric emptying. Since food buffers the effect of the acid; then pain increases with an empty stomach.

10.25 ③ In diabetes insipidus, a potential complication following a craniotomy, one of the first signs is a significant increase in urine output and pale colored urine. Option #1 is incorrect because the specific gravity is decreased, and foul smelling urine usually indicates infection. Option #2 is incorrect because intake is normal. Option #4 may be associated with client receiving antibiotics, but is not a priority over option #3.

10.26 ① Before teaching or client learning can occur, the client must identify thoughts about his/her current status including concerns, fears, anxieties, etc. Option #2 is not a priority because the nurse is processing instead of the client. Option #3 is important, but is not a priority over #1. Option #4 will be done at a later time.

10.27 ① Option #1 is correct. Options #2, #3, and #4 are incorrect. Option #3 should be downward over the stump and to the back of the leg. Option #4 should be so that it narrows toward the distal end.

10.28 ③ Adequate fluids will help maintain regular bowel function. Options #1 and #4 are unnecessary. Option #2, while beneficial, will not promote bowel function.

10.29 ④ Second-degree burns create a lot of pain for the client. Option #1 would be a priority within the first few hours for upper extremity burns. However, these are on the lower body. Option #2 is a concern, but not a priority to pain. Option #3 is a major concern initially after the burns, but should be resolved in 72 hours.

10.30 ② It is important to prevent nausea and vomiting as this would increase the intraocular pressure and could cause damage to the area repaired. Option #1 would not be effective. Option #3 refers to an eye infection. This would be important after the initial operative day. Option #4 is incorrect because eye irrigations are not common following this procedure.

10.31 ② Option #2 is correct for the CN XI (spinal accessory). Option #1 is evaluation of the CN I (olfactory). Option #3 is evaluation of the CN II (optic). Option #4 is evaluation for the CN XII (hypoglossal).

10.32 ② A characteristic of this condition is the intense facial pain experienced along the nerve tract. Nursing care should be directed toward preventing stimuli to the area and decreasing pain. Option #1 does not occur with this condition. Option #3 describes Ménière's disease. Option #4 may occur, but option #2 is a priority.

10.33 ④ This method aids wound debridement. Option #1 would not be effective. Option #2 will prevent adherence of gauze to wound debris and limit debridement. Option #3, wetting again before removal, will defeat the purpose of wound debridement.

10.34 ④ The nurse should always speak when entering the room of a client with decreased vision. This makes the client aware of the nurse's presence. Options #1, #2, and #3 are incorrect because the client will become more confused with sensory deprivation.

10.35 ③ The parents need to understand the importance of monitoring and reporting signs of increased intracranial pressure. Vomiting is a sign of IICP. Signs of infection would also be important to report. Options #1 and #2 are incorrect positions. In option #4, parents need to understand how to pump the shunt in order to maintain patency.

10.36 ③ This procedure takes approximately 1½ hours, and there is a lot of noise associated with the test. Option #1 is incorrect because there is no dye used for an MRI. Option #2 is incorrect because the client is not anesthetized for this procedure. Option #4 is inappropriate for this situation.

10.37 ④ The client has increased muscle fatigue and needs more assistance towards the end of the day. Option #1 is incorrect because the client does not experience vertigo. Option #2 is incorrect because though fluid and electrolytes are important, they are not a priority over option #4 in this clinical situation. Option #3 is incorrect because increased intracranial pressure is not associated with myasthenia gravis.

10.38 ① Option #1 is correct. TEF is a medical condition in the neonate that the proximal end of the esophagus ends in a blind pouch, and the lower segment connects to the trachea. As a result of this pathophysiology, there may be an overflow of secretions into the larynx which can lead to laryngospasms. This leads to an obstruction to inspiration stimulating the contraction of the accessory muscles of the thorax to assist the diaphragm in breathing. As a result of this, substernal retractions are produced in addition to tachypnea. (Normal RR—30 to 50/min). When secretions are removed from the oropharynx, the laryngospasms resolve quickly. A brassy cough that can occur in the infant with TEF is a result of the constant laryngeal narrowing, usually secondary to edema. This is not indicative of the need to suction infant. This infant is the priority due to the immediate need to relieve the airway of the secretions. Option #2 is presenting with possible otitis media and does need to be assessed soon, but is not a priority over option #1 who has an airway complication. Option #3 includes expected clinical findings for a school-age child 2 hours-post-operative for a tonsillectomy and adenoidectomy. The HR is within normal range for this age. A small amount of blood that is partially digested, and is dark brown may be present with the emesis during the post-operative period. Option #4 is incorrect since this is an expected finding for a child with cystic fibrosis. Children with cystic fibrosis (CF) have poor digestion and absorption of foods, especially fats, which can result in frequent bowel movements that are bulky, large, and foul-smelling. These stools contain large amounts of fat which is referred to as steatorrhea.

10.39 ③ Option #3 is the safety with airway. Options #1 and #4, while correct, are not a priority to option #3. Option #2 is incomplete. Documentation should also include during and after the seizure.

10.40 ② Avoiding sudden motion of the head will reduce incidence of vertigo, nausea, and vomiting. Option #1 is incorrect because salt should be restricted. Option #3 is incorrect because fluids should not be restricted. Option #4 is incorrect because cotton will not help the condition.

10.41 ② Eye pain and nausea may be indicative of increased intraocular pressure. Option #1 is for a client with hypertension and atherosclerosis. Option #3 is incorrect because the client may not experience any improvement in vision, but further deterioration may be prevented. Option #4 is incorrect because the eye drops may be continued indefinitely.

10.42 ④ Option #4 is correct. A deep vein thrombosis is a venous complication with marked leg swelling and dependent edema. Skin may become discolored with slightly painful ulcers. The area on the calf may be warm to touch. Peripheral pulses will be normal. Option #1 is incorrect since this would be more indicative of an arterial complication. With the arterial insufficiency the skin on the legs will be shiny and smooth. The extremity will have pallor on elevation. The peripheral pulses will be weak. The temperature will be cool to touch. A classic symptom of arterial insufficiency is intermittent claudication. Option #2 is incorrect since this is indicative of an arterial complication as reviewed in the rationale for option #1. Option #3 is incorrect since this represents intermittent claudication which is also an arterial versus a venous insufficiency.

I CAN HINT: Three of the options indicate a complication with arterial insufficiency versus the one that is focused on the DVT.

10.43 ① When teaching paralyzed clients how to transfer themselves, it is important for them to understand that the strong side leads. Options #2, #3, and #4 are ineffective.

10.44 ④ These are symptoms of compartmental syndrome which must be relieved as soon as possible. The only action within the scope of practice for the nurse is to document assessments and secure the health care provider's intervention immediately. Option #1 is an inappropriate response to the symptoms assessed. Option #2 is not typically ordered q 45 min., and it is only palliative. This action would be ignoring the fact that the client did not receive any pain relief from the previous dose. This ongoing pain is very indicative of compartmental syndrome. Option #3 is beyond the scope of practice, though bivalving is desirable.

10.45 ③ Options #3 and #4 are correct. Nasogastric
④ losses are isotonic, containing both sodium and potassium. Since these electrolytes are being pulled out, the clinical findings would be related to hypokalemia and hyponatremia. Other signs and symptoms of hypokalemia may include: fatigue, muscle weakness, nausea in addition to the flat T waves on the ECG monitor and muscle cramps. Hyponatremia may present with tachycardia, hypotension, hypoactive bowel sounds, anorexia, headache, muscle weakness, lethargy, confusion, seizures, coma. None of these are included in any of the options. Options #1, #2, and #5 are incorrect since these are clinical findings consistent with hypocalcemia and do not occur with nasogastric tube suctioning.

10.46 ② Option #2 is correct. It is done to decrease risk of aspiration. Options #1, #3, and #4 are incorrect. While the nurse may implement option #1, it is not a priority to option #2.

10.47 ② Option #2 is the answer. There is no cure for Raynaud's phenomenon. Treatment is based on symptoms, so there is a need for further teaching with this statement. Raynaud's phenomenon consists of intermittent episodic spasms of the arterioles typically in the fingers and toes. Spasms are not necessarily correlated with peripheral vascular problems. Symptoms are precipitated by emotional upset, exposure to cold, and nicotine and caffeine intake. Options #1, #3, and #4 are correct statements and indicate an understanding of this condition.

10.48 ② The surgical inflammation can cause some temporary leg pain after disc excision. Option #1 is incorrect because early ambulation should be encouraged and sitting for long times is contraindicated. Option #3 may occur, but a prediction is not made at this time. Option #4 is inaccurate.

10.49 ③ Option #3 is correct. This clinical finding could result in a compromised airway. Option #1 is not a priority over #3. Option #2 is a concern, but is not a priority over #3. Option #2 is a psychosocial need, and does not require immediate care. Option #4 is an expected finding for this client.

10.50 ② With myxedema, there is a slowing of all body functions. Options #1, #3, and #4 are associated with hyperthyroidism.

10.51 ① The crutches should be positioned about 2" under the axillary area to prevent nerve damage to the brachial plexus area which would result in arm paralysis or numbness. Options #2, #3, and #4 are incorrect positions.

10.52 ① The prone position provides maximum extension of the hip joint and prevents hip flexion contracture. If hip flexion contracture occurs, then it is very difficult to correctly fit or utilize prosthesis. Option #2 contains incorrect information. Option #3 is not a priority. Option #4 can result in contractures.

10.53 ① Option #1 is correct. After aspirating fluid from the client, the volume decrease may have resulted in a decrease in the blood pressure causing a decrease in cerebral perfusion. This can lead to syncope with the client complaining of a feeling of passing out. Option #2 is incorrect. After the procedure, the shirt should feel looser due to the aspiration of fluid. With this change, the abdominal girth should decrease; however, even if there was no change option #1 still is the priority due to the safety involved and risk for falls. Option #3 is expected and would not mandate immediate evaluation. The nurse would not ignore the statement, but this would not require immediate evaluation. Option #4 is not a priority since the client most likely voided prior to the procedure. This is simply a distractor and does not present a safety issue to the client.

10.54 ③ This will prevent atrophy of the flexor and extensor muscle groups which will result in optimizing mobility. Options #1 and #2 are inappropriately restraining the client which will result in complications of immobility. Option #4 should say "encourage independence" versus "as much assistance."

10.55 ③ Thyroid hormone replacement is usually continued for life. A sudden discontinuing of the medication may cause a myxedema crisis. Option #1 is a correct statement because thyroid hormones may produce hyperglycemia due to the increased rate of carbohydrate breakdown. Option #2 is a correct statement because taking it before breakfast will prevent insomnia. Option #4 is a correct statement because thyroid hormones enhance toxic effects of digoxin preparations.

10.56 ③ Tetany is the major sign of hypoparathyroidism. Options #1 and #2 are important to monitor, but are not top priority. Option #4 is incorrect because bone deformities are most frequently observed with hyperparathyroidism.

10.57 ① Option #1 is correct. Remember, "Side up with puncture." Option #2 is incorrect. The client needs fluids to flush out the dye. Option #3 is incorrect. The voice should not be hoarse. Option #4 is incorrect since this is an expected finding, does not present a safety issue to the client; therefore, no need to notify the health care provider.

10.58 ② Overexposure to heat or cold may cause damage related to the changes in sensation. Options #1 and #3 are incorrect because the client is encouraged to ambulate as tolerated and participate in an exercise program to include ROM, stretching, and strengthening exercises. Option #4 is incorrect because a client with multiple sclerosis is encouraged to continue usual activities as much as possible, including social activities.

10.59 ① Option #1 is correct. Lispro (Humalog) has an onset of less than 15 min. and peaks within 0.5 to 1 hr. It is imperative that food is at the bedside, so client does not experience any complications with hypoglycemia due to the rapid onset. Option #2 is incorrect. There is no need to hold this medication. Option #3 is incorrect; the standard of practice is to administer it subcutaneously. Option #4 is incorrect since there is nothing in the stem of the question that would cause the nurse to question if this was an appropriate order. If the AM glucose was low or the client was presenting with clinical assessments indicating hypoglycemia, then this would be an appropriate action.

10.60 ① If steroids are taken at night, they may cause sleeplessness. Option #2 is incorrect because the dosage has to be regulated according to stress. Option #3 is incorrect because the client with Addison's disease can have hyperkalemia. Option #4 is incorrect because steroids can cause fluid retention which can increase the blood pressure.

10.61 ③ This statement does not indicate the client realizes that there is an increased susceptibility to infections. Option #1 is a correct statement. Option #2 is a correct statement because these clients may develop hypertension related to sodium and water retention. Option #4 is a correct statement since the diet should be low carbohydrate, low sodium, and high protein.

10.62 ① Option #1 is correct. This intervention evaluates the Allen's test. If the pinkness returns to the hand quickly, this indicates patency of the radial artery. This action may also be repeated for the ulnar artery in order to evaluate its patency. Option #2 is incorrect. This evaluates the Tinel's sign which is most specific for carpal tunnel syndrome. Option #3 is incorrect. This nursing action is not specific for this identified exam. It is simply a distractor. Option #4 is incorrect. This is evaluating capillary refill. This is an assessment for determining hypoxia; it is not specific to radial artery patency.

10.63 ① Hypertension is a major symptom associated with pheochromocytoma. While diaphoresis, glycosuria, and weight loss are also symptoms, an elevation in the blood pressure is the priority clinical finding that must be monitored (making Options #2 and #4 incorrect). Option #3 is not necessary, since hematuria is not associated with this medical condition.

10.64 ③ Option #3 is correct. Buck's traction is a skin traction and assessment is needed to make sure circulation is not being compromised. Option #1 is incorrect because Buck's traction is a type of skin traction. Therefore, there are no pins. This would be appropriate for a client in skeletal traction. Option #2 is incorrect because skin traction has no need for topical ointment. Option #4 is incorrect because the skin is not lubricated under the bandages.

10.65 ④ A position of abduction should be maintained. Flexion beyond 60 degrees and internal rotation should be avoided in the early post-operative period. Options #1, #2, and #3 are incorrect.

CHAPTER 11
Basic Care and Comfort

Let us never consider ourselves finished nurses... we must be learning all our lives.
— FLORENCE NIGHTINGALE

✔ Clarification of this test ...

There have been no changes in percentages. This chapter still represents 6–12% of exam items. The minimum standards include: providing direct basic care and comfort, including elimination, mobility/immobility, performing skin assessment, and implement measures to maintain skin integrity and prevent skin breakdown; implement procedures necessary to safely admit, transfer, or discharge a client; measures to promote circulation, nutrition, non-pharmacological comfort interventions; promoting activities of daily living; complementary and alternative therapies; and promoting client ability to perform activities of daily living, rest, and sleep.

- Assess client for pain and intervene as appropriate.
- Perform skin assessment and implement measures to maintain skin integrity.
- Evaluate client intake and output and intervene as needed.
- Provide non-pharmacological comfort measures.
- Assess client performance of activities of daily living and assist when needed.
- Assist client to compensate for a physical or sensory impairment (e.g., assistive devices, positioning).
- Assess and manage client with an alteration in bowel and bladder elimination.
- Implement measures to promote circulation (e.g., active or passive range of motion, positioning and mobilization).
- Evaluate the client's nutritional status and intervene as needed.
- Assess client sleep/rest pattern and intervene as needed.
- Provide client nutrition through tube feedings.
- Apply, maintain or remove orthopedic devices.
- Recognize complementary therapies and identify potential benefits and contraindications (e.g., aromatherapy, acupressure, supplements).
- Perform irrigations (e.g., of bladder, ear, eye).
- Perform post-mortem care.

Adapted from: © National Council of State Boards of Nursing, Inc. (NCSBN). (2022). 2021 *RN Practice Analysis: Linking the NCLEX-RN® Examination to Practice*. Chicago: Author.

Adapted from: © National Council of State Boards of Nursing, Inc. (NCSBN). (2023) *Next Generation NCLEX® NCLEX-RN® Test Plan. Chicago*: Author.

Chapter 11: BASIC CARE AND COMFORT

11.1 What interventions are important for the nurse to include in the plan of care for prevention of pressure ulcers in an elderly client? **Select all that apply.**
① Turn and reposition every 1-2 hours.
② Keep skin moist with alcohol-based lotions.
③ Encourage diet with decreased calories.
④ Promote fluid intake of 2000 - 3000 mL per day unless contraindicated.
⑤ Dry skin briskly after bathing.
⑥ Discuss importance of receiving adequate amounts of protein and vitamin A and C.

11.2 What nursing interventions are important to prevent complications of immobility for a client in Buck's traction? **Select all that apply.**
① Use incentive spirometer every 2 hours while awake.
② Limit caloric intake to avoid weight gain.
③ Administer stool softener as ordered.
④ Adjust weights to maintain traction.
⑤ ROM on the unaffected extremities 2-3 times per day.

11.3 Which of these clinical findings indicate a desired outcome for an immobile client who is currently taking an anticholinergic medication and has been started on a high fiber diet?
① Urine output – 85 mL/hour
② Urine specific gravity 1.028
③ Bowel movement daily
④ Two to ten bowel sounds per minute

11.4 Which dietary plan is important to include in the nursing care for a client on lithium therapy?
① Restricted sodium diet with increased fluid intake.
② High calorie diet with sodium and potassium restriction and adequate fluid intake.
③ Regular diet with normal sodium and fluid intake of 1,500-3,000 mL.
④ Reduced calorie diet with an increased sodium and reduced fluid intake.

11.5 The nurse has admitted an elderly client to the medical unit with poor capillary refill, lethargy, and urinary incontinence. What plan will the nurse include in the plan of care?
① Document characteristics of lips, mucous membranes, and skin turgor.
② Evaluate client for skin breakdown.
③ Initiate active range of motion per hospital protocol.
④ Monitor intake and output.

11.6 What is the priority clinical finding that requires intervention for an older adult client 3 days post-op receiving Morphine via a PCA pump?
① Requires tactile stimulation to arouse.
② A respiratory rate from 28 breaths/min to 24 breaths/min.
③ Urine output from 90 mL/hr to 68 mL/hr.
④ Last bowel movement was four days ago.

11.7 Which nursing intervention is most important for the nurse to implement after assessing a stage I pressure ulcer on the right heel of a client's foot?
① Wound irrigation as prescribed.
② Wet-to-dry dressing.
③ Antibiotic therapy as prescribed.
④ Pressure-relieving device.

11.8 What is the best initial treatment plan for a sleep disorder in an elderly client?
① Discuss the importance of including naps daily in the plan of care.
② Discuss the importance of decreasing noise and light in the environment.
③ Review the importance of taking trazodone as prescribed.
④ Review the importance of taking amitriptyline as prescribed.

11.9 The nurse is getting the client out of bed to the chair who is partial weight bearing. (Place the sequence of steps in chronological order for this task. All options must be included.)

| ① Instruct client to pivot on the foot further from the chair. |
| ② Assist client to sit on the side of the bed. |
| ③ Assist client to rock to a standing position. |
| ④ Apply the transfer belt. |
| ⑤ Along the client's sides, grasp the transfer belt. |

| |
| |
| |
| |
| |

11.10 Which of these interventions for a client with Addison's disease can be delegated to the unlicensed assistive personnel (UAP)?

① Provide frequent stimulation.
② Record intake and output.
③ Provide client with low calorie diet.
④ Report skin that is hot and dry to the RN.

11.11 Which of these actions indicate the client understands the appropriate and safe use of the cane? **Select all that apply.**

① The cane and the unaffected leg move together.
② The cane is used on the side opposite of the affected leg.
③ The cane is placed approximately 3 feet in front.
④ The cane and the affected leg move together.
⑤ The cane is placed on the affected side and moved with the affected leg.

11.12 Which of these statements made by the daughter of an older adult (mother) indicates an understanding of safe skin care for the mother?

① "I will apply sunscreen lotions with a sun protection (SPF) of 11 when I take mom out in the sun."
② "I will apply perfumed skin lotions daily to keep mom's skin moist."
③ "I will avoid skin products that contain alcohol."
④ "I will use a strong detergent when washing mom's clothing in order to remove the odors and stains."

11.13 Which of these interventions would be appropriate for an older client with a diagnosis of glaucoma to decrease complications of incontinence? **Select all that apply.**

① Teach client how to perform Kegel exercises daily.
② Review the importance of taking the newly prescribed dicyclomine as ordered.
③ Review the importance of avoiding or decreasing the intake of caffeine.
④ Discuss the importance of increasing the use of a daily vitamin.
⑤ Review the rationale for avoiding alcohol consumption.

11.14 A client presents to the ED following a motor vehicle accident with a HR—118 bpm, RR—26/min, BP—94/62, Hgb—7 g/dL (70 g/L), and urine specific gravity 1.029. Which of these nursing actions by the UAP would require immediate intervention by the charge nurse?

① Places the client in the Fowler's position.
② Places the client in the supine position.
③ Places the client in the Trendelenburg position.
④ Hangs Lactated Ringer's solution.

11.15 While coordinating with rehabilitation, what would be the priority of care for a client who is post-op following a hip replacement?

① Instruct the client to lift the leg upward from a lying position.
② Encourage client to elevate the knee when sitting.
③ Keep abductor pillow in place while client is in the bed.
④ Review exercises with client on how to flex hip 90 degrees or more to prevent stiffness.

11.16 Which of these nursing actions indicate the nurse understands how to safely use a walker for an older-adult client who has been unsteady and requires assistance with ambulation after stretching a muscle in the right leg while exercising? **Select all that apply.**
① Advise to advance "affected" lower limb, then move unaffected limb forward.
② Discuss with client that wrists are even with the handgrips on the walker when arms are dangling downward.
③ Instruct client to wear nonskid slippers.
④ Review the importance of advancing the walker approximately 16 inches (40.64 cm).
⑤ Teach client the importance to advance walker with the "affected" lower limb.

11.17 An older client, who is being seen on the medical unit by the health care provider, complains of having difficulty sleeping at night. Which of these plans would be appropriate to include in the plan of care for this client? **Select all that apply.**
① Advise client to have a cup of warm tea 1 hour prior to going to bed.
② Avoid all caffeinated beverages.
③ Advise to drink a glass of water 20 minutes prior to going to bed.
④ Limit naps throughout the day.
⑤ Recommend the routine bath that is taken at home in the evening.

11.18 An older client with chronic pain from osteoarthritis asks the nurse what would be a recommended alternative therapy to use along with the prescribed rehabilitation plan. What statement made by the nurse is the most appropriate response?
① "Discuss with your health care provider the possibility of starting acupuncture."
② "Discuss with your health care provider the need to change the NSAID client is currently taking."
③ "I am not able to discuss this question with you since it is not within my scope of practice."
④ "I recommend you add some music therapy to your daily routine to assist with pain control."

11.19 Which of these lab values would be a priority to report to the provider of care for a client who is receiving Lactulose for the diagnosis of encephalopathy, secondary to cirrhosis?
① Serum ammonia level 200 µg/dL (117.4 µmol/L)
② Serum potassium level 4.8 mEq/L (4.8 mmol/L)
③ pH:—7.29; HCO_3—20 mEq/L (20 mmol/L)
④ AST—60 units/L; ALT—40 units/L

11.20 Place in chronological order the steps for placing a nasogastric tube in a client. All options must be used.

① Aspirate gently to collect gastric contents and test pH.
② Gradually insert the tube and when tubing reaches the mark, anchor the tube using tape.
③ Measure the tubing from the tip of the nose, to the tip of the ear lobe, to the tip of the xiphoid, and mark it with adhesive tape.
④ Explain procedure to client and assist client to high-Fowler's position if possible.
⑤ Put on gloves and Lubricate the tip.

11.21 Which actions will the nurse include in the plan for a client with cirrhosis who has ↑ ammonia, AST, ALT levels & ↓ platelets? **Select all that apply.**
① Apply mittens on both hands of the client.
② Move client frequently in bed by having him bend legs and push up in bed.
③ Maintain the dynamap BP reading ongoing to monitor trends in changes with the reading.
④ Verify the appropriateness of a new intramuscular medication order.
⑤ Report a new symptom of a course tremor of the wrists and fingers.
⑥ Monitor the level of consciousness.

11.22 What is the priority of care for a client with a score of 23 on the Braden scale?
① Initiate a plan for the prevention of pressure-ulcer development due to being in the high-risk category.
② Document and continue with current prevention plan for pressure ulcers since client is not in a high-risk category.
③ Continue to assess and monitor the measurement of the pressure ulcer.
④ Discuss treatment plan with nursing team to prevent any further skin breakdown.

11.23 Which of these documentations indicates the nurse understands how to accurately evaluate the client's stool for occult blood?
① Collected stool and placed in a clean container to examine for pathological organisms.
② Remained on regular diet prior to test being done.
③ Stool sample obtained from one area of the stool.
④ Guaiac tested positive for occult blood. Paper turned blue.

11.24 Which of these interventions indicates safe practice for a client with chronic renal disease?
① Administers Milk of Magnesia for complications with gastroesophageal reflex disease.
② Administers lisinopril for BP 160/90.
③ Administers spironolactone for the increase in edema.
④ Encourages client to include green leafy vegetables in diet.

11.25 A client with chronic cancer pain has been receiving meperidine 100 mg PO q4h PRN for pain, without much relief. Which change in narcotic pain management would be the most valid suggestion to make to the health care provider?
① Decrease to twice a day.
② Decrease to every 6 hours PRN.
③ Give every 4 hours around the clock.
④ Give every 2 hours PRN.

11.26 In a 7-month-old infant, which is the best way to detect fluid retention?
① Weigh the child daily.
② Test the urine for hematuria.
③ Measure abdominal girth weekly.
④ Count the number of wet diapers.

11.27 What would be a priority in establishing a bladder retraining program?
① Provide a flexible schedule for the client to decrease anxiety.
② Schedule toileting on a planned time schedule.
③ Teach client intermittent self-catheterization.
④ Perform the Crede maneuver tid.

11.28 How many milliliters (mL) should be documented indicating the total amount of fluid loss for an infant who had 12 soiled diapers weighing 5 grams at the end of a 10-hour shift? One dry diaper weighed 0.2 grams.

_____ mL

11.29 What would be the priority of care for a client who had a laparoscopic cholecystectomy 24 hours ago and is now calling the hospital to report right shoulder pain?
① Advise client that this discomfort is from how he was positioned during procedure.
② Discuss the importance of moving shoulder; performing ROM two times/day.
③ Eliminate any activity to the shoulder for next 24 hours.
④ Recommend client to sit upright in a chair and apply heat to the right shoulder 15 minutes every hour.

11.30 During report, the nurse indicates that the client's nasogastric tube (NG tube) quit draining over the last hour. Prior to that, it was draining 110 mL of fluid q 2 hr. Which plan would best assist this client?
① Place in a new NG tube.
② Reposition the tube to promote drainage.
③ Order a chest X-ray to determine placement.
④ Force 50 mL of normal saline down the tube.

11.31 A client has a bovine graft inserted into the left arm for hemodialysis. During the immediate post-operative period, what would be the priority plan to prevent complications?
① Restart the IV above the level of the graft.
② Take blood pressures only on the right arm.
③ Elevate the left arm above the level of the heart.
④ Check the radial pulse on the left arm q4h.

11.32 A client is experiencing gastric upset after taking his phenazopyridine hydrochloride. Which nursing action is most appropriate?
① Tell client to seek treatment for probable pyelonephritis.
② Notify physician if urine turns red.
③ Discontinue medication if urine becomes cloudy.
④ Instruct client to take the drug with food.

11.33 A client has been transferred from a nursing home to the hospital with an indwelling urinary catheter. The urine is cloudy and foul-smelling. Which nursing measure would be most appropriate?
① Clean the urinary meatus every other day.
② Encourage the client to increase fluid intake.
③ Empty the drainage bag every 2–4 hours.
④ Irrigate the Foley catheter every 8 hours to maintain patency.

11.34 Which of these clinical assessments for a client who is post-prostatic resection (TURP) require further intervention by the nurse?
① Urine output is light red to red during the first post-operative day.
② Urine output has 2 blood clots during the first post-operative day.
③ Urine output is very dark red 2nd post-operative day.
④ Urine output is pale pink the 3rd post-operative day.

11.35 Which instruction would be included in the teaching plan of a client taking sulfasalazine?
① Restrict fluids to 1500 mL per day.
② Explain to client that the stool may turn to a clay color.
③ The medication should be continued even after symptoms subside.
④ If diarrhea occurs, the client should discontinue the medication.

11.36 What is the priority of care after the urinary catheter is removed?
① Encourage client to decrease fluid intake.
② Document size of catheter and client's tolerance of procedure.
③ Evaluate client for normal voiding.
④ Document client teaching.

11.37 The nurse is caring for a client with a perforated bowel secondary to a bowel obstruction. At the time the diagnosis is made, which nursing priority would be most important in the care plan?
① Maintain the client in a supine position.
② Notify the client's next of kin.
③ Prepare the client for emergency surgery.
④ Remove the nasogastric tube.

11.38 A client returns to his room following a ureterolithotomy with a left ureteral catheter in place. Which instruction concerning the catheter would be included in the nursing care plan?
① The catheter may be clamped for short periods of time.
② Teach the client that the urine from this catheter should be clear.
③ Gently advance catheter if there is no drainage for 2 hours.
④ The catheter should be irrigated every 2 hours to maintain patency.

11.39 A client with a peptic ulcer had a partial gastrectomy and vagotomy (Billroth I). In planning the discharge teaching, which instruction to the client should be included?
① Sit up for at least 30 minutes after eating to reduce peristalsis.
② Avoid fluids between meals to promote the transit of food from the stomach to the jejunum.
③ Increase the intake of high carbohydrate foods to prevent dumping syndrome.
④ Avoid eating large meals that are high in simple sugars and liquids.

11.40 Which statement made by a client scheduled to have a TURP would indicate a need for further teaching?
① "If I have this surgery, I will become impotent."
② "I will call the nurse if my bladder feels like it is full."
③ "A catheter will be in place to drain my bladder."
④ "At first my urine may be somewhat bloody."

11.41 Which of these nursing actions indicate the licensed practical nurse (LPN) and unlicensed assistive personel (UAP understand how to safely position a client who had a lumbar laminectomy?
① Position client in the semi-Fowler's position.
② Position client in the Trendelenburg position.
③ Position client in the reverse Trendelenburg position.
④ Position a small pillow under the client's head, positioned in the supine position with knees slightly elevated.

11.42 The nurse would anticipate which assessment findings in a client who has developed a lower intestinal obstruction?
① Nausea, vomiting, abdominal distention
② Explosive, irritating diarrhea
③ Abdominal tenderness with rectal bleeding
④ Mid-epigastric discomfort, tarry stool

11.43 A client is beginning peritoneal dialysis. During the first infusion of dialysate, the client experiences mild abdominal discomfort. What would be the next nursing action?
① Stop the infusion.
② Decrease the total infusion volume.
③ Inform the client that the discomfort will subside after a few exchanges.
④ Notify the physician.

11.44 Which of these laboratory findings would be a priority concern for a client with the diagnosis of cystitis?
① Serum hematocrit 36%
② Serum WBC 6,000/mm^3
③ Urine bacteria 105,000 colonies/mL
④ Urinalysis with 2–3 WBCs present

11.45 Which method would be the best to assess a client's understanding of colostomy care prior to discharge?
① Review teaching materials.
② Have client explain irrigation procedure.
③ Have client demonstrate colostomy care.
④ Observe colostomy film.

11.46 For a client receiving total parenteral nutrition (TPN), the nurse reviews the following lab values:

Glucose	=	72 mg/dL (4 mmol/L)
Chloride	=	98 mEq/L (98 mmol/L)
Sodium	=	138 mEq/L (138 mmol/L)
Potassium	=	3.0 mEq/L (3.0 mmol/L)

Based on this assessment, which nursing action is appropriate?
① Discontinue TPN administration.
② Notify health care provider and obtain order for potassium supplement.
③ Administer IV glucose immediately.
④ Check client vital signs immediately.

11.47 Which nursing action is most appropriate for a 2-month-old infant with reflux?
① Hold the next feeding.
② Teach the mother CPR.
③ Maintain normal feeding schedule.
④ Elevate the head of the bed.

11.48 A client is taking metoclopramide hydrochloride orally for nausea secondary to chemotherapy. In reference to the timing of the medication, when would the nurse instruct the client to take the medication?
① With each meal
② Thirty minutes before meals
③ One hour after each meal
④ At the same time each day

11.49 Which dietary modifications are important to include in a teaching plan for a client with cirrhosis of the liver?
① Decrease in calories and increase in protein.
② Decrease in carbohydrates and vitamin B.
③ Increase in carbohydrates and calories.
④ Increase in protein and fats.

11.50 A 3-month-old infant is scheduled for a barium swallow in the morning. Prior to the procedure, what would be the most appropriate nursing action?

① Offer the infant only clear liquids.
② Make the infant NPO for 3 hours.
③ Feed the infant regular formula.
④ Maintain NPO for 6 hours.

11.51 A nurse is obtaining a health history from a mother of a child with failure to thrive. Which assessment would provide the most pertinent data?

① Weight and height
② Urine output
③ Type of feedings
④ Mother-child interactions

11.52 What instructions would a nurse give a diabetic client who has been vomiting for 24 hours and is concerned about blood glucose levels?

① Take only half of the regular insulin dose.
② Attempt to maintain a regular diabetic diet.
③ Limit intake of sweets and sugar.
④ Drink liquids as often as possible.

11.53 Which of these nursing actions are most appropriate to delegate for a school-age child with Cystic Fibrosis?

① The unlicensed assistive personnel (UAP) would encourage fluids throughout the day.
② The licensed practical nurse (LPN) would give the child a diet including a lettuce salad with low fat dressing and limit to three crackers.
③ The licensed practical nurse (LPN) would administer the pancreatic enzymes on an empty stomach 40 min. following a meal.
④ The unlicensed assistive personnel (UAP) would discuss importance of child wearing a medic alert bracelet and review CPR with parents.

11.54 The nurse is preparing a teaching plan for feeding an infant post-operative repair of a cleft lip. In order to prevent complications, what is the priority to teach the mother?

① Feed the infant with a newborn nipple while holding him in the recumbent position.
② Clean the suture site with a cotton dipped swab soaked in Betadine.
③ Place the infant in prone position after feeding.
④ Feed the infant with a rubber-tipped syringe and bubble frequently.

11.55 Which assessment would be most important to report to the next shift for a client who received 6 units of regular insulin 3 hours ago?

① Kussmaul's respirations and diaphoresis
② Anorexia and lethargic
③ Diaphoresis and trembling
④ Headache and polyuria

11.56 A 3-year-old is admitted with nausea and vomiting. The nurse would offer which foods for initial PO intake?

① Ice cream
② Apple juice
③ Orange juice
④ Pudding

11.57 Organize these steps in chronological order for a client who is having a nasogastric tube removed.

| ① Assist client into semi-Fowler's position. |
| ② Ask client to hold her breath. |
| ③ Assess bowel function by auscultation for peristalsis. |
| ④ Flush tube with 10 mL of normal saline. |
| ⑤ Withdraw the tube gently and steadily. |

| |
| |
| |
| |
| |

11.58 Which of these clinical observations would be most important for the UAP to report to the RN for a client with a C3 fracture?
① Unable to assist with ROM and move lower extremities.
② No bowel movement for 48 hours.
③ High pressure alarm going off on ventilator during respiratory therapy.
④ Client does not want to see any visitors today.

11.59 Which instructions would be given to an adult client in preparation for a plasma cholesterol screening?
① Eat a vegetarian diet for one week before the test.
② Limit alcohol intake to two glasses of wine the day before the test.
③ Abstain from dairy products for 48 hours before the test.
④ Only sips of water should be taken for 12 hours before the test.

11.60 What would be the priority of care for a client who has a blood sugar of 200 mg/dL (11.10 mmol/L) at 7:00 AM?
① Increase the PM dose of NPH insulin.
② Increase the AM dose of regular insulin.
③ Wake the client up at 3:00 AM and evaluate the blood sugar.
④ Decrease the PM dose of NPH insulin.

11.61 In working with an overweight adolescent with hypertension, what is the most helpful suggestion the nurse can make regarding long-term health promotion and maintenance?
① Avoid participating in organized sports.
② Join an adolescent weight-reduction support group.
③ Limit socialization with non-overweight friends.
④ Adhere to a 1,000-calorie, low-fat diet.

11.62 A client has a nasogastric tube in place after extensive abdominal surgery and is complaining of nausea. The client's abdomen is distended, and there are no bowel sounds. What would be the first nursing action?
① Administer the PRN pain medication and antiemetic.
② Irrigate the nasogastric tube with normal saline.
③ Replace with a new nasogastric tube.
④ Check the placement and patency.

11.63 The nurse would plan on administering levothyroxine by mouth at which time of day?
① Prior to breakfast
② With lunch
③ At bedtime
④ Two hours after eating the main meal of the day

11.64 What is an appropriate plan of care for a client admitted in the acute stage of Hepatitis C? **Select all that apply.**
① Encourage intake of oatmeal, whole grains, strawberries, and apples.
② Instruct client to avoid alcohol.
③ Instruct client that after 3 months they may donate blood.
④ Encourage periods of rest initially followed by gradual increase in activity.
⑤ Administer acetaminophen for mild discomfort.

11.65 Which of these plans would be appropriate for a client requiring ostomy care? **Select all that apply.**
① Change pouch system daily.
② Eliminate popcorn, peanuts, and/or unpeeled vegetables for clients with an ileostomy.
③ Empty pouch when ¾ full.
④ Irrigate colostomy that is with the descending colon at approximately the same time daily.
⑤ Review the importance for the family to be included in the teaching plan and remain responsible for the home care.

Answers & Rationales

11.1 ① Options #1 is important to decrease pressure
④ on the skin and maintain skin integrity.
⑥ Option #4 is important to minimize risk for urinary tract infections and constipation. Option #6 will assist in decreasing skin breakdown. Options #2, #3, and #5 can contribute to skin breakdown.
I CAN HINT: Apply the clinical judgment/cognitive skill, take-action (first-do priority interventions), to the care for the elderly client.
NCLEX® Standard: Perform skin assessment and/or implement measures to maintain skin integrity and prevent skin breakdown.

11.2 ① Option #1 is correct. Immobility can result
③ in alteration in oxygenation, so it is imperative
⑤ to implement option #1 to assist in lung expansion. Option #3 is important to prevent alteration in elimination (constipation) that can result from immobility. Option #5 needs to be implemented to prevent contractures, skin breakdown, foot drop, etc. Options #2 and #4 (not in scope of practice for RN) are incorrect..
I CAN HINT: Apply the clinical judgment/cognitive skill, take-action (first-do priority interventions), to the care for the immobilized client. Priority of care for clients in traction include preventing circulatory impairment, respiratory complications, urinary retention, constipation, foot drop, skin breakdown, and care of the traction. It goes back to the concept of immobility.
NCLEX® Standard: Provide pulmonary hygiene (e.g., incentive spirometry, etc.). Manage client with an alteration in elimination. Implement measures to promote circulation.

11.3 ③ Option #3 is correct. These drugs can result in: Can't Pee, See, Spit, and Sh*t. Since the client has been taking fiber, a positive outcome would be a bowel movement daily. Options #1, #2, and #4 do not address the question. Urine is within the desired range. Specific gravity is on the higher side, but it does not address the fiber. Option #4 does not support the information in the question.
I CAN HINT: Apply the clinical judgment/cognitive skill, evaluate outcomes, for a client taking an anticholinergic.
NCLEX® Standard: Manage client with an alteration in elimination.

11.4 ③ Lithium is a salt. Adequate fluid intake should be consumed to prevent complications from the polyuria, diarrhea, N/V, and mild thirst that can occur as side effects from lithium. Option #1 is incorrect. Sodium intake should not be increased or decreased; it should remain at the normal level. Option #2 is incorrect due to the sodium restriction. If part of an answer is incorrect, the entire option is incorrect. Option #4 is incorrect due to calorie reduction, increase in sodium, and reduced fluid intake.
I CAN HINT: Apply the clinical judgment/cognitive skill, generate solutions (first-do priority plans), for the client taking lithium.
NCLEX® Standard: Evaluate client intake and output and intervene as needed.

11.5 ② Option #2 is correct. The key words in the question are "poor capillary refill, lethargy, and incontinence". The poor capillary refill indicates decrease in perfusion. The client is not active since question indicates lethargy and is incontinent. Option #2 is a priority concern with the decrease in perfusion and incontinence. Option #1 is a concern, but skin turgor is not a valid assessment for the elderly client due to the loss of elasticity. Option #3 does not answer the question and option #4 is not priority over option #2..
I CAN HINT: Apply the clinical judgment/cognitive skill, generate solutions (first-do priority plans), for the elderly client.
NCLEX® Standard: Perform skin assessment and/or implement measures to maintain skin integrity and prevent skin breakdown.

11.6 ④ Option #4 is correct. Morphine is an opioid agonist. Decreased GI peristalsis is an undesirable effect and can result in constipation. Option #1 is not priority. An effect from the drug is drowsiness. This does not read noxious stimuli; it simply reads tactile

stimulation, so is not correct over option #4. Options #2 and #3 are not significant enough to be a priority.
I CAN HINT: Apply the clinical judgment/cognitive skill, recognize cues (system-specific assessments), to the opioid agonist, Morphine. "Droopy Deuteronomy" in the book, *Pharmacology Made Insanely Easy*, by Manning and Rayfield, outlines the undesirable effects around the "6 D's": Drowsiness, Dizziness, Depressed respirations, Decreased GI peristalsis and urine output, Decreased blood pressure, and Drug dependence.
NCLEX® Standard: Manage client with an alteration in elimination.

11.7 ④ The initial treatment is to minimize pressure from the heel. Pressure can restrict flow of blood and may result in ischemia to underlying tissue. The outcome is a pressure ulcer. Stage I pressure ulcers still has skin that is intact, redness, and does not blanch with external pressure. Options #1, #2, and #3 are not appropriate for a stage I pressure ulcer on the heel of client's foot.
I CAN HINT: Apply the clinical judgment/cognitive skill, take-action (first-do priority interventions), for preventing pressure ulcers. Priority care for decreasing altered skin integrity include the following:
"PRESSURE": Position and turn every 1-2 hours; Remember nutrition and fluid intake are important. Eliminate pressure by special pressure relieving devices such as mattresses, Sheepskin pads also protect skin (clean and dry skin, wrinkle free linens, sun protection). Silicone gel pads placed under buttocks if in wheelchair. Use active and passive exercises to promote circulation. Rehydrate client. Eliminate rubbing excessively and hot water. Use soft towel, especially following toileting to keep skin clean and dry. Evaluate skin frequently, especially bony prominences.
NCLEX® Standard: Perform skin assessment and/or implement measures to maintain skin integrity and prevent skin breakdown.

11.8 ② Option #2 is correct. The initial plan would be to correct environmental factors and treatment of underlying iatrogenic and medical conditions to incorporate with the initial treatment plan. Option #1 is incorrect; actually, eliminating naps throughout the day may be useful in facilitating sleep. Option #3 is incorrect. Even though trazodone may be useful if sleep deprivation is prominent, it would not be the initial treatment plan. Option #4 is incorrect. Amitriptyline may cause excessive somnolence.
I CAN HINT: Apply the clinical judgment/cognitive skill, generate solutions (first-do priority plans), for the elderly client with a sleep disorder.
NCLEX® Standard: Assess client sleep/rest pattern and intervene as needed.

11.9

| ②Assist client to sit on the side of the bed. |
| ④Apply the transfer belt. |
| ⑤Along the client's sides, grasp the transfer belt. |
| ③Assist client to rock to a standing position. |
| ①Instruct client to pivot on the foot further from the chair. |

11.10 ② Option #2 is correct. The key to answering this question is an understanding that Addison's disease is a result of insufficient hormonal solution of mineralcorticoids and glucocorticoids which result in increased water excretion. This client may experience hypovolemia and hypotension. This is why it is important for the UAP to record the I&O, so the nurse is able to monitor and evaluate for any potential complications with fluid deficit. Option #1 is not correct and has no connection with this endocrine diagnosis. Option #3 is not correct; calories should be increased and may even need supplemental glucose. Option #4 is not correct; these are symptoms of hyperglycemia and clients with Addison's disease may experience hypoglycemia. Hypoglycemia may present with "cold and clammy skin". *"Hot and dry; my blood sugar is high, but cold and clammy; I need some candy."*

11.11 ② Options #2 and #4 are correct. The cane is
④ used on the side opposite of the affected leg for safety reasons. It provides more balance. Option #4 is correct; the cane and affected leg should be moved together. This will provide the necessary support for the balance due to one leg being weaker or not able to provide much support and will assist in the prevention of falls. Option #1 is not correct based on the rationale above. Option #3 is too far in front. Option #5 is not correct; correct rationale is in previous options.

I CAN HINT: "CANE" will assist you in organizing this information to assist with making clinical decisions regarding the use of a cane.

Cane is used on the side opposite the affected leg.

Affected leg and cane move together.

Note that the cane should be advanced simultaneously with the opposite affected lower limb.

Evaluate for correct size of cane … Measure from the wrist to the floor.

11.12 ③ Option #3 is correct. Since alcohol is drying to the skin, it should be avoided. Age-related skin changes of the elderly include fragile and dry skin. Option #1 is not correct, since it should have an SPF of 15 or greater to protect against sunburn. Option #2 is not correct. Skin lotions should be used without perfume since perfume in the lotions may increase skin irritation and increase the risk of injury to the skin resulting in skin breakdown. Option #4 is not correct.

11.13 ① Options #1, #3, and #5 are correct. Urinary
③ incontinence is a significant factor to
⑤ falls, fractures, depression, and altered skin integrity, especially in older adult clients. There are six major types of urinary incontinence. These include: stress, urge, overflow, reflux, functional, and total incontinence. Part of the collaborative care for these clients include: teaching how to perform Kegel exercises daily, reviewing the importance of avoiding or decreasing the intake of caffeine, and reviewing the rationale for avoiding alcohol consumption. Specific medications may result in the stimulation of voiding. Vaginal cone therapy may be used to strengthen pelvic muscles for clients with stress incontinence. Option #2 is not correct. While dicyclomine (Bentyl) may be used to decrease urgency for a client with a neurogenic or overactive bladder, if the client has a diagnosis of glaucoma and if this medication is taken an increase intraocular pressure may occur, so dicyclomine should not be administered to this client. The order should be verified due to inappropriateness for this client with glaucoma. Option #4 is not correct. The vitamin is not prescribed to decrease incontinence.

11.14 ① Option #1 is correct. This client is presenting with a rapid heart rate, low blood pressure and low hemoglobin with an increase in the specific gravity. This client is dry and with the Hgb being < 8 g/dL, the conclusion is the client has lost some blood or has an active bleeding occurring. Now, with this in mind, would you want the UAP to sit the client in the Fowler's position? You are so correct! The answer is NO! This would cause the blood pressure to decrease even more. The nurse needs to intervene, so client does not get more hypotensive.

11.15 ③ Option #3 is correct. This is the standard of care for the client in the post-op period following a hip replacement. Options #1 and #2 can pop the prosthesis out of the socket. Option #4 is incorrect. This can also result in prosthesis displacement.

11.16 ① Option #1 is correct. This indicates safe
② practice. Option #2 is correct. This does
⑤ indicate an understanding of safe practice with walker care. Option #3 is incorrect. The standard of care should be to have the client wear safe shoes. Option #4 is incorrect. The walker should only be advanced approximately 12 inches (30.5 cm). Sixteen inches (40.6 cm) are too much and may result in a fall. Option #5 is correct practice and demonstrates an understanding of safe walker care.

11.17 ④ Options #4 and #5 are correct. Clients may
⑤ be instructed with the following to assist in developing a bedtime routine. In addition to limiting naps throughout the day and continuing with routines from home, such as an evening bath, older clients can be

encouraged to exercise regularly at least 2 hours prior to bedtime. Organize the sleep environment for comfort. Caffeine, alcohol, and nicotine should be limited at least 4 hr prior to bedtime. Fluids should be limited to 2 to 4 hours prior to bedtime. If client is anxious or stressed, engage in muscle relaxation. If someone is available for a back rub 15 min. prior to going to bed, this can also be very therapeutic. Warm milk and crackers can be soothing prior to going to bed. Options #1, #2, and #3 are incorrect for assisting with sleep.

11.18 ④ Option #4 is correct. Music therapy has been proved by research that it will assist in clients' daily living activities and provide a different and new focus. Option #1 is incorrect. This must be performed by a skilled practitioner. Option #2 does not include an alternative therapy. Option #3 is incorrect. The nurse is able to answer this question and provide recommendations to the client.
I CAN HINT: In reviewing these options, notice that options #1, #2, and #3 are focused on someone other than the client. The correct option focuses on what the client can do. If you have no idea what the answer is, a great decision making strategy is to focus on the client.

11.19 ③ Option #3 is the correct answer. As you read the question, you want to ask yourself how does this medication work? If you only remember, that it works by binding with the protein which is then excreted through the stools then this will help you be successful! If the client experiences too many stools, then the complication of metabolic acidosis may occur. These labs, pH and HCO_3 indicate a complication with metabolic acidosis. Option #1 is an expected finding in liver disease. This is the reason the client is receiving the medication. The normal serum ammonia levels should be 15 to 45 mcg/dL (8.81–26.42 μmol/L). Option #4 is also an expected finding with a client who has a diagnosis of cirrhosis or hepatitis. The normal ranges for these are: AST—5 to 40 units/L; ALT—7 to 56 units/L. Option #2 is a normal value. Normal serum potassium level is 3.5 to 5.0 mEq/L (3.5 to 5.0 mmol/L).

11.20

④Explain procedure to client and assist client to high-Fowler's position if possible.
③Measure the tubing from the tip of the nose, to the tip of the ear lobe, to the tip of the xiphoid, and mark it with adhesive tape.
⑤Put on gloves and Lubricate the tip.
②Gradually insert the tube and when tubing reaches the mark, anchor the tube using tape.
①Aspirate gently to collect gastric contents and test pH.

11.21 ① Option #1 will minimize scratching that
④ could lead to bleeding. Option #4 should be
⑤ avoided due to the low platelet count.
⑥ Option #5 is consistent with hepatic encephalopathy and requires further intervention. Option #6: mental fogginess, mild confusion, etc., may be the result of the ammonia levels that have crossed the blood-brain barrier into the brain tissue. Option #2 could result in skin breakdown. Option #3 could result in bleeding from the ongoing tightness of the cuff squeezing on the arm.

11.22 ② Option #2 is correct. The Braden scale is a tool for predicting pressure sore risk which includes six subscales: sensory perception, moisture, activity, mobility, nutrition, and friction and shear. Each of the subscales rates factors within the above schema from 1 (least favorable) to 4 (most favorable), for a total of 23 points. A score of 16 to 18 points or less is the cut off for adults in predicting risk. This client does not have one point off of the scale. The care would be to document findings and continue the prevention plan. It is obviously working out with great outcomes. Option #1 is incorrect since the no. on the scale does not indicate the high risk category. Option #3 is incorrect since this scale does not measure the pressure ulcer status over time. The Braden scale evaluates the risk assessment for developing a pressure ulcer. The Pressure Ulcer Scale for Healing (PUSH Tool) is the tool that was developed by the National Pressure Ulcer Advisory Panel (NPUAP) as a quick, reliable tool to monitor the change in pressure ulcer status over time. Option #4 is incorrect since there is no need for a treatment plan.

11.23 ④ Option #4 is correct. Options #1, #2, and #3 are incorrect. Option #1 should be in a sterile container. Option #2, client may be on a specific type of diet prior to test being done to minimize false results. Option #3 should be collected from various areas of stool.

11.24 ④ Option #4 is correct. These are high in folic acid that is important due to lack of erythropoietin. Option #1 is incorrect. This is unsafe, since magnesium can be elevated with this medical condition. Options #2 and #3 may be contraindicated due to risk of hyperkalemia.

11.25 ③ Research shows that around-the-clock (ATC) administration of analgesics is more effective in maintaining blood levels to alleviate the pain associated with cancer. Options #1 and #2 actually decrease the amount of pain medication. Option #4 might be too frequent an interval.

11.26 ① Option #1 is correct. Fluid retention is best detected by weighing daily and noting a gaining trend. Options #2 and #3 are incorrect and will not provide information regarding fluid retention. Option #4 can provide an estimation of the amount of urine output, but not about fluid retention.

11.27 ② This is a priority when establishing a program. Option #1 is incorrect. Option #3 may not always be necessary in all programs. Option #4 would only be appropriate for a client with overflow incontinence.

11.28 **57.6 mL**

Step One: Determine the amount of fluid loss. (One gram of dry weight is equal to 1 mL of fluid loss)
12 diapers x 5 grams = 60 grams

Step Two: Determine the weight the dry diapers.
12 x 0.2 grams = 2.4 grams

Step Three: Determine total mL lost by infant.
60 grams − 2.4 grams = 57.6 grams

I CAN HINT: Remember: 1 gram of dry weight is = to 1 mL of fluid. Remember to subtract the weight of each dry diaper prior to documenting fluid loss from the infant.

11.29 ④ Option #4 is correct. During the diagnostic procedure, the abdomen is insufflated with CO_2 to assist the laparoscope to be inserted and assist in visualization. This CO_2 may result in shoulder discomfort. Option #1 is incorrect. Option #2 is not reported in research to demonstrate any evidence that this would alter this type of pain. Option #3 is incorrect. This action is unrelated to this type of pain from the procedure.

11.30 ② This will be the best plan to minimize trauma and be effective. Option #1 is not necessary in this situation. Option #3 is inappropriate. Option #4 is incorrect since fluid should never be forced down any tube.

11.31 ② Blood pressures should always be taken on the arm opposite the one used for hemodialysis. Option #1 is incorrect because IVs should not be started in the grafted arm. Option #3 is not necessary after surgery. Option #4 would not necessarily prevent complications which is what the question is asking.

11.32 ④ Phenazopyridine (Pyridium) should be taken with food to minimize gastric distress. Option #1 is not a typical symptom of pyelonephritis. Option #2 is incorrect because this drug normally turns the urine red. Option #3 is incorrect because this drug does not make urine cloudy.

11.33 ② Increasing fluids is an appropriate independent nursing action that facilitates the removal of concentrated urine. Options #1 and #3 are incorrect because they do not address the problem of the client's urine. Option #4 is incorrect and cannot be performed without a physician's order.

11.34 ③ Option #3 is correct. This would be a concern as the expected outcome for 48 hours following a TURP would be the urine should be pink in color, not dark red. Option #1 is incorrect. There is no need for further intervention since this is an expected finding for the first post-operative day. Option #2 is also an expected outcome and would not be a concern. Option #4 is incorrect. This is a desired outcome on day 3 and would not require further intervention.

11.35 ③ Sulfonamides need to be given with lots of fluids to prevent crystallization in the kidney tubules. The client should continue on the medication even after the symptoms subside. They may turn the urine an orange-red color temporarily. If the client has ulcerative colitis, medication would be continued even with diarrhea; HCP should be notified. Options #1, #2 and #4 contain incorrect information.

11.36 ③ Option #3 is a priority. Within 24 hours client should be voiding normally. Options #1, #2, and #4 are incorrect. Option #1 should be increased. Option #2 is not totally correct. The size of the catheter should have been documented when it was placed. Option #4 is important but is not a priority for this question.

11.37 ③ When the bowel perforates as a result of increased intraluminal pressure within the gut, intestinal juices are released into the peritoneum leading to peritonitis. Option #1 is incorrect because the client is kept in semi-Fowler's position. Option #2 is correct but is not a priority action. Option #4 is incorrect because it would be unwise to remove the nasogastric tube.

11.38 ② After surgery, a small amount of blood-tinged urine is normal. However, the client is taught that the urine should be clear. Options #1, #3, and #4 are incorrect because ureteral catheters are not to be clamped, advanced, or irrigated due to the small size of the ureter and the potential for trauma.

11.39 ④ The basic guidelines to teach a post-gastrectomy client are measures to prevent dumping syndrome. Option #1 is incorrect because the client is taught to lie down for 30 minutes after meals. Options #2 and #3 are incorrect because the client is taught to limit the intake of fluids, avoid highly spiced foods, and avoid high carbohydrate foods during meals.

11.40 ① Following TURP, the client will not have physiological impotency. Option #2 is correct because this could be an early indication of urinary retention. Options #3 and #4 are correct and indicate the client understands his post-operative management.

11.41 ④ Option #4 is correct. The procedure is a surgery on the lower back area. Alignment and stability are the priority in the care. Options #1, #2, and #3 do not provide the appropriate alignment and stability needed for this procedure.

11.42 ① There is distention above the level of obstruction and initially hyperactive bowel sounds. Options #2, #3, and #4 are incorrect because there would be no stool as motility distal or below the obstruction would cease. Therefore, no diarrhea, rectal bleeding, or a tarry stool would be present.

11.43 ③ Option #3 is correct. Mild discomfort is expected with the first few exchanges until the peritoneal space has expanded to accommodate fluid. This will subside after several exchanges. Option #1 is unnecessary unless the client experiences acute pain. Option #2 is incorrect. This will interfere with the effectiveness of the dialysis. Option #4 is not necessary at this time.

11.44 ③ Option #3 is a priority due to count indicating infection. Option #1 is slightly low but is not a priority concern. In Option #2 the WBC is within normal limits. Option #4 is not a priority.

11.45 ③ A return demonstration is the most reliable method to evaluate the effectiveness of teaching. Options #1 and #4 are effective as initial presentation methods when teaching. Option #2 is not as effective as option #3.

11.46 ② The normal plasma potassium level is 3.5–5.0 mEq/L (3.5–5.0 mmol/L). This client's potassium is low and needs replacement. Options #1, #3, and #4 do not address the problem.

11.47 ④ An infant with reflux should be maintained in an upright position. The head of the bed should be raised at a 30-degree angle. Option #1 may not be necessary, if positioning is effective. Option #2 is an action for the mother versus the infant. Option #3 is incorrect because the client's feedings should be changed to small volume, frequent feedings.

11.48 ② Since metaclopramide (Reglan) facilitates gastric emptying, it must be taken before meals. Options #1 and #3 do not promote optimum effects of the medication. Option #4 is incorrect because the time of administration should be changed to give with the client's meals.

11.49 ③ Option #3 is an appropriate diet for a client with cirrhosis of the liver. Options #1, #2, and #4 are inappropriate for this disorder.

11.50 ② An infant should be NPO 3 hours prior to the procedure. Options #1 and #3 are inappropriate. Option #4 is incorrect because it is not necessary for an infant to be NPO for 6 hours.

11.51 ① This provides the most pertinent data in assessing actual growth. Option #2 is inappropriate for this situation. Options #3 and #4 are important assessments but are not a priority to Option #1.

11.52 ④ Diabetic ketoacidosis is frequently associated with dehydration. Fluids should be encouraged. Option #1 is incorrect because a diabetic should alter the dose according to serial glucose checks. Option #2 is incorrect because the client is not tolerating PO foods. Option #3 is incorrect because sweets can be used as calories in this situation.

11.53 ① Option #1 is correct. Cystic Fibrosis primarily affects the lungs, pancreas, and sweat glands. In the pulmonary system, the thick mucus provides an excellent medium for bacterial growth and secondary respiratory tract infections. Fluids are an excellent action to decrease the viscosity and assist with expectorating and this is within the scope of practice for the UAP. Option #2 is incorrect since the diet should be high-calorie; high-protein; fats as tolerated; increase salt intake. Option #3 is incorrect since the enzymes should be taken with meals. Option #4 is incorrect since this is not within the scope of practice for the UAP. The UAP does not teach.

11.54 ④ The rubber tip can be placed in from the side of the mouth to avoid the operative area and to prevent sucking on the tubing. Infants with cleft lip swallow excessive amounts of air so they require frequent bubbling. Options #1 and #3 are unsafe due to the risk for aspiration. Option #2 is incorrect because the site should be cleansed with saline or hydrogen peroxide.

11.55 ③ Regular insulin peaks in 2–4 hours. These are signs of hypoglycemia which may occur. Option #1 is incorrect because Kussmaul's respirations are signs of hyperglycemia. Options #2 and #4 are not indicative of hypoglycemia.

11.56 ② Clear liquids should be offered first. As child tolerates these fluids, then full liquids may be offered. Options #1, #3, and #4 are all part of a full liquid diet.

11.57

③ Assess bowel function by auscultation for peristalsis.
① Assist client into semi-Fowler's position.
④ Flush tube with 10 mL of normal saline. *Flushing will ensure that the tube doesn't contain stomach contents that could irritate tissues during tube removal.*
② Ask client to hold her breath. *This is to close epiglottis.*
⑤ Withdraw the tube gently and steadily.

11.58 ② Option #2 could result in a complication with autonomic dysreflexia. This would be a medical emergency, so intervention is imperative to prevent this from occurring. Option #1 is an expected behavior with the diagnosis. Option #3 is expected during respiratory therapy. Option #4 is important, but is not going to result in a medical emergency.

11.59 ④ Only sips of water are permitted for 12 hours before plasma cholesterol screening for accurate results. Options #1 and #3 are incorrect because a normal diet should be eaten the week before the test. Option #2 is incorrect because alcohol intake will interfere with test results.

11.60 ③ It is important to know what the 3:00 AM blood sugar is to determine if the hyperglycemia is from the somogyi effect. Options #1 and #4 will be adjusted after knowing if the AM blood sugar is the accurate reading or a rebound response to a low blood sugar at 3:00 AM. Option #2 is incorrect.

11.61 ② This is an excellent means of obtaining information and support while helping the client. Option #1 is incorrect because properly supervised physical activity is desirable, not to be avoided. Option #3 is incorrect because peer relationships are important, not to be avoided. Option #4 is not enough calories for an adolescent, and a diet too low in calories is hard to comply with and may set the adolescent up for failure.

11.62 ④ The first assessment in determining problems with nasogastric tubes is to determine tube placement and patency. Option #1 may be implemented after the placement and patency of the tube are determined. Option #2 would be completed only after option #4 was completed. Option #3 is inappropriate without further assessment.

11.63 ① Option #1 is correct since administering levothyroixine (Synthroid) prior to breakfast will reduce the possibility of insomnia, and the body avoids the need to fight the digestion of food with the digestion of the medication due to the 50–80% absorption rate associated with oral forms of this drug. Option #2 is contraindicated because the body will digest the food slowing the absorption rate of the medication. Option #3 is incorrect because insomnia is associated with this drug. Consequently, administration at bedtime will heighten the chances of sleep disruption. Option #4 is incorrect.

11.64 ① ② ④ Options #1, #2, and #4 are correct. Option #1 includes foods that increase the carbohydrate in the diet, which would be recommended for a client with hepatitis. Option #2 is correct since the diseased liver is unable to metabolize potential toxins like alcohol. Option #4 is correct because rest is important during the acute stages of the disease, so the metabolic demands on the liver are decreased and there is time for healing. As the client improves, they can increase their activity, but pace it with rest periods. Option #3 is incorrect because a client with a history of hepatitis should never give blood. Option #5 is incorrect. Acetaminophen is hepatoxic, so it should be contraindicated for this client.

11.65 ② ④ Option #2 is correct. High-fiber food can cause severe diarrhea for clients with an ileostomy. Clients with a colostomy should resume the regular diet gradually. Foods that were a problem preoperatively should be introduced cautiously. Option #4 is correct. Clients with descending-colon colostomies can irrigate to provide control over effluence. Clients should irrigate at approximately the same time daily. Clients should use warm water (cold or hot water may cause cramping). Clients should wash around the stoma with lukewarm water and a mild soap. Commercial skin barriers may be purchased for home use. Foods in diet that cause offensive odors can be eliminated. Option #1 is incorrect. The pouch system should be changed every 3 to 7 days. Option #3 is incorrect. The pouch should be emptied when it is one third to one half full. Option #5 is incorrect. Although the family definitely should be included in the teaching plan regarding ostomy care, the client is ultimately responsible for own care.

Notes

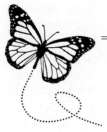

CHAPTER 12
Pharmacological and Parenteral Therapies

> Words of course are the most powerful drugs used by mankind.
> — UNKNOWN

✔ Clarification of this test ...

Note: this percentage has increased to 13–19% with the new NCLEX-RN®. Clarification of this test includes performing and directing activities necessary for safe administration of medications (adverse effects, dosage calculation, expected effects/outcomes, contraindications and side effects, blood and blood products, pharmacological interactions, pain management, and TPN).

- ☛ Prepare and administer medications using rights of medication administration.
- ☛ Handle and maintain medication in a safe and controlled environment.
- ☛ Evaluate client response to medication.
- ☛ Review pertinent data prior to medication administration (e.g., contraindications, lab results, allergies, potential interactions).
- ☛ Evaluate appropriateness and accuracy of medication order for client.
- ☛ Monitor intravenous infusion and maintain site.
- ☛ Handle and administer controlled substances within regulatory guidelines.
- ☛ Administer medications for pain management.
- ☛ Educate client about medications.
- ☛ Dispose of medications safely.
- ☛ Handle and administer high-risk medications safely.
- ☛ Access and/or maintain central venous access devices.
- ☛ Perform calculations needed for medication administration.
- ☛ Titrate dosage of medication based on assessment and ordered parameters.
- ☛ Participate in medication reconciliation process.
- ☛ Administer parenteral nutrition and evaluate client response.
- ☛ Administer blood products and evaluate client response.

Adapted from: © National Council of State Boards of Nursing, Inc. (NCSBN). (2022). 2021 *RN Practice Analysis: Linking the NCLEX-RN® Examination to Practice*. Chicago: Author.
Adapted from: © National Council of State Boards of Nursing, Inc. (NCSBN). (2023) *Next Generation NCLEX® NCLEX-RN® Test Plan. Chicago*: Author.

12.1 The nurse is finishing shift report. Which client would the nurse intervene with first after report and administer the prescribed medication?
① A client with myasthenia gravis with a prescription for neostigmine.
② A post-operative GI client who is requesting pain medication with pain rated a 6 on a 1 to 10 pain scale.
③ A client presenting with a temperature of 101.4° F (38.56° C) who has a prescription for cephalexin.
④ A client with Addison's disease and has a prescription for a steroid.

12.2 What plan will the nurse include in care for the client who is newly diagnosed with type 2 diabetes mellitus (DM) and has been prescribed metformin?
① Monitor and report creatinine level 1.2 mg/dL (106.1 μmol/L).
② Monitor and report a HbA1C 7%.
③ Monitor and report a respiratory rate of 30 breaths/min and muscle aches.
④ Monitor a weight loss of 1 pound in 1 week.

12.3 The LPN is administering medications to a group of clients. Which of these clinical situations should the charge nurse intervene with immediately?
① Lispro insulin is administered to a client when the breakfast tray arrives.
② Metoprolol is administered prior to surgery for a client with pheochromocytoma.
③ Propranolol is administered to a client with hyperthyroidism.
④ Metformin HCL is administered to a client with a creatinine of 3.8 mg/dL (335.93 μmol/L).

12.4 What is the priority clinical assessment finding that the nurse should report to the health care provider for a client taking chlorpromazine?
① Complaints of dizziness when rising quickly from the supine position.
② Complaints of a sore throat.
③ Presents with a skin rash.
④ Presents with a dry mouth.

12.5 What is the most important for the nurse to monitor while administering metoprolol? Select all that apply? **Select all that apply.**
① Serum glucose - 50 mg/dL
② Blood pressure - 98/62
③ Heart rate - 90 bpm
④ Heart block
⑤ Ventricular tachycardia
⑥ Heart rate - 58 bpm

12.6 What information will the nurse include in plan of care for a client with a new prescription for lovastatin?
① Instruct client that lipids will decrease within 7-10 days.
② Review the importance of taking acetaminophen daily for muscle pain.
③ Advise to take on an empty stomach at 8 AM.
④ Review the importance of not taking lovastatin with grapefruit juice.

12.7 Which plan will the nurse include in the nursing care for a client taking topotecan for ovarian cancer?
① Report nausea and vomiting.
② Report oozing of blood around IV site.
③ Advise client to expect to experience a sore throat.
④ Review the importance taking the influenza vaccination in the fall.

12.8 Which order should the nurse verify if appropriate for a client admitted to the Emergency Department with a diagnosis of acute diverticulitis?
① Administer morphine as prescribed for pain.
② Administer meperidine as prescribed for pain.
③ Insert a nasogastric tube.
④ Start intravenous fluid of D_5W at 115 mL/hour.

12.9 Which of these clinical assessment findings require the nurse to immediately intervene following shift report for a violent client who has received multiple injections of PRN haloperidol to control behavior? **Select all that apply.**
① 8 AM: T - 99. 1° F; 9 AM: T-103.6° F.
② 8 AM: HR- 88 bpm; 9 AM: HR- 128 bpm.
③ 8 AM: BP- 140/80; 9 AM: BP - 110/68.
④ 8 AM: Eating diet; 9 AM: complaining of nausea and vomiting.
⑤ 8 AM: Dry skin; 9 AM: diaphoresis

12.10 A nurse is closely monitoring the client in the Intensive Care Unit who is receiving amiodarone by intravenous drip. The nurse understands that the infusion must be stopped if any of these EKG changes occur. **Select all that apply.**
① Sinus bradycardia
② Atrioventricular (AV) block
③ Ventricular tachycardia
④ Atrial fibrillation
⑤ Q-T prolongation
⑥ Premature atrial contractions

12.11 The team consists of a registered nurse (RN) and licensed practical nurse (LPN/VN). Which of these assignments would be most appropriate to delegate to the LPN/VN?
① A toddler admitted to the Pediatric Oncology Unit for IV chemotherapy and needs evaluation of response to chemotherapy.
② A preschool child with asthma who has a new order for albuterol via metered-dose inhaler—2 inhalations q 4 to 6 hours that needs a plan of care developed.
③ A young adult with cancer who needs a subcutaneous injection of filgrastim subcutaneous as prescribed.
④ A middle-aged adult admitted for a blood transfusion of 1 unit of packed red blood cells over 4 hours.

12.12 Which of these clinical findings would be priority for the nurse to question a new prescription for acetaminophen 650 mg every 4 hours PRN pain?
① HR – 88 bpm
② Blood pressure – 140/89 mm Hg
③ Currently takes atorvastatin for hypercholesterolemia
④ Joint discomfort

12.13 During the discharge teaching for a client with a diagnosis of asthma who has an order to take albuterol with a meted-dose inhaler (MDI), which order should the nurse teach client to use when taking the MDI safely and appropriately? Place in chronological order. Use all of the options and reorder this list of answers using drag and drop. (1 is the first step and 5 is the last step.)

| ① Breathe out through the nose. |
| ② Activate the MDI when inhaling. |
| ③ Wash hands. |
| ④ Hold breath for 5 to 10 seconds and then exhale. |
| ⑤ Shake the inhaler. |

| |
| |
| |
| |
| |

12.14 Which of these actions by the client who is using a metered-dose inhaler (MDI) for taking albuterol indicates an appropriate understanding of safe use of the MDI? **Select all that apply.**
① When two puffs are needed, the client allows for 1 minute elapse between the two.
② The activation of the MDI is coordinated with expiration.
③ Special care is taken not to shake the inhaler prior to using.
④ When using the MDI, the client inspires slowly.
⑤ Client understands that albuterol is used on a continuous basis in the absence of symptoms.

12.15 What is the priority of care for a client with a new prescription order for enoxaparin IM daily?
① Leave the bubble in the syringe when administering enoxaparin.
② Identify the client prior to administering the medication.
③ Rub the site gently after administering.
④ Notify the provider of care and question the appropriateness of the order.

12.16 Prior to administration of raloxifene, which data would be most pertinent for the nurse to review?
① Results from Dual-energy Xray absorptiometry (DEXA) scan.
② Past medical history with attention to risks for blood clots.
③ Most recent hematocrit and hemoglobin.
④ Client's ability to remain upright for 30 minutes after administration.

12.17 Which of these interventions would be included in the plan of care for a client presenting to the emergency department with a diagnosis of Diabetic Ketoacidosis (DKA)? **Select all that apply.**
① Administer Novolin N insulin IV as prescribed.
② Obtain IV access for 0.9 Normal Saline bolus.
③ Monitor for potassium greater than 5.0 mEq/L (5.0 mmol/L).
④ Review ABG for pH—7.48; HCO_3—29 mEq/L (29 mmol/L); pCO_2—44 mm Hg.
⑤ Review urinalysis results for ketones.

12.18 Which of these plans would be important for a client with a new order for Sumatriptan? **Select all that apply.**
① Review with client the importance of notifying the health care provider for continuous or severe chest pain.
② Review the importance of taking isocarboxazid with this medication.
③ With the initial dose, monitor the blood pressure 2 to 4 hours before and after.
④ In addition to the medication, encourage client to lie down in a quiet, dark room to assist in decreasing complications from the migraine.
⑤ Advise not to drive until medication effect has been established.

12.19 Which is the best action by the nurse who has drawn 2 mg of Morphine Sulfate into a syringe, and the client refuses the medication?
① Label the syringe and send it back to the pharmacy.
② Waste the medication with another RN witness and document.
③ Explain to the client that the medication is drawn up and needs to be administered.
④ Label the medication with the date and time, and save it for the next scheduled dose.

12.20 A client has an order for Humulin N 70/30 insulin 18 units every morning subcutaneously plus the following sliding scale for Humulin Regular U-100 insulin before meals and at bedtime subcutaneously?

Blood Glucose Level	
(mg/dL)	Regular Insulin
Less than 70 mg/dL (3.89 mmol/L)	Call MD
70-120 mg/dL (3.89-6.66 mmol/L)	0 units
121-175 mg/dL (6.72-9.71 mmol/L)	2 units
176-225 mg/dL (9.77-12.49 mmol/L)	4 units
226-275 mg/dL (12.54-15.26 mmol/L)	6 units
276-325 mg/dL (15.32-18.04 mmol/L)	8 units
325-375 mg/dL (18.04-20.82 mmol/L)	10 units
376-425 mg/dL (20.87-23.59 mmol/L)	12 units
Greater than 426 mg/dL (23.65 mmol/L)	Call MD

At 0800, the client's blood sugar is 384 mg/dL (21.31 mmol/L). Shade in the amount the nurse will administer.

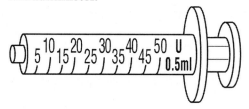

12.21 The nurse is caring for an older adult client who is 3 hours post-op total hip replacement with a history of COPD, and receiving Hydromorphone via PCA pump. The morning assessment reveals HR—62 bpm; RR—7 per min, client cannot be aroused from sleep. Which is the priority action by the nurse?
① Position the client in high-Fowler's.
② Administer oxygen at 8 liters via simple face mask.
③ Call the health care provider.
④ Administer naloxone 1 mg slow IV push.

12.22 Which is the best indication that Hetastarch is effective for a client who has a serum lactate level of 54 mg/dL (6 mmol/L); temperature—103°F (39.4°C); and heart rate of 128 bpm?
① BP increase to 118/78
② Urine output = 160 ml over the past 4 hours
③ PT = 35 seconds, aPTT = 102 seconds, INR = 3
④ Temperature = 98.5°F (36.9°C)

12.23 The RN is delegating tasks for the day. Which task would the RN assign to the LPN?
① Administer carbamazepine po to a client with a carbamazepine level = 2.1 mg/L and reassess medication level over time.
② Develop a nutritional plan for a client on long-term phenytoin therapy.
③ Trend changes in ALT/AST and assess for bleeding in a client who takes phenobarbitol.
④ Implement second teaching session to reinforce proper gum care for a client taking phenytoin.

12.24 Which laboratory data is most important for the nurse to review before discharging a 17-year-old female with a new prescription for isotretinoin?
① BUN and Creatinine
② CBC with differential
③ Serum HCG
④ Wound culture

12.25 Which of the following medications requires the nurse to caution the client about exposure to the sun? Select all that apply.
① Trimethoprim and Sulfamethoxazole
② Tetracycline
③ Cephalexin
④ Azithromycin
⑤ St. John's Wort

12.26 What instruction from the nurse should be included in the teaching plan for a client who is taking pramlintide for type 1 diabetes mellitus?
① "Administer medication with the AM dose of insulin in the same syringe."
② "Freeze unused vials of pramlintide."
③ "Administer oral medications 1 to 2 hours after injection of pramlintide."
④ "Recognize that the solution is cloudy, and this is an expected finding."

12.27 During the administration of Amphotericin B, what is the priority of nursing care?
① Assess for a spiked T-wave and report to health care provider.
② Monitor for a low digoxin level.
③ Encourage a diet low in calories and protein.
④ Evaluate the IV site for phlebitis.

12.28 What is the priority of care before pushing a medication via a heparin lock?
① Change the angiocath every 48 hours.
② Change the dressing every 24 hours.
③ Check for a flashback prior to administering the medication.
④ Flush the heparin lock with 25 mL fluid prior to administering the medication.

12.29 A client is being treated with Lorazepam 5 mg IV q hour. Which nursing action is a priority after administration?
① Have naloxone at the bedside and ready for administration.
② Obtain a baseline pulse oximetry reading.
③ Do a complete neurological exam every shift.
④ Check respiratory status every 15 minutes.

12.30 Which action would be appropriate for a client receiving a continuous infusion of heparin with a PTT greater than 150 seconds?
① Slow the heparin drip.
② Stop the heparin and notify the health care provider.
③ Maintain the heparin at the current infusion rate.
④ Increase the infusion rate and notify the health care provider.

12.31 Which medication would the nurse question?
① Carvedilol for a client with COPD
② Enalapril for a client being discharged post MI
③ Hydrochlorothiazide for a client with stage 1 hypertension
④ Digoxin for an adult patient with a heart rate of 64

12.32 What would the nurse teach a client who is being discharged with sublingual nitroglycerin?
① Take the medication 5 minutes after the pain has started.
② Stop taking the medication if a burning sensation is present.
③ Take the medication on an empty stomach.
④ Avoid abrupt changes in posture when taking nitroglycerin.

12.33 While monitoring a client receiving pain relief from client-controlled analgesia (PCA), what should be the priority care for this client?
   ① Set the pump's hourly infusion rate to equal total mL/hour needed to control pain.
   ② Evaluate the client for orthostatic hypotension.
   ③ Monitor the respiratory rate for tachypnea.
   ④ Inform the client that all of his pain can be controlled by simply pushing a button.

12.34 What would be the most appropriate nursing action for a child after administering Dimetane-DC cough syrup and noting the child has become excitable and restless?
   ① Report the child's behavior to the health care provider.
   ② Decrease the dose by half in the future.
   ③ Have the child drink a glass of warm milk to dilute the medication.
   ④ Chart the client's response to the medication and alert the next shift.

12.35 An elderly client experiencing diarrhea for 4 days has been taking Kaopectate at home. Which nursing assessment indicates a complication of kaolin and pectin mixtures?
   ① Itching
   ② Fecal impaction
   ③ Nausea
   ④ Dysrhythmia

12.36 Which assessment finding indicates a side effect of meperidine and hydroxyzine hydrochloride for an elderly client?
   ① Tachypnea
   ② Lethargy
   ③ Hypertension
   ④ Disorientation

12.37 What is the priority of care for a postpartum client who has Ibuprofen 600 mg ordered Q 6 hours ATC (around the clock) and has been complaining of cramping and bleeding that has been heavy since delivery, 4 hours ago? Labs drawn on admission (pre-delivery) are as follows: WBC—14,000 mm^3; HGB—10.8 g/dL; HCT—28.6%; Platelets—120,000/mm^3?
   ① Start a pad count.
   ② Start a calorie count.
   ③ Substitute Aleve for Ibuprofen.
   ④ Hold the Ibuprofen; consult with the health care provider.

12.38 The nurse is preparing to start a blood transfusion of 250 mL packed cells to the client. Which would be most important for the nurse to consider during this process?
   ① Hang D_5W for flushing blood tubing.
   ② Start transfusion at 60 mL per hour.
   ③ Warm the blood in the microwave.
   ④ Start transfusion with a 19-gauge needle.

12.39 Which observation indicates the most common side effect of trimethoprim-sulfamethoxazole?
   ① Hypotonia
   ② Loss of hearing
   ③ Hypotension
   ④ Urticaria

12.40 Before beginning a dopamine infusion on a client, what is the priority assessment?
   ① Urine output
   ② Weight
   ③ Patency of IV
   ④ Pulmonary artery pressures

12.41 The nurse is assessing a client who is scheduled to receive diltiazem. What is the priority of care after the nurse reviews the chart below?

Vital Signs		
Date	8/4/15	8/5/15
Time	8 AM	8 AM
Temp.	97.8°F (36.6°C)	98.2°F (36.8°C)
Heart Rate	86	58
Respirations	20	22
BP	124/88	118/72

   ① Administer the medication as prescribed.
   ② Administer and advise the UAP to monitor the blood pressure every 2 hours.
   ③ Hold the medication and notify the provider of care.
   ④ Discuss the undesirable effect of this medication with the client.

12.42 Which of these clients would be seen initially after shift report?
① A client with an order for interferon 2A, but the RN refuses to administer due to a history of egg allergy.
② A client who is receiving doxorubicin and complaining of nausea and vomiting.
③ A client with cancer who is receiving vincristine and is complaining of discomfort at IV site.
④ A client with cancer who is receiving bleomycin and is beginning to present with alopecia.

12.43 Which of these nursing actions from a nurse who is admitting an older client to the medical unit with a history of diabetes mellitus, asthma, and hypertension require further intervention by the charge nurse?
① The nurse requests the family members to be involved with the medication reconciliation.
② The nurse is reconciling any written medication that the client has been taking prior to admission.
③ The nurse is reconciling medication orders only written by the health care provider (HCP).
④ The nurse explains to the client and family that medication reconciliation is a Joint Commission National Patient Safety Goal.

12.44 An adult client is admitted to the outpatient clinic to receive 2 units of blood for a hemoglobin of 7.0 g/dL. Which of these actions is vital to administering the blood safely? **Select all that apply.**
① Follow protocol and check client identity with blood label by two nurses.
② Place client in a private room near the nurse's station in case of allergic reaction.
③ Administer the blood slowly at 15 gtts/minute for the first 15 minutes.
④ Check client BP, pulse, and temperature every 15 minutes during the first hour for possible indications of blood transfusion reaction.
⑤ Discontinue the blood immediately and keep the vein open with D_5W if there is a documented reaction.

12.45 What is the priority action before administering terbutaline to a client in labor who has a HR—144 bpm?
① Withhold the medication.
② Decrease the dose in half.
③ Administer the medication.
④ Wait 15 minutes; recheck the pulse rate.

12.46 The nurse is administering morning medications to assigned clients. Which of the following clients would the nurse with hold the medication and contact the health care provider?
① The client on furosemide that had a urine output of 60 mL/hour over the past 12 hours.
② The client on Digoxin who has a heart rate that is 98 and regular.
③ The client on Digoxin with a potassium of 3.8 mEq/L (3.8 mmol/L).
④ The client on an enalapril that is complaining of swollen lips.

12.47 Which of these clinical findings indicate effectiveness of treatment after the administration of Nitroprusside IV drip to a client in the Intensive Care Unit?
① Heart rate decreased to 60 from 120 beats per minute.
② Blood pressure decreased from 190/120 to 136/78 within minutes.
③ Chest pain decreased from sharp and stabbing level 10 to mild and level 5.
④ Relief of nausea and vomiting.

12.48 What is the most appropriate nursing action for a client with a new order from the provider of care for an intramuscular injection of neostigmine to a client with a history of asthma?
① Administer the medication.
② Check blood pressure and pulse.
③ Notify the health care provider, so the medication can be changed.
④ Ask the pharmacist if the medication can be given by mouth.

12.49 A client has been taking perphenazine by mouth for two days and now displays the following:
- head turned to the side and arched at an angle
- stiffness, and
- muscle spasms in neck.

Which PRN medication would the nurse give?

① Promazine
② Biperiden
③ Thiothixene
④ Haloperidol

12.50 Which statement by a client reflects a correct understanding of alprazolam?

① "I can take it whenever I feel upset."
② "I should not take this with anything but water."
③ "I need to quit drinking white wine."
④ "This medication will help me forget and go on."

12.51 The nurse administers meperidine 50 mg IM for pain as per physician's orders. Three hours later, the client again complains of pain, and the nurse administers a second injection of meperidine. Which statement describes the nurse's liability?

① The nurse administered the medication appropriately; there is no liability.
② The nurse violated the narcotic law in not having an order to administer the meperidine a second time.
③ The client was not injured. Therefore, the nurse is not liable.
④ The nurse should have waited at least 4 hours then there would be no liability.

12.52 Which response would the nurse recognize as the desired outcome to levodopa in the treatment of Parkinson's Disease?

① Dyskinesia
② Complete remission of symptoms
③ Less rigidity
④ Decrease in fine motor tremors

12.53 What is the priority action for a client who is receiving vancomycin 500 mg IV over 30 minutes and develops a flushed neck and face?

① Decrease the rate of the vancomycin.
② Discontinue the infusion.
③ Evaluate the client's temperature and vital signs.
④ Notify provider of care for an order for an antihistamine.

12.54 What is the best plan for the administration schedule for an adult taking a psychostimulant, such as methylphenidate?

① Breakfast and bedtime
② Early morning, late afternoon
③ Breakfast time—not after 2:00 PM
④ Late afternoon, dinner time

12.55 Which of these prescriptions would the nurse clarify appropriateness with the provider of care for a client who had just undergone a craniotomy for sustained increased intracranial pressure (ICP)?

① Dexamethasone
② Morphine sulfate
③ Ondansetron
④ Phenytoin

12.56 A client who weighs 75 kilograms has an order for heparin, 5,000 units, subcutaneously every 12 hours. The vial contains 5,000 units/mL and the medication administration record (MAR) indicates that the client will receive 2 milliliters (2 mL). What is the priority nursing intervention?

① Question the order.
② Administer the 2 milliliters as ordered.
③ Perform a stool hemocult on the client prior to administration.
④ Check the lab values prior to administration.

12.57 Which of these statements made by the client indicate an understanding of misoprostol?

① "I will take a magnesium-based antacid with this medication."
② "I should not experience any NSAID-induced ulcers."
③ "I can expect to find some blood in my stool and emesis."
④ "I can still take this medication if I am pregnant."

12.58 The physician orders heparin, 7,000 units, subcutaneously every 8 hours for a client with deep vein thrombosis. The heparin available is 20,000 units per 1 mL. How many milliliters of heparin should the nurse administer?

_____ milliliters

12.59 Which observations indicate the client is experiencing a side effect(s) of prednisone?
① Decreased sodium levels and increased urinary output
② Vomiting small amounts of bile-stained fluid
③ Bleeding gums with a decrease in clotting time
④ Ecchymosis and an increase in the retention of fluids

12.60 A client is brought to the ER by his family after severe, extensive burn injury. Which of these orders will the nurse question?
① Begin Lactated Ringers infusion stat.
② Give furosemide 80 mg IV push stat.
③ Give morphine sulfate 2 mg IV push stat.
④ Insert Foley catheter.

12.61 Prior to the administration of hydralazine, the nurse will evaluate for which symptom?
① A decrease in the pulse pressure
② Pulse rate in excess of 110
③ A significant decrease in blood pressure
④ Presence of confusion and disorientation

12.62 Which response is the desired client response to hydroxyzine?
① Decrease in anxiety, and control of nausea and vomiting.
② Control of diarrhea by direct action on intestinal nerve endings.
③ Edema is decreased due to the increased excretion of water.
④ Inflammation in joint is decreased; pain is reduced.

12.63 What nursing action is most appropriate when inserting a vaginal suppository?
① Remove the suppository from the wrapper and lubricate it with Vaseline.
② Instruct client to place in tampon after inserting the vaginal medication.
③ With an applicator on the forefinger of your free hand, insert the suppository about 2 inches (5 cm) into the vagina.
④ Direct the applicator up initially and then down and forward.

12.64 Which of these statements made by the new graduate nurse indicates a need for further teaching about medication reconciliation?
① "It is the process of comparing a client's medication orders to all of the medications that the client has been taking."
② "It is a process that has been standardized across health care organizations with the implementation of electronic health records."
③ "It is done to avoid medication errors such as omissions, duplications, dosing errors, or drug interactions."
④ "It should be done at every transition of care in which new medications are ordered or existing orders are rewritten."

12.65 Which observation is a sign of impending toxicity from an aminoglycoside antibiotic such as gentamycin sulfate?
① Decrease in blood pressure
② Pulse rate drops from 140 to 90
③ Decrease in agitation
④ Hearing loss

Answers & Rationales

12.1 ① Option #1 is correct. Anticholinesterase medications such as neostigmine must be administered in a timely manner for clients with myasthenia gravis to optimize functioning of the muscles. The primary muscle that is always a concern for these clients is the upper respiratory tract muscles. Options #2, #3, and #4 all need to be seen and medications administered but are not priority over option #1.
I CAN HINT: Apply the clinical judgment/cognitive skill, take-action (first-do priority medications), when comparing to several clients. The priority will typically be if the medication needs to be administered in a timely manner; if client is experiencing an emergency (respiratory, cardiac, seizure, etc.); if client is experiencing an adverse effect from a medication; if a client has an unsafe medication level; or if a nurse is preparing to make an error in administering medication.
NCLEX® Standard: Prioritize the delivery of client care.

12.2 ③ Option #3 is correct. Toxic effects: lactic acidosis with clinical presentation of hyperventilation, muscle aches, fatigue, and lethargy. There is a 50% mortality rate with this complication. Severe lactic acidosis can be treated with hemodialysis. Clients with renal insufficiency should not use metformin due to accumulation to toxic levels can occur quickly. Options #1 and #2 need to be monitored, but these are within the current reference range and do not need to be reported. Option #4 is a good clinical finding.
I CAN HINT: Apply the clinical judgment/cognitive skill, generate solutions (first-do priority plans), for the client taking metformin who is presenting with toxic effects.
NCLEX® Standard: Evaluate client response to medication.

12.3 ④ Option #4 needs an immediate intervention. Clients with renal insufficiency should not use metformin due to the risk in development of lactic acidosis can occur quickly. Options #1, #2, and #3 are correct nursing actions and do not require immediate intervention.
I CAN HINT: Apply the clinical judgment/cognitive skill, take-action (first-do priority medications), when providing care for a client taking metformin.
NCLEX® Standard: Review lab results prior to medication administration. Protect client from injury.

12.4 ② Option #2 is correct. A sore throat is an assessment finding for agranulocytosis, an undesirable effect from this medication and other first-generation antipsychotic medications. Option #1 can occur to any of us when rising quickly from the supine position. Option #3, a skin rash does not occur with the first-generation antipsychotic medications. Option #4 can occur due to the anticholinergic effects but is not a priority over agranulocytosis..
I CAN HINT: Apply the clinical judgment/cognitive skill, analysis of cues (analysis), when providing care for a client taking the antipsychotic medication, first generation, chlorpromazine. "STANCE" in the book, *Pharmacology Made Insanely Easy*, by Manning and Rayfield, provides an easy approach to remembering each of the undesirable effects for each generation of this drug classification.
NCLEX® Standard: Evaluate client response to medication.

12.5 ①②④⑥ Options #2, #4, and #6 are correct due to the effect of contractility on the heart. Option #1, serum glucose is a concern due to the risk of hypoglycemia. Options #3 and #5 are incorrect. The concern would be with bradycardia.
NCLEX® Standard: Evaluate client response to medication.

12.6 ④ Option #4 is correct. Grapefruit juice suppresses CYP3A4 and can result in ↑ statin levels. Clients taking statins should avoid grapefruit and grapefruit juice. Option #1 is incorrect. It may take several weeks for cholesterol to decrease. This medication is used in combination with diet, exercise, weight reduction, etc. Option #2 is incorrect. Muscle pain should be reported to the health care provider. Rhabdomyolysis is a condition that can occur in which damaged muscle breaks down rapidly. Symptom may include muscle pains, weakness, vomiting, and confusion. Tea colored urine or an irregular heart rate may be a result of this condition. Option #3 is incorrect. Lovastatin should be administered with evening meals. Evening dose is best because most cholesterol is synthesized during the night.
I CAN HINT: Apply the clinical judgment/cognitive skill, generate solutions (first-do priority plans), for the client taking lovastatin.
NCLEX® Standard: Educate client about medications.

12.7 ② Option #2 is correct. Client must be monitored for bleeding due to risk of thrombocytopenia when taking the Topoisomerate Inhibitor, topotecan. Option #1 is an expected finding, so ondansetron (Zofran), the anti-emetic will be administered to minimize vomiting. Option #3 is incorrect. This finding should be reported. A sore throat may be indicative of neutropenia secondary from the chemotherapy. Option #4 is incorrect. No vaccinations should be taken without consulting the provider of care due to the risk for immunosuppression from the chemotherapy.
I CAN HINT: Apply the clinical judgment/cognitive skill, generate solutions (first-do priority plans), for the client taking the Topoisomerate Inhibitor, topotecan.
NCLEX® Standard: Educate client about medications.

12.8 ① Option #1 is correct. Morphine is contraindicated because it can increase pressure in the colon, exacerbating symptoms. The analgesic of choice is option #2, meperidine. This medication does not increase colon pressure and is safe for this client. Option #3 does not need to be verified. A nasogastric tube will be appropriate to assist in decompressing the bowel and assist in removing hydrochloric acid. Option #4 is an appropriate plan to assist in preventing dehydration. This client will need to remain NPO.
NCLEX® Standard: Verify the appropriateness/accuracy of a medication order.

12.9 ① Options #1, #2, and #5 are correct. These are
② clinical findings for neuroleptic malignant
⑤ syndrome which can be a life-threatening medical emergency. These undesirable effects from haloperidol include fever, tachycardia, diaphoresis, dysrhythmias, muscle rigidity, and changes in the level of consciousness. Options #3 and #4 are incorrect. These do not require immediate intervention.
I CAN HINT: Apply the clinical judgment/cognitive skill, analysis of cues (analysis), when providing care for a client taking the antipsychotic medication, first generation, haloperidol. "STANCE" in the book, *Pharmacology Made Insanely Easy*, by Manning and Rayfield, provides an easy approach to remembering each of the undesirable effects for each generation of this drug classification.
NCLEX® Standard: Recognize changes and intervene.

12.10 ① Options #1, #2, and #5 are correct.
② Amiodarone Antidysrhythmic (class III)
⑤ prolongs the duration of action potential and effective refractory and noncompetitive alpha and beta adrenergic inhibition. This increases PR and QT intervals resulting in a decrease in the sinus rate and a decrease in peripheral vascular resistance. Options #3, #4, and #6 are incorrect because these clinical findings are inconsistent with the action of this medication.

12.11 ③ Option #3 is correct. Subcutaneous injection of figrastim (Neupogen) is within the scope of practice for the LPN. Option #1 is not correct, since there are many undesirable effects with chemotherapy, and the LPN/VN does not evaluate in isolation of the RN. This would be done collaboratively with the RN. Option #2 is not correct due to the fact it is a new order with risks of undesirable effects, and there is a need to make new assessments and ongoing evaluations regarding the effectiveness of the medication. The LPN/VN does not plan the care in isolation of the RN. Option #4 would not be appropriate due to the unexpected outcomes that may occur with the transfusion. The LPN/VN would need to make initial assessments regarding potential complications with hemolytic, allergic, and/or febrile reactions.

12.12 ③ Option #3 is correct. Both drugs (acetaminophen and atorvastatin) are metabolized in the liver and could result in hepatotoxicity. Options #1, #2, and #4 do not require the nurse to question the order.
NCLEX® Standard: Verify the appropriateness/accuracy of a medication order.

12.13

| ③Wash hands. |
| ⑤Shake the inhaler. |
| ②Activate the MDI when inhaling. |
| ④Hold breath for 5 to 10 seconds and then exhale. |
| ①Breathe out through the nose. |

12.14 ① ④ Options #1 and #4 are correct. Option #2 is not correct, since this is coordinated with inspiration. Option #3 is not correct, since the inhaler should be shaken up prior to use to provide an adequate amount of inhalation medication. Option #5 is not correct. Albuterol (Proventil) is used for short-term relief of acute reversible airway problems. This is not used on a continuous basis in absence of symptoms.

12.15 ④ Option #4 is correct. Enoxaparin should only be administered subcutaneously and never intramuscular. This is a violation of one of the rights of medication administration, "Right Route." Option #1 is incorrect even though the bubble should be left. With the order to administer IM which is not included in the standard of care, it is a priority to question the order. Option #2 is incorrect. While this is important, it is not a priority over option #4 since the nurse should not get to the bedside with this inappropriate order. The order needs to be changed to a safe route first prior to even considering administering to the client. Option #3 is incorrect. No rubbing is the correct procedure, but before the nurse can consider the correct procedure the correct medication order remains the priority.

12.16 ② Option #2 is correct. Raloxifene (Evista) is an estrogen modifier and just like birth control pills (which also affect estrogen/progesterone) the risk for blood clots is high. If the client has a history of blood clots, this medication is contraindicated and must not be administered. Option #1 is incorrect. While the DEXA scan results would be nice, it is not a priority over option #2. Option #3 is incorrect since the hct and hgb are not considerations with this medication. Option #4 is incorrect for this medication. It is with the bisphosphonates (all end in "*dronate*") that the client should remain upright.

12.17 ② ③ ⑤ Options #2, #3, and #5 are correct. 0.9 Normal Saline (isotonic solution) bolus is necessary to dilute the glucose in the intravascular space; this will stop cellular dehydration. In the presence of metabolic acidosis, the potassium increases and must be monitored. The nurse should review the lab data including urinalysis looking for ketones (indicating ketoses). Option #1 is incorrect because only regular insulin (Novolin R) can be given by the IV route and NPH (Novolin N) is an intermediate insulin with an onset of at least 1 hour. Option #4 indicates metabolic alkalosis. Clients who are experiencing DKA will present with metabolic acidosis.

12.18 ① Options #1, #4, and #5 are correct. Option #1,
④ coronary artery vasospasms/angina;
⑤ chest pressure (heavy arms or chest tightness must be reported. These are undesirable effects and must be further evaluated. Option #4 can be therapeutic for clients with migraines. Option #5 is a safety precaution for this medication until the effect has been established. Option #2 is incorrect. Sumatriptan (Imitrex) should not be administered within 2 weeks of stopping MAOIs since this may lead to MAOI toxicity. Option #3 is incorrect. The BP should be evaluated 1 hour before and after administration.

12.19 ② Option #2 is the correct option. All other options are not appropriate. A narcotic must be wasted immediately if the client refuses the medication, and this action must be witnessed by another RN and documented.

12.20 The correct dosage is 18 units for the regular morning dose plus 12 units for the sliding scale giving a total of 30 units in the syringe.

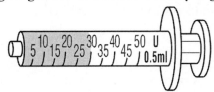

12.21 ④ Option #4 is correct. This client has opioid overdose. The age puts client at risk for toxicity and the vital signs coupled with the decreased level of consciousness (LOC) are key assessments for opioid overdose. Option #1 is incorrect. The high-Fowler's position is not only contraindicated for post total hip replacement, but it would not help the underlying issue of opioid overdose. Option #2 is incorrect. It would not be safe to place a client with COPD on this much oxygen via face mask. Option #3 is incorrect. The health care provider should be called after the naloxone (Narcan) is administered and the client is reassessed.

12.22 ① Option #1 is correct. Hetastarch is a plasma expander used to increase blood pressure (shift fluid into the intravascular space) for clients in hypovolemic shock. The increase in BP is the best indicator that this medication is working. Option #2 is incorrect. The urine output is still too low (40 mL/hr) to indicate effectiveness. Option #3 is incorrect. Hetastarch does have an anticoagulant affect, but these values do not indicate a therapeutic effect. Option #4 is incorrect. Hetastarch will not affect the temperature.

12.23 ④ Option #4 is correct. The key to this answer is that this is a second teaching session to reinforce gum care. An undesirable effect of phenytoin (Dilantin) is gingival hyperplasia and requires meticulous oral hygiene. If the teaching session was the first one, then it would need to be the RN initiating the teaching based on the scope of practice for the LPN and RN. Option #1 is incorrect. While the LPN can administer po medications, it would not be safe for the LPN to track the level over time. Option #2 is incorrect because LPNs do not develop nutritional plans. Planning should be done in collaboration with the RN. Option #3 is incorrect because LPNs do not analyze lab changes that are connected with side effects (Phenobarbitol can adversely affect the liver, resulting in failure).

12.24 ③ Option #3 is correct. Isotretinoin (Accutane) is a known teratogenic agent, and the client must have a negative pregnancy test with each new refill of the prescription (every 30 days). The other options are incorrect for this medication.

12.25 ① Options #1, #2, and #5 are correct. These
② medications increase the risk for sunburn due
⑤ to the undesirable effect of photosensitivity. Options #3 and #4 would not need to have the same caution included.

12.26 ③ Option #3 is correct. Oral medications may be delayed in absorption. Options #1, #2, and #4 are incorrect for this medication. Insulin and pramlintide should not be in the same syringe. Option #2 is incorrect. This should never be frozen. Option #4 is incorrect. Do not administer if solution is cloudy. It may have difficulty concentrating.
I CAN HINT: Symlin acts as a synthetic analogue of amylin, an endogenous pancreatic hormone that helps to control postprandial hyperglycemia. It slows gastric emptying, suppresses glucagon secretion and regulates food intake. "**DOSING**" will assist you in remembering some of the important facts for NCLEX® regarding this medication.

Dosing must be careful; it is available 0.6 mg/ml; dosing is in mcg, and insulin syringe for administration is in units.

Osteoporosis, thyroid disease, or alcoholism—use with caution.

Solution is cloudy—do NOT mix.

Insulin and pramlintide (Symlin) must be in SEPARATE syringes.

Not to freeze.

Give oral meds 1-2 hours after injection of pramlintide (Symlin).

12.27 ④ This anti-fungal medication is very irritating to the vein. The IV site must be evaluated frequently for phlebitis. Option #1 is incorrect, since the problem that can occur is hypokalemia which would present in a depressed T wave. Option #2 is incorrect, since the concern with this medication would be with digoxin toxicity. Option #3 should be small, frequent feeding of diet high in calories and protein.

12.28 ③ Checking for a flashback is a priority before administering any medication via a heparin lock. Another alternative would be to flush the lock, but 25 mL is too much fluid. Options #1, #2, and #4 are inappropriate.

12.29 ④ Benzodiazepines cause respiratory depression, especially by IV route. Option #1 Narcan is only for opioids. Option #2 would need to be accomplished BEFORE administration. Option #3 is correct; however, neuro exams need to be more often than once per shift.

12.30 ② The client is excessively anticoagulated. The heparin should be stopped immediately and the physician notified for further action. Option #1 is incorrect because the client is still receiving the drug, and it should be stopped. Options #3 and #4 are inappropriate actions.

12.31 ① Option #1 is correct. Carvedilol is a nonselective beta blocker medication. It will affect the beta fibers in the lungs causing bronchoconstriction. Option #2—Enalapril is an ACE inhibitor—appropriate post MI. HCTZ—Option #3—is often a first-line treatment for HTN. Option #4—Digoxin should be held if pulse <60.

12.32 ④ Nitroglycerin can cause hypotension. The client should avoid changing positions quickly to decrease the chances of falling. Option #1 is incorrect because the client should be taught to take medication with the onset of pain. Option #2 is incorrect because a burning or stinging sensation indicates the medication is working. Option #3 is incorrect because the client should be taught to place the medication under the tongue and let it melt, not swallow it.

12.33 ② Orthostatic hypotension and respiratory depression may occur from the PCA. Option #1 should read mg/hour. Option #3 is incorrect, and Option #4 may not relieve all the pain.

12.34 ① While this type of response to antihistamines is not uncommon in young children, it is undesirable and must be reported to the health care provider, so a change in drug therapy can be initiated. Option #2 is not within the realm of the nurse's scope of practice. The health care provider, physician, nurse practitioner, or physician's assistant must order dose changes. Option #3 will not affect the medication. Option #4 is incorrect because the health care provider must be alerted, so a preventive action can be taken.

12.35 ② Kaolin and pectin may cause constipation which, although transient, may lead to fecal impaction, especially in the elderly. Options #1, #3, and #4 are not complications of Kaopectate.

12.36 ④ The elderly are prone to paradoxical reactions and can become agitated and disoriented. Options #1 and #3 are inappropriate. Option #2 is an expected finding.

12.37 ④ Option #4 is correct. Ibuprofen (Motrin) can cause or exacerbate GI bleed, GI ulceration/perforation, thrombocytopenia (low platelet count) and various forms of anemias (aplastic & hemolytic). When answering the question, begin with the labs that are included in the question. The hemoglobin/hematocrit and platelets are all decreased. The WBC count is elevated. Range for WBC include 5,000–10,000 mm³; hgb—12 to 16 g/dL; hct 37–47% (or 3x hgb), and platelets—150,000–400,000/mm³. The concern is with the signs of bleeding and the blood count. Option #1 would not be a priority over Option #4. While Option #1 needs to be evaluated, it will not fix the complication of bleeding. Option #2 is a distractor and does not address the bleeding. Option #3 is incorrect. These medications have the same undesirable effects, so Aleve will not solve the problem with bleeding.

12.38 ④ This is necessary to prevent hemolysis of the cells. Option #1 should read normal saline. Option #2 is too fast at the beginning. Option #3 should NEVER be done.

12.39 ④ Mild to moderate rashes are the most common side effects of Bactrim. Options #1, #2, and #3 are not side effects of Bactrim.

12.40 ③ A serious side effect of dopamine, if extravasation occurs, is sloughing of the surrounding skin and tissue. A patent IV is essential to prevent serious side effects. Option #2 contains correct information, but is not a priority over option #3. Options #1 and #4 are not critical assessments at this time.

12.41 ③ The correct answer is option #3 since the HR has decreased from 86 to 58 bpm. This is a calcium channel blocker and the action is to cause a decrease in the contractility and decrease conductivity of the heart. As a result, the client may experience bradycardia. The blood pressure can also become too low, but this is not the situation with this client. The provider of care needs to know how client is responding. Option #1 would be unsafe nursing practice. Option #2 is ignoring the decrease in the HR in the above vital signs. Option #4 is important, but not a priority based on the vital signs.

12.42 ③ Option #3 is correct. Vincristine (Oncovin) is a vesicant and can be very damaging to the tissue. If client is complaining of discomfort at the site, the nurse needs to go and assess client immediately. Many times there will be a protocol for administration of antidotes and application of heat or cold prior to administering this drug. Option #1 is good practice since interferon is grown in eggs, and if there is an allergy there is a risk for the client to develop a hypersensitivity reaction. This is a good practice not to administer, and notify health care provider. Options #2 and #4 are expected outcomes, so would not be a priority over option #3.

I CAN HINT: An easy way to remember the undesirable effect with vincristine (Oncovin) is to remember the "V". Vesicants damage the veins Very much if extra Vasation occurs. These drugs include Vincristine, Vinblastine, and Vinorelbine. When you see a question on these with a focus on discomfort at the IV site, you can safely know that this is a priority due to the damage that can occur.

12.43 ③ Option #3 is correct. A National Patient Safety Goal of The Joint Commission is to accurately and completely reconcile all medications across the continuum of care. The goal is to compare the medications the client is currently taking with those that have been ordered while client is hospitalized. During transition into a new facility, transitions across settings, services, providers, or levels of care, there is an increased risk for client to miss medications due to not being ordered. Option #3 needs further intervention since the nurse is only reconciling orders written by the health care provider and the over-the-counter meds must also be included in the reconciliation process. Option #1 is a correct statement because the client's family, along with the client, are an important part of this medication reconciliation; so there is no need for further intervention. Option #2 is a correct statement. There is no need for further intervention. Option #4 is a correct statement and does not require further intervention.

I CAN HINT: "RECONCILE" will assist you in organizing this information.

Regimen for all meds the client is taking

Evaluate and obtain all meds

Compare list of all meds

Over-the-counter meds

Note: herbs, vitamins, vaccinations, nutritional supplements, etc. due to drug interactions

Compare with what client is taking both prescription and nonprescriptions

Identify meds at time of admission, transfers, inpatient discharge

Lists of drugs

Evaluate and determine meds for post discharge

12.44 ①③④ Options #1, #3, and #4 are all safe procedures for blood product administration. Option #2 is not necessary, and option #5 is incorrect. The vein should be kept open with Normal Saline rather than with D_5W.

12.45 ① Maternal tachycardia is a side effect of Brethine. Other side effects include nervousness, tremors, headache, and possible pulmonary edema. Fetal side effects include tachycardia and hypoglycemia. Terbutaline (Brethine) is usually preferred over ritodrine (Yutopar) because of minimal effects on the blood pressure. Options #2 and #3 could be harmful. Option #4 is incorrect because the pulse is unlikely to decrease enough to give terbutaline (Brethine).

12.46 ④ Option #4 is correct. The client with the complaints of swollen lips may be experiencing the side effect of angioedema caused by ACE inhibitors in some clients. This swelling can be detrimental and spread to the throat, causing the client to experience difficulty breathing. Option #1 is incorrect because adequate hourly urine output is at least 30-50 mL/hour, so this is a good urine output for a client on a diuretic. The client on Digoxin has a heart rate that is acceptable to administer digoxin, therefore option #2 is incorrect. Option #3 is incorrect because the potassium level is within normal limits.

I CAN HINT: enalapril (Vasotec) is an ace inhibitor. Refer to *Pharmacology Made Insanely Easy* for a strategy to remember this category of medication.

12.47 ② Option #2 is correct. Nitroprusside sodium (Nitropress) is the drug of choice for clients in a hypertensive crisis with a systolic BP over 180 and diastolic between 120-130. It is given IV and immediately lowers the blood pressure due to its potent vasodilating effect, immediate onset and short half-life. The heart rate significantly decreased after administration; option #1 is incorrect. Options #3 and 4 are incorrect because this medication does nothing to correct chest pain or nausea and vomiting.

12.48 ③ Cholinergics such as neostigmine can cause bronchoconstriction in asthmatic clients which may precipitate an acute asthmatic attack. The health care provider will need to order an appropriate medication. Option #1 is unsafe due to adverse effects of bronchoconstriction. Option #2 is secondary to option #3. Option #4 does not address the question that has a focus on the asthma and new medication order.

12.49 ② This medication is an anti-parkinsonian agent used to counteract the extrapyramidal side effect the client is experiencing. Options #1, #3, and #4 are antipsychotic medications which would not relieve the adverse effects.

12.50 ③ Sedative-type drugs should not be taken with alcoholic beverages. Option #1 is unsafe because maximum dose is 4 mg/day. Option #2 is incorrect because GI upset can be reduced if the medication is taken with food. Option #4 is an untrue statement. This drug is given for anxiety disorders or panic attacks.

12.51 ② The order does not state PRN. Therefore, the nurse only had an order for the first injection and not the second one. Options #1, #3, and #4 do not address the fact there was no order for the meperidine (Demerol) to be repeated.

12.52 ③ The drugs of choice to treat rigidity are the dopaminergics which include levodopa (L-Dopa). Option #1 is inaccurate and is an adverse side effect of L-Dopa. Option #2 is inaccurate. Option #4 is incorrect because anticholinergic drugs, such as benztropine mesylate (Cogentin) are beneficial for a client whose primary symptom is tremors.

12.53 ① Option #1 is correct. "Red Man Syndrome" occurs when the vancomycin is infused too quickly. Vancomycin should be infused in, over at least 60 minutes. Option #2 is incorrect. Option #3 is not the appropriate action for this clinical situation. Option #4 may help decrease the flushing, but option #1 is the priority.

12.54 ③ The psychostimulant, methylphenidate (Ritalin) generates increased vigilance and attention in the medically ill, depressed client. However, with this comes hyperalertness, insomnia and tremors. Restricting the hours of scheduled administration can help to diminish the medication's side effects related to insomnia. Administering the last dose at least 6–8 hours before bedtime is preferred.

12.55 ② Option #2 is correct. This should be questioned since it is a narcotic and can mask the neurological assessment for this client. Options #1 and #4 may be administered to this client if indicated. Option #1 is a steroid and may be prescribed for inflammation and cerebral edema. Option #4 is an anticonvulsant and may be prescribed if client was to be at risk for seizures. Option #3 is an antiemetic and is used predominantly for nausea and vomiting following chemotherapy or surgery. It would not present a risk to this client. Due to the actions of the medications in options #1, #3, and #4, there would be no reason to clarify the appropriateness of the order.

I CAN HINT: Remember any drug that masks the neurological assessment would be inappropriate. "Droopy Deuteronomy" in the book *Pharmacology Made Insanely Easy*, outlines the effects from morphine ... For a quick review it can result in **d**rowsiness, **d**izziness, **d**ecreased respirations, **d**ecreased GI peristalsis and urine output, **d**ecreased blood pressure, and **d**rug dependence. Just remember the "Six Ds"!

12.56 ① Option #1 is correct. If 2 milliliters are given, the client will receive 10,000 units of Heparin. The order reads for 5,000 units to be administered. This would be an overdose. Questioning the order is the safe action to take. Option #2 would be an unsafe dose. Options #3 and #4 should have been performed prior to approving the medication for administration. Even if they had not been performed, the priority still remains with option #1 due to an unsafe order.

12.57 ② Option #2 is correct. Options #1, #3, and #4 are incorrect. Option #1 can lead to an increased risk in diarrhea. Option #3 should be reported to the provider of care. Option #4 is incorrect and should not be taken when pregnant.

I CAN HINT: Misoprostol (Cytotec) acts as an endogenous prostaglandin in the GI tract to decrease acid secretion, increase the secretion of bicarbonate and protective mucus, and to produce vasodilation to maintain submucosal blood flow. These actions will help to prevent gatric ulcers.

12.58 0.35 milliliters

$$\frac{20,000 \text{ U}}{1 \text{ mL}} \quad \frac{7,000 \text{ U}}{X}$$

$$20,000 \text{ U}/x = 7,000 \text{ U/mL}$$

$$X = \frac{7,000 \text{ mL}}{20,000}$$

$$X = 0.35 \text{ mL}$$

12.59 ④ Steroids such as prednisone have many side effects such as ecchymosis (large, bruised areas of the skin) and edema. Option #1 is incorrect because the sodium levels would be increased and the urine output decreased. Option #2 would indicate a problem with the gall bladder or liver. Option #3 is incorrect though bleeding gums may occur due to thrombocytopenia. The drugs will not cause a decreased clotting time.

12.60 ② Furosemide (Lasix) is a loop diuretic and would contribute to intravascular fluid volume deficit after burn injury. Option #1 is correct. Fluid resuscitation is a priority as severe burns cause fluid shift from the intravascular to the interstitial space. Option #3 is correct as IV morphine is the preferred drug and route for pain management after severe burn. Option #4 is correct as a way to monitor renal function and the effectiveness of fluid resuscitation.

12.61 ③ Prior to administering an antihypertensive medication, it is important to assess the client for a decreased blood pressure. Option #1 is expected in a medication that has vasodilating effects like Apresoline. Option #2 would be consistent with a diagnosis of hypertension. Option #4 would indicate a decrease in oxygenation to the brain.

12.62 ① Hydroxyzine (Vistaril) is an antihistamine with CNS depressant, anticholinergic, and antispasmodic activities. Option #2 might refer to a medication like Imodium. Option #3 is often associated with the action of diuretics. Option #4 refers to an anti-inflammatory medication.

12.63 ③ Option #3 is correct. Option #1 is incorrect. It should be lubricated with a water-soluble lubricant. Option #2 should not be done because the tampon would absorb the medication and decrease the effectiveness. Option #4 should read to direct the applicator down initially (toward the spine), and then up and back (toward) the cervix.

12.64 ② Option #2 is correct. There is a lack of standardization in the process of medication reconciliation across health care organizations. This lack of standardization results in a variation in the historical information gathered, sources of information used, comprehensiveness of medication orders, and how information is communicated among health care providers. Options #1, #3, and #4 are accurate statements with regard to the process of medication reconciliation.

12.65 ④ Ototoxity (hearing loss) is a major adverse reaction from this drug. Other reactions include rash, urticaria, nephrotoxicity, nausea. and vomiting. Options #1, #2, and #3 are incorrect.

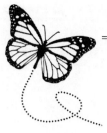

Notes

CHAPTER 13
Post-Test #1

The genius thing that we did was,
we didn't give up!
— JAY Z

> The three post-tests are comprehensive, integrated exams and are comparable to the pretest. We suggest you complete the other chapters prior to taking the post-tests and practice test.

13.1 Which of these clients requires the charge nurse to intervene with the LPN who is providing care for these clients, and review the standard of care for the hospitalized client?
① Setting a bed exit alarm for an older adult client exhibiting memory problems.
② Positioning a middle-aged client on the right side following a liver biopsy.
③ Allowing an older adult surgical client to smoke outside the front door of the hospital.
④ Allowing an older adult client with a steady gait to ambulate in the hallway unassisted.

13.2 A client is learning how to manage insulin dependent diabetes mellitus when experiencing sick days. Which instructions would be included in the client education to decrease the risk of developing complications? **Select all that apply.**
① The client should decrease the amount of insulin to half the ordered units on the days when sick.
② The client should test the serum glucose every 3 to 4 hours, and notify the health care provider for a serum glucose over 300 mg/dL (16.65 mmol/L).
③ The client should eat soft food such as soup, gelatin, or pudding 6 to 8 times a day if unable to eat typical food.
④ The client should notify the health care provider if unable to keep liquids down due to vomiting or diarrhea.
⑤ The client should test ketones in the urine only if unable to eat less than three meals per day while sick.

13.3 A client is admitted with a diagnosis of a head injury. Which clinical finding are most important for the nurse to report to the provider of care four hours after admission? **Select all that apply.**
① Confused regarding person, place and time.
② Glasgow Coma Scale has increased from 7 to 12.
③ Heart rate—88 beats per minute; BP—122/78.
④ Left pupil constricts when bright light is shined into right pupil.
⑤ Projectile vomiting.

13.4 Which of these assessments is most important to report to the health care provider for the wife of a rehab client who has sustained a C4 fracture spinal cord injury?
① The wife indicates to the nurse a feeling of a potential need for counseling to help cope with the current situation.
② The wife has elicited the support of family and friends in helping to provide care for her husband after discharge.
③ The wife has lost 10 lbs. (4.5 kg) since the accident, and shares with the nurse feelings of hopelessness about the future have resulted in the inability to sleep at night.
④ The wife reports going to bed one hour earlier to get needed rest to assist in handling the current situation of the husband.

13.5 Which of these orders would the nurse question for a client receiving prednisone?
① Administer varicella zoster vaccine.
② Taper drug when discontinuing.
③ Notify provider of care of sore throat.
④ Monitor the sodium level.

13.6 After a client has a positive Chlamydia trachomatis culture, she and her husband return for counseling. Which question would the nurse ask during the assessment?
① "Do you have contacts to identify?"
② "What is your understanding regarding how Chlamydia is transmitted?"
③ "Do you have questions about the culture and its validity?"
④ "Do you have allergies to the medications?"

13.7 Based on the Standards of Practice for a client with an acute myocardial infarction which plans would be appropriate for this client? **Select all that apply.**
① Bed rest
② Supplemental oxygen
③ Clear liquid diet
④ Continuous cardiac monitoring for an elevated ST segment and/or dysrhythmias
⑤ Evaluate the serum amylase level

13.8 Which of these clinical assessment findings would alert the nurse to intervene due to complications from bleeding following a GI surgery? **Select all that apply.**
① Urine output from 60 mL/hour to 38 mL/hour
② BP—140/95
③ HR from 80 bpm to 120 bpm in 1 hour
④ Increase in state of alertness
⑤ Mucous membranes dry and pale

13.9 What are the priority nursing actions for a client who is being admitted to the medical unit with new clinical presentations of a diffuse macular rash and a fever? The health care provider suspects rubella. **Select all that apply.**
① Notify the infection control practitioner.
② Check the immunization status of the employees on the unit.
③ Place the client on protective precautions.
④ Place the client on droplet precautions.
⑤ Place the client on contact precautions.

13.10 What is the best response to a client with cardiomyopathy who asks how will he know if he is "over-doing it" when he gets home?
① "Fatigue is a good guide."
② "The health care provider will advise you on specific do's and don'ts."
③ "If you begin coughing up increased amounts of sputum, you have overdone it."
④ "It is best to let others do as much as possible for you."

13.11 Which comment made by a client who is hospitalized for treatment of uncontrollable aggressive impulses is most important to record to establish a baseline of data before beginning a behavior-modification plan?
① Client tells each nurse that she is his favorite.
② Client has been flirtatious with female members of the staff.
③ Client threatened to hit two clients within a 2-hour time span.
④ Client appears to be insincere and superficial in his interactions.

13.12 The health care provider (HCP) orders an analgesic to be administered to a woman in labor who is 9 cm dilated and having contractions every 3 minutes lasting for 50 seconds. Which nursing action is the most important?
① Identify client prior to administering medication.
② Calculate the amount of medicine to be administered.
③ Hold the medication and document in nursing notes.
④ Notify the physician regarding the status of the contractions.

13.13 A mother is admitted to the labor and delivery unit in a sickle cell crisis. Which nursing action is a priority?
① Administer oxygen.
② Turn to right side.
③ Provide adequate hydration.
④ Start antibiotics.

13.14 Which statement made by an older client indicates more health promotion regarding safely taking NSAIDs is needed?
   ① "I will take the NSAIDs on an empty stomach."
   ② "I will inform my dentist prior to surgery that I am taking NSAIDs."
   ③ "I will report tinnitus to my physician."
   ④ "I will inform my physician if my stool becomes dark and tarry."

13.15 Which of these plans indicate an understanding of the Standard of Care for an infant admitted with a new diagnosis of pertussis?
   ① The nurse wears a surgical mask when 3 feet from child.
   ② The nurse puts on gloves and a gown when entering the room.
   ③ The nurse uses only Standard Precautions during care.
   ④ The nurse assigns child to be in room with a child with tuberculosis.

13.16 The nurse is managing an oxytocin drip. Which clinical findings will require the nurse to stop the medication? **Select all that apply.**
   ① Fetal heart rate of 140
   ② Contractions lasting 2 minutes
   ③ Inadequate uterine relaxation
   ④ Early decelerations on the fetal monitor
   ⑤ Late decelerations with a decrease in variability

13.17 Which comment made by a client indicates an understanding for safe care during the last trimester of pregnancy?
   ① "I will report any shortness of breath to my health care provider."
   ② "I will report any headaches or blurred vision to my health care provider."
   ③ "I will limit my fluid intake after 3 PM."
   ④ "I will limit my salt intake during this time."

13.18 A client with a history of Myasthenia Gravis is presenting with a HR of 112 bpm, R 24/min with accessory muscle use, anxiety and restlessness. Which of these are appropriate immediate nursing interventions? **Select all that apply.**
   ① Elevate the head of the bed.
   ② Administer furosemide 40 mg IV.
   ③ O_2 per health care provider (HCP) orders.
   ④ Teach the importance of wearing a medical identification bracelet.
   ⑤ Apply a lubricating eye drop.

13.19 How would the nurse position the ear of a toddler while initiating ear drops?
   ① Pull the ear up and back.
   ② Pull the ear down and back.
   ③ Open the canal with an otoscope.
   ④ Position the client's head off the bed.

13.20 What is the priority nursing action for a confused elderly client who is to receive a medication, but does not have on an armband?
   ① Ask another nurse who has floated to the unit to identify client.
   ② Ask client to state name and social security number.
   ③ Ask the roommate to identify client.
   ④ Review the chart for a photo of client.

13.21 What would be the priority of care for a client admitted to the emergency room in severe emotional distress with Respirations—42/min and the blood gas pH—7.5 and pCO_2—34 mm Hg?
   ① Instruct the client to breathe into a paper bag.
   ② Start an IV of D_5W STAT.
   ③ Administer O_2 immediately.
   ④ Place the client's head between the knees.

13.22 Which statement, made by the client during the admission interview, is most indicative that this client is in an abusive relationship?
   ① "My husband does not need to know that I am pregnant."
   ② "I will give my prescription to my husband to be filled."
   ③ "I got this bruise when I fell off the step ladder."
   ④ "My husband and father don't get along so I am not allowed to visit my family."

13.23 During a non-stress test (NST), the nurse observes a decrease in fetal heart rate with any fetal movement. Which nursing action is the most appropriate?

① Reposition the mother on her right side.
② Notify the physician for further evaluation.
③ Document results in the nursing notes.
④ Stop the oxytocin immediately.

13.24 An elderly client constantly screams out. The nursing staff is planning a behavior modification technique to deal with the screaming. Which initial nursing assessment is necessary in establishing a successful program?

① Monitor ability to complete activities of daily living (ADL).
② Assess levels of pain and correlate with response to analgesia.
③ Observe behavior at regular intervals to obtain baseline information related to the screaming.
④ Ask why the client is screaming and document it on the nursing assessment record.

13.25 A preschool child is unable to go to sleep at night in the hospital. Which nursing interventions may best help promote sleep for the child?

① Turn out the room light and close the door.
② Tire the child during the evening with play exercises.
③ Identify the child's home bedtime rituals and follow them.
④ Encourage visitation by friends during the evening.

13.26 During a nursing history with an adolescent client, she states that she drinks "lots" of fluids and still feels thirsty. What additional information is particularly important for the nurse to obtain at this time?

① An overall pattern of weight loss or gain for the past three months
② Use of narcotic medication and over-the-counter drugs
③ Medication and food allergies
④ Menstrual history and current menstrual status

13.27 Which of these clinical findings for a client receiving magnesium sulfate require immediate intervention? **Select all that apply.**

① Blood pressure from 140/90 to 120/78
② Hyperactive with complaints of insomnia
③ Hyper-reflexic deep tendon reflexes
④ Respirations from 26/min to 14/min
⑤ Urine output ↓ from 80 mL/hr to 40 mL/hr

13.28 What would be the priority assessment for a client who is taking a sulfonylurea and prednisone?

① Monitor hemoglobin
② Monitor platelets
③ Monitor photosensitivity
④ Monitor serum glucose

13.29 The nurse observes a school-age client who has leukemia with a new, large arm burn that appears oily. The client states it was burned on an iron and the client's mother put cooking fat on it, so it would not blister. What is the priority nursing action?

① Document the findings in the chart and suggest the mother to use an ointment next time.
② Call the provider of care immediately to advise of the injury.
③ Teach the client that oil holds germs and infection is more likely.
④ Wash the burn with soap and water to remove the oil.

13.30 Which statement made by the parent of a preschool child with sickle cell anemia indicates a need for further teaching?

① "When she complains of pain, I give her baby aspirin."
② "I try to keep her away from people with infections."
③ "I sometimes have to give her meperidine for pain."
④ "I encourage her to drink a lot of water."

13.31 The nurse administers oxycodone to a post-operative client. After 30 minutes, what would the nursing priority action be?

① Change the client's position in bed.
② Elevate the client's head and put a pillow under shoulders.
③ Observe the client for nonverbal behaviors indicating comfort.
④ Ambulate the client.

13.32 There is an order for starting regular insulin sliding scale.

Blood glucose levels:	Insulin order:
< 170 mg/dl (9.44 mmol/L)	No insulin
170-240 mg/dl (9.44-13.32 mmol/L)	10 units regular insulin S.C.
241–300 mg/dl (13.38-16.65 mmol/L)	20 units regular insulin S.C.
>300 mg/dl (16.65 mmol/L)	Notify provider of care for order.

The AM blood glucose level is 178 mg/dl (9.88 mmol/L). Point and click on the syringe, the appropriate amount that should be administered.

① 10
② 20
③ 30
④ 40

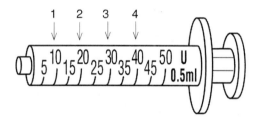

13.33 A client is intubated and is receiving oxygen by T-piece at 50% FiO_2. The nurse notices that the client has an increase in secretions, becoming more anxious, and RR—42/min. What would be the first nursing action?

① Call the health care provider.
② Increase the FiO_2.
③ Administer a sedative as ordered.
④ Assess lung sounds, suction PRN.

13.34 A health care provider has written an order for an HIV-positive infant to receive oral polio immunization. Which nursing actions are most appropriate?

① Wear gloves and a gown when administering the immunization.
② Administer the immunization as the infant is being discharged.
③ Call the health care provider and discuss the rationale for the immunization.
④ Administer the medication in the same manner as you would any other infant.

13.35 An adult client who is NPO with a nasogastric tube has orders to receive acetaminophen 650 mg PRN for a temperature greater than 101°F (38.3°C). Which measure would be included in the administration of this drug?

① The tablets should be swallowed carefully with sips of water.
② The medication should be withheld until the nasogastric tube is removed.
③ Placement of the nasogastric tube should be checked prior to giving medication.
④ Powdered medication should be used and mixed with water to form a solution.

13.36 An elderly client tells the nurse that he is worried about the wife's impending colostomy surgery. What is the most appropriate response to the husband?

① Review the wife's surgical procedure with the husband.
② Offer the client the option to take a class explaining the discharge care.
③ Encourage the husband to discuss how he feels and his fears about the surgery.
④ Explain the importance of the husband attending the teaching sessions offered by the interstomal therapist.

13.37 What is the nursing priority while planning care for an infant with congenital heart disease who becomes easily fatigued and vital signs increase during feedings?

① Give small, frequent feedings.
② Change diapers before feeding.
③ Increase the caloric content of the feedings.
④ Mix rice cereal in the formula.

13.38 A 4-month-old infant, who had a temperature of 100.3°F (37.9°C) following the last DTP (Diphtheria, Tetanus, and Pertussis) vaccine, is seen in the clinic for another immunization administration. Prior to administering the DTP, which nursing action is a priority?

① Withhold the immunization.
② Give half the dose in this injection.
③ Consult with the physician on giving Pediatric DP (Diphtheria and Tetanus).
④ Instruct the parents to give acetaminophen following administration of the full dose of DTP.

13.39 During an examination with a mother in her last trimester, the nurse would identify which sign to indicate placenta previa?
① Painful vaginal bleeding
② Fetal bradycardia
③ Painless vaginal bleeding
④ Irritability of the uterus

13.40 Following the administration of an incorrect dose of medication, which statement best describes the incident on a incident report?
① Due to illegible physician order, 9 mg of gentamycin was given IV at 0200 instead of 7 mg IV.
② At 0200, gentamycin 9 mg was given IV instead of 7 mg IV as ordered.
③ At 0200, client received 2 mg more of gentamycin than was ordered.
④ Gentamycin 9 mg IV was given at 0200. Physician's order to decrease dose was not transcribed to the Kardex by previous shift RN.

13.41 What would be the priority nursing evaluation of the neurological status for a newly admitted client who has suffered a cerebral vascular accident?
① Equality of pulses in all four extremities.
② Orientation to person, place, and time.
③ Regularity of neuromuscular claudication.
④ Decrease in the pulse pressure and tachycardia.

13.42 Which laboratory test result suggests that the anorexic client is at risk for developing renal calculi?
① High serum calcium levels
② Low serum potassium
③ High serum osmolality
④ AST elevation

13.43 Following the initiation of an IV oxytocin drip, which is the most appropriate nursing action?
① Assess vital signs every 15 minutes.
② Check the frequency and duration of contractions.
③ Determine blood pressure every 4 hours.
④ Monitor urine output for polyuria.

13.44 What is most important to teach a client who is being discharged on home peritoneal dialysis?
① Drink only distilled water.
② Cap the Tenchkoff catheter when not in use.
③ Boil the dialysate one hour prior to a pass.
④ Clean the arteriovenous fistula site with hydrogen peroxide daily.

13.45 What is most important to include in the teaching plan regarding what to avoid for a client who is receiving a monoamine oxidase inhibitor (MAOI) medication for treatment of depression?
① Tropical vacations
② Aged cheeses and Chianti wine
③ Ice cream sundaes
④ Driving a car

13.46 Which action describes the best method for obtaining an infant's vital signs?
① Take an axillary temperature first because this is the most important measurement.
② Count respirations for 15 seconds and multiply the number by 4.
③ Count respirations for a minute prior to arousing the infant.
④ Use a stethoscope with a one and a half inch diaphragm for counting the apical pulse.

13.47 Which plan would be priority for a hypertensive client on captopril?
① Encourage client to take medicine with meals.
② Discuss the need for a potassium supplement.
③ If client misses a dose, take 2 doses at next scheduled time.
④ Instruct client to take this drug one hour before meals.

13.48 What is most important to include in the teaching plan regarding when to notify the health care provider for a client taking trifluoperazine?
① Nasal stuffiness
② Heat intolerance
③ Hand and arm tremors
④ Weight loss and diarrhea

13.49 Which statement made by the parents of a school-age child with an ostomy indicates they are providing quality home care?
① "We change the bag at least once a week, and we carefully inspect the stoma at that time."
② "We change the bag every day so we can inspect the stoma and the skin."
③ "We encourage our daughter to watch TV while we change her ostomy bag."
④ "We only have to change the ostomy bag every ten days."

13.50 Which statement by the client best indicates an emotional readiness for surgery?
① "I know the physician isn't telling me everything, but at this point, I can't do anything about it."
② "I've never heard of this specialist before. Does he do much work here?"
③ "I'm glad the trapeze is on my bed so I can start working on my exercises as soon as I wake up."
④ "Can you please check my record to be sure it says I'm diabetic?"

13.51 To prepare an adolescent client for a lumbar puncture, which instruction would the nurse include in the teaching?
① General anesthetic will be used.
② Fluids will be restricted for 8 hours before the test.
③ The client will need to remain flat in bed for 8 hours after the test.
④ A compression bandage will be in place for 10 hours after the test.

13.52 What is the priority nursing care in assisting a client in diffusing escalating, aggressive/violent behavior?
① Utilizing an organized team to place the client in seclusion.
② Leaving the client alone in their room to identify feelings of anger.
③ Redirecting the client to a quiet activity to divert their attention and not disturb the other clients.
④ Assisting the client in identifying and expressing their feelings of increasing anxiety, frustration and anger.

13.53 Which medication can be given intravenously to reverse the effects of a narcotic overdose?
① Hydromorphine
② Disulfiram
③ Benztropine
④ Naloxone

13.54 Two days after the placement of a pleural chest tube, the chest tube is accidentally pulled out of the intrapleural space. What would be the nursing priority?
① Replace the tube, using sterile gloves.
② Apply a dressing immediately over the site, taping on 3 sides.
③ Instruct the client to cough to expand the lung.
④ Auscultate lung to determine if it is collapsed.

13.55 Metoprolol 12.5 mg is prescribed and available are 50 mg tables. Point to the correct dosage.

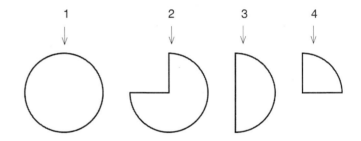

13.56 An older client uses a walker for ambulation support and is receiving a diuretic and must use the bathroom several times during the night. Which of these actions is a priority in promoting safety for this client?
① Maintain the side rails in the upward position.
② Leave the bedroom light on at all times.
③ Hold the diuretic medication.
④ Provide the client with a bedside commode.

13.57 In preparing the teaching plan for a prenatal client who is eight week's gestation with a positive VDRL, which instruction is most appropriate for the nurse to include?
① Refrain from taking any medications to prevent damage to the fetus.
② Take the penicillin for the prescribed time.
③ Refrain from sexual activity.
④ Maintain the confidentiality of sexual partners.

13.58 Which nursing action offers the most support to a child and family in the terminal stage of the child's illness?
① Encourage the family to avoid any reference to death so the child does not get upset.
② Limit the amount of visiting time so the child does not become over-exhausted.
③ Assure the ongoing participation of all disciplines in the child's care, even after discharge if needed.
④ Limit the amount of information and explanations given to parents who are already overloaded at this time.

13.59 What is a priority assessment for a geriatric client diagnosed with diabetes mellitus and is being discharged with a treatment plan that includes a 1500-caloric diabetic diet, insulin, and regular exercise by walking 30 minutes a day?
① Does the client have adequate vision and manual dexterity to administer own insulin?
② Does the client understand the impact diabetes will have on lifestyle?
③ Since the client is living alone, is there a need for Home Health Care to check on client daily?
④ Does the client understand how to perform daily urinary sugar and acetone determinations?

13.60 Which plan is a priority for a newly admitted client with meningitis due to Hemophilus influenza?
① Place in reverse isolation for at least 24 hours.
② Monitor vital signs and neurological checks every 4 to 6 hours.
③ Dim lights in the room and minimize environmental stimuli.
④ Encourage PO fluids to decrease the fever.

13.61 Prior to discharging a client after a mastectomy, the documentation in the chart would indicate that the client has been educated regarding which plan?
① Use a heating pad under the shoulder every other night.
② Wear a sling on the affected forearm for 4 weeks after surgery.
③ Attend the support group RESOLVE.
④ Avoid use of the affected arm for blood pressure evaluation or for any needle sticks.

13.62 The charge nurse notices that whenever a client is admitted with a history of sexual abuse, the 3–11 nurse, subtly and sometimes overtly, verbally attacks the client. Further investigation reveals that the 3–11 nurse was sexually abused as a child. What is the priority plan in making assignments?
① Assign the nurse to this client to promote therapeutic feedback to the client about the behavior from someone who has been "on the other side."
② Assign the nurse to the client and insist that the nurse begin therapy to work on unresolved feelings.
③ Assign someone else to the client because the nurse is not ready to cope with this and may be detrimental to the client.
④ Assign someone else to the client, but do not inform the nurse of your rationale for doing so.

13.63 Several clients are admitted to the medical unit at the same time. Each client has an order for an IV to be started. Which case would the manager assign as priority for an IV start?
① A client with abdominal pain.
② A client with vaso-occlusive cell crisis.
③ A client with mild dehydration.
④ A client with surgery scheduled in the morning.

13.64 What is the priority nursing action prior to removing a nasogastric tube and the nurse aspirates 350 mL of fluid?
① Return the 350 mL through the tube to the client's stomach.
② Remove the tube and have the client drink 350 mL of a clear liquid.
③ Chart the findings after removing the tube.
④ Notify the health care provider after removing the tube.

13.65 Which factor is most important for the rehabilitation nurse to assess during the admission of a new client?
① The client's expectations of family members.
② The client's understanding of available supportive services.
③ The client's personal goals for rehabilitation.
④ The client's past experiences in the hospital.

13.66 Two days after admission, a client's sputum culture is reported as positive for tuberculosis. While awaiting orders from the provider of care, what would be the priority nursing intervention?
① Initiate measures to transfer the client to a tuberculosis unit.
② Institute measures to initiate standard/airborne precautions in the hospital.
③ Arrange for all of the client's personal items to be decontaminated.
④ Notify the client's family that they have been exposed to a highly contagious disease.

13.67 Which plan is a priority for the elderly client who lives in an assisted living center?
① Encourage verbalization of feelings regarding the relationship with family who initiated his assisted living center placement.
② Help client express favorite pastimes and enjoyable activities.
③ Orient client to present time and assist in being alert when family visits.
④ Direct conversations to assist client to reminisce and talk about important past events in his life.

13.68 A client with peptic ulcer disease (PUD) is seen in the clinic for pain associated with gout. Which medication order would be questioned by the nurse?
① colchicine
② allopurinol
③ probenecid
④ indomethacin

13.69 A client has an order for antacids for his peptic ulcer disease (PUD). Which statement by the client indicates an understanding of how to take antacids?
① "I will take them with food."
② "I will take them thirty minutes before and after meals."
③ "I will take them one hour after meals."
④ "I will take them with my other medications."

13.70 Which interventions will be most appropriate when obtaining urine from an indwelling catheter for culture and sensitivity?
① Unclamp the drainage spout from the urine bag, wipe it with alcohol, and collect the specimen in a sterile container.
② Clamp the catheter tubing, swab the injection port with alcohol, and aspirate urine into a syringe.
③ Remove the indwelling urinary catheter, insert a new one and obtain urine from the new sterile bag.
④ Don sterile gloves, disconnect the catheter from the drainage tubing, and drain the urine directly into a sterile container.

13.71 Which assistive care device would the nurse plan on having available for an elderly client who has a below-the-knee amputation?
   ① Crutches
   ② 4-point walker
   ③ A cane
   ④ Wheelchair

13.72 Prior to administering aspirin, the nurse will notify the health care provider if a client has which medical diagnosis?
   ① Peptic ulcer disease (PUD)
   ② CVA
   ③ Osteoarthritis
   ④ Rheumatoid arthritis

13.73 The nurse would identify which situation as an indication for the unlicensed assistive personnel (UAP) to participate in a clinical skills lab?
   ① Securing a Foley catheter bag on the side of the bed rail
   ② Elevating the head of the bed for a client receiving a tube feeding
   ③ Using gloves to empty urine from a graduated cylinder
   ④ Turning a client who is bedridden every two hours to prevent skin breakdown

13.74 A client with CVA begins to choke and cough on a piece of meat. Which action is the nursing priority?
   ① Provide blows to the back.
   ② Assist with expelling the meat immediately.
   ③ Avoid interfering with his attempt to expel the meat.
   ④ Administer 5 abdominal thrusts followed by a blind finger sweep.

13.75 A school-age child with a history of asthma arrives in the ER wheezing and reports a difficult time breathing for the last couple of hours. The client's albuterol aerosol x 4 has not helped. What would be the nursing priority based on protocol?
   ① Start an IV and prepare for administration of epinephrine.
   ② Walk the boy to x-ray stat for chest x-ray.
   ③ Administer a po fluid challenge stat.
   ④ Administer a breathing treatment with nebulizer and prepare for chest x-ray stat.

Category Analysis—Post-Test #1

1. Management of Care
2. Reduction of Risk Potential
3. Reduction of Risk Potential
4. Psychosocial
5. Management of Care
6. Health Promotion
7. Physiological Adaptation
8. Physiological Adaptation
9. Safety and Infection Control
10. Health Promotion
11. Psychosocial
12. Health Promotion
13. Health Promotion
14. Pharmacology
15. Safety and Infection Control
16. Pharmacology
17. Health Promotion
18. Reduction of Risk Potential
19. Pharmacology
20. Pharmacology
21. Physiological Adaptation
22. Psychosocial
23. Physiological Adaptation
24. Psychosocial
25. Health Promotion
26. Basic Care and Comfort
27. Pharmacology
28. Pharmacology
29. Safety and Infection Control
30. Health Promotion
31. Pharmacology
32. Pharmacology
33. Physiological Adaptation
34. Health Promotion
35. Pharmacology
36. Psychosocial
37. Basic Care and Comfort
38. Pharmacology
39. Health Promotion
40. Management of Care
41. Reduction of Risk Potential
42. Basic Care and Comfort
43. Pharmacology
44. Safety and Infection Control
45. Pharmacology
46. Basic Care and Comfort
47. Pharmacology
48. Pharmacology
49. Basic Care and Comfort
50. Psychosocial
51. Reduction of Risk Potential
52. Psychosocial
53. Pharmacology
54. Physiological Adaptation
55. Pharmacology
56. Reduction of Risk Potential
57. Safety and Infection Control
58. Psychosocial
59. Health Promotion
60. Reduction of Risk Potential
61. Management of Care
62. Management of Care
63. Management of Care
64. Basic Care and Comfort
65. Psychosocial
66. Safety and Infection Control
67. Psychosocial
68. Basic Care and Comfort
69. Basic Care and Comfort
70. Basic Care and Comfort
71. Reduction of Risk Potential
72. Pharmacology
73. Safety and Infection Control
74. Management of Care
75. Physiological Adaptation

Chapter 13: POST-TEST #1

Directions

1. Determine questions missed by checking answers.
2. Write the number of the questions missed across the top line marked "item missed."
3. Check category analysis page to determine category of question.
4. Put a check mark under item missed and beside content.
5. Count check marks in each row and write the number in totals column.
6. Use this information to:
   - identify areas for further study.
   - determine which content test to take next.

We recommend studying content where most items are missed—then taking that content test.

Number of the Questions Incorrectly Answered

Post-Test	Items Missed													Totals
C Management of Care														
O Safety and Infection Control														
N Health Promotion and Maintenance														
T Psychosocial Integrity														
E Physiological Adaptation: Fluid Gas														
N Reduction of Risk Potential														
T Basic Care and Comfort														
Pharmacology and Parenteral Therapies														

Answers & Rationales

13.1 ③ Option #3 is correct. Allowing a post-op client to smoke is a violation of the standard of care for client's health and to the hospital policy. Option #1 is incorrect. The bed exit alarm would be appropriate for this client with memory problems who may be at risk for falls and does not require a review of the standard of care. Option #2 is incorrect. There is no need to intervene and review the standard of care when this is the correct position following a liver biopsy. This position provides pressure on the biopsy site which will decrease the risk of bleeding. Option #4 is incorrect. A client who ambulates steadily, even if client is an older adult, should be allowed to ambulate unless there is any contraindication due to medications, diagnostic tests, surgery, or if there is an order for immobility. There is no need to review the standard of care with the nurse since there is no indication of any risks.

13.2 ② ③ ④ Options #2, #3, #4 are correct. Option #2 is correct. The nurse must explain the "sick day rules" emphasizing that the client should take insulin agents as usual and test their blood sugar and urine ketones every 3 to 4 hours. In fact, insulin-requiring clients may need supplemental doses of regular insulin every 3 to 4 hours. The client should report elevated glucose levels (greater than 240 mg/dL (13.32 mmol/L) or as otherwise instructed) or urine ketones to the health care provider. Option #3 is correct. If the client is not able to eat normally, client should be instructed to substitute soft foods such a gelatin, soup, or pudding. Option #4 is correct. If vomiting, diarrhea, or fever persists, the client should have an intake of liquids every 1/2 hour to 1 hour to prevent dehydration. Fluid loss is dangerous: nausea, vomiting, and diarrhea should be reported to the health care provider. Clients with type 1 diabetes who cannot retain oral fluids may need hospitalization to avoid diabetic ketoacidosis and possibly a coma. Options #1 and #5 are not correct for the standard of care for the "sick day rules" for a diabetic client. The client should continue to take insulin or oral antidiabetic agents as ordered. The urine should be tested for ketones and reported to provider if they are abnormal (level should be negative to small). Clients need to learn the signs and symptoms of hypoglycemia (tachycardia, irritable, restless, diaphoresis, shakiness, weakness, headache, nausea, chills, confusion) and hyperglycemia (hot, dry skin, fruity breath).

13.3 ① ⑤ Options #1 and #5 are correct. Confusion is one of the earliest symptoms of increased intracranial pressure. These both may be indications that the client is experiencing an increase in the cerebral edema or bleeding from the head injury. Option #2 indicates a positive outcome. The neurological status for this client is improving, so there is not a need to report this to the provider of care. The best possible Glasgow Coma Scale (GCS) is 15. The total scores of the GCS correlate with the degree or level of coma. Less than 8 is associated with a severe head injury and coma. A score of 9-12 indicates a moderate head injury. Greater than 13 reflects minor head trauma. Option #3 is not a correct answer since there is no indication of a change in these readings, and these values are considered to be normal. Option #4 is an expected finding. There is no need to report this finding.

13.4 ③ Option #3 is correct. This question is evaluating the ability for you to "*Recognize impact of illness on individual/family.*" This statement identifies several risk factors for this client that must be addressed. These include the weight loss, a feeling of hopelessness, and insomnia. There is a need for intervention on behalf of the wife. Option #1 indicates self awareness and does not require the nurse to report the finding to the health care provider. Option #2 is not correct since she has elicited support on her own which is very healthy. Option #4 is not correct. There is no need to report this when this is also a very healthy behavior.

13.5 ① Option #1 is correct. Prednisone (Deltasone) may result in immunosuppression of the body. A small number of people who get the vaccine may still get chickenpox. However, they usually have a milder case than persons who did not receive the vaccine. If taken with prednisone (Deltasone) the client may become infected with varicella. This order should be questioned in order to decrease this risk of an infection and provide safe client care. Options #2, #3, and #4 are appropriate for this medication and do not need to be questioned. It is important not to abruptly discontinue the prednisone (Deltasone). Option #3 is a statement that does not need to be questioned. This sore throat may indicate the client is experiencing an infection from being immunosuppressed and unable to fight off an infection, so the provider of care will need to be notified. Option #4 should be monitored. This does not need to be questioned. Clients taking this medication may experience an increase in the sodium level.

I CAN HINT: *An easy way to remember the lab changes that may occur when taking this med. is the little saying, "Some People Get Cold." Take the first letter of each of these words: S in "Some" is now sodium and the P in "People" is now potassium and the G in "Get" is now glucose and the C in "Cold" is now calcium. Remember to start with the arrow going up and then each one will be the opposite, so in other words the sodium is ↑, potassium is ↓, glucose is ↑, and calcium is ↓. This will help you remember this information FOREVER! See you CAN do this!*

13.6 ② The transmission of Chlamydia may or may not have been made clear to both partners so the nurse would have to assess this first. Chlamydia is a reported sexually-transmitted disease. Option #1 may be part of the follow-up. Option #3 is a possibility, but most cultures used today have few false positives. Option #4 would be done later in the nursing assessment.

13.7 ① ② ④ Options #1, #2, and #4 are correct. Following an acute myocardial infarction, the client to be on bed rest with supplemental oxygen to decrease the stress on the heart. The ECG pattern that occurs with a myocardial infarction is an elevated ST segment. Remember, with an MI the ST segment is high. Option #5 is not correct. This would be for pancreatitis. Troponin and CPK-MB would be evaluated and monitored for the client who had a myocardial infarction.

13.8 ① ③ ⑤ Options #1, #3, and #5 are correct. The key to answering this question is to recognize client is bleeding and the findings would indicate a complication from the bleeding. Option #1 is correct since it is trending down. An intervention needs to be implemented prior to urine output decreasing any more. Option #3 is correct. The elevated HR indicates the heart is working hard to pump out the blood that is being lost from the bleeding. Option #5 is correct. This occurs from the blood loss. Option #2 is not correct. Hypertension is not a complication from bleeding; the complication would be with hypotension. Option #4 is not correct. The complication would be lethargy and a decrease in alertness.

13.9 ④ ⑤ The correct responses are options #4 and #5. Rubella (German measles) presents with a low-grade fever and a rash that begins on the face and spreads to the body. It is transmitted by direct droplets when an infected person breathes, coughs, or sneezes (Droplets larger than 5 micrometers). Measles can remain infectious in the air for up to 2 hours after an infected person leaves an area. Direct contact is another way it is spread, so contact transmission precautions should also be implemented. Option #1 is necessary, but in this case is not a priority. Option #2 will require the assistance of employee health to check immunization records. Option #3 is incorrect, since there is no indication of the client being immunosuppressed.

13.10 ① Option #1 is correct. Fatigue is a useful guide in gauging activity tolerance in clients with decreased cardiac output. Option #2 is incorrect. The client is not asking for specific do's and don'ts, but rather a general guide to use for activity in general. This may indicate that the nurse is abdicating client-teaching responsibilities. Option #3 may indicate developing pulmonary edema, and the client should discontinue activity at this point. Option #4 is inaccurate and may cause the client to lose independence.

13.11 ③ This is the most concrete evidence of aggressive behavior. Options #1, #2, and #4 are less directly related to aggression.

Chapter 13: ANSWERS & RATIONALES

13.12 ④ The information indicates the woman is in transition phase. Analgesics cause depressed respirations in the baby. Options #1 and #2 contain correct information but not for this situation. Option #3 does not address the immediate problem.

13.13 ③ Adequate hydration is a priority for any client in sickle cell crisis. Option #1 may be correct for the situation but is not a priority to Option #3. Options #2 and #4 are not priority actions for this client.

13.14 ① More health promotion is necessary since these medications should be taken with meals because they can cause GI distress. Option #2 is imperative since NSAIDs reduce platelet adhesiveness predisposing clients to bleeding, especially after surgery. Routinely, clients will stop the NSAIDs two weeks prior to surgery. There is no need for more teaching. Option #3 must be reported. It is an adverse reaction from these medications. There is no indication for more teaching. Option #4 indicates the client understands this is a problem. Dark and tarry stools indicate blood or bleeding from the GI tract.

13.15 ① Option #1 is correct. When providing care for infants with pertussis, infection control guidelines for droplet precautions should be implemented. These guidelines require a surgical mask within 3 feet of the client. Option #2 is not necessary for this medical condition. These personal protective equipment (PPE) would be appropriate for an infant who needed to be in contact precautions which would include: MRSA, Clostridium difficile, VRE, cellulites, etc. Option #3 would be included in addition to the droplet precautions for this infant. This is currently incorrect because it states that "ONLY" Standard Precautions should be used. This is incorrect since pertussis is transmitted as a droplet. Option #4 is incorrect since TB requires a different type of isolation precautions. It requires airborne precautions including a negative pressure room and an N95 mask.

I CAN HINT: It is important to know that if clients must be put in a room with another person that the isolation precautions should be the same. This is a great clinical decision making strategy that will help you in the future with these type of questions. The one exception is MRSA, VRE and Clostridium difficile. MRSA and VRE should not be put in the same room as a client with Clostridium difficile.

13.16 ② ③ ⑤ Options #2, #3, and #5 are correct. Oxytocin (Pitocin) is used to induce labor or to help labor progress. It can be dangerous to the baby and can cause fetal distress as well as uterine rupture in extreme cases. Option #2 can result in a ruptured uterus if the drip continues. Option #3 is correct since this can also result in a risk for ruptured uterus and complications with the fetus from hypoxia and/or potential fetal/maternal death. Option #5 is correct. The infusion would need to be discontinued due to symptoms of hypoxia to the fetus as indicated by the late decelerations from uteroplacental insufficiency and the decrease in variability. Option #1 would be a normal finding. The normal FHR is 120–160. Option #4 may indicate head compression, but no complication with either fetal or maternal hypoxia that would mandate stopping the medication.

13.17 ② Signs of advanced pregnancy induced hypertension are headaches, blurred vision, and epigastric pain which are imperative to report to the provider of care. Option #1 is expected due to the enlarged uterus causing pressure on the lungs. Options #3 and #4 are not appropriate for this client.

13.18 ① ③ Options #1 and #3 are correct. Elevating the head of the bed will assist with lung expansion. Option #3 addresses the clinical symptoms of hypoxia. Option #2 is incorrect. There is no indication of fluid overload. Options #4 and #5 are not immediate needs.

13.19 ② The correct positioning of the child's ear while instilling ear drops is to pull the ear down and back. This will assist in accessing the auditory canal. Option #1 is correct for an adult client. Options #3 and #4 contain inaccurate information.

13.20 ④ Option #4 is correct. You may think to yourself that there usually is not a photo on the chart where you work, but remember if it is in the option it is available to you. You simply have to make a decision if this is the best option for this client. Many acute-care settings are requiring a photo of client in the chart to prevent errors due to lack of client identification. Option #1 is incorrect. This is not the correct way to identify the client. Option #2 is not correct because the client is confused. Option #3 is not an appropriate way to identify the client.

13.21 ① Because of hyperventilation, the client is in respiratory alkalosis so having the client re-breathe their own CO_2 will reverse the blood gases. Option #2 does not address the problem. Option #3 is incorrect because the client is not hypoxic. Option #4 is for a client who feels faint.

13.22 ④ Option #4 is correct. This is indicative that the client is secluded from family which is a sign of abuse. Option #1 is the client's right to privacy. Option #2 is not indicative of abuse. Option #3 is not an indicative sign of abuse.

13.23 ② A decrease in the fetal heart rate (FHR) during the NST should be immediately evaluated by the physician. Options #1 and #3 do not resolve the immediate problem. Option #4 is incorrect because Oxytocin (Pitocin) is not used for the non-stress test.

13.24 ③ In designing an effective behavior modification program, an accurate baseline data about the target behavior in relation to frequency, amount, time, and precipitating factors must first be collected. Options #1 and #2 are incorrect because each option assesses only one area of behavior that may be related to the target behavior of screaming and does not provide comprehensive data for developing a behavior management program. Option #4 will most likely give inaccurate information.

13.25 ③ Preschool-aged children require bedtime rituals which should be followed in the hospital if possible. Option #1 would increase child's fear. Options #2 and #4 would not promote sleep.

13.26 ① Excessive thirst and weight loss are two notable symptoms of diabetes mellitus. Options #2, #3, and #4 do not provide useful information related to the assessment information.

13.27 ④ Options #4 and #5 are trending down and
     ⑤ need intervention. Option #1 is an expected finding with this medication. Options #2 and #3 do not support signs of toxicity. These indicate the client would need more medication, but do not require immediate intervention.

13.28 ④ An undesirable effect of prednisone may be hyperglycemia. It is important to monitor the glucose since prednisone is working in direct opposition to the action of sulfonylureas. Sulfonylureas stimulate insulin release from the beta cells in the pancreas resulting in a lower serum glucose. Options #1, #2, and #3 are incorrect.

13.29 ④ Since clients with leukemia are immuno-suppressed, they are more susceptible to infections. Cooking fat applied to an open wound increases the possibility of infection. Burns should be immediately rinsed with tap water to reduce the heat in the burn. Options #1 and #3 do not address the immediate problem of cleansing the wound. Option #2 is not necessary at this time based on the information presented.

13.30 ① Aspirin can cause hemorrhage during a sickle cell crisis and definitely indicates a need for further teaching. Options #2 and #4 are important aspects in the care of a sickle cell client to prevent sickling crisis. Option #3 is an appropriate medication used to decrease the client's pain.

13.31 ③ In evaluating the effectiveness of pain medication, the nurse must first identify actual outcomes of the client's sense of well-being and comfort. Options #1 and #2 would be helpful in promoting comfort for the client. However, the priority is to determine pain medication effectiveness. Option #4 would be done after the client has some pain relief.

13.32 ① The correct answer is Option #1: 10.

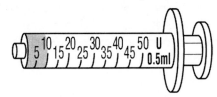

13.33 ④ Additional assessment data helps define the problem. Suctioning can relieve distress and restore airway patency. Option #1 will delay nursing intervention to treat the problem. Option #2 will not be useful if the airway is not patent. Option #3 is inappropriate and could lead to further CO_2 retention.

13.34 ③ Polio is a live virus and should not be given to children who are immunocompromised. Options #1, #2, and #4 do not address the identified problem of the compromised immune system.

13.35 ③ Liquid acetaminophen may be administered via the nasogastric tube after tube placement has been checked. Option #1 is incorrect because the client is NPO so nothing can be taken orally. Option #2 is incorrect since medication should not be withheld. Option #4 is incorrect because Tylenol does not come in powdered form at this time.

13.36 ③ This is a common cause related to anxiety. Encouraging the husband to talk about his fears will assist in alleviating this anxiety. Other options are secondary.

13.37 ① Feeding small amounts more frequently will not cause as much fatigue and cardiovascular stress. Option #2 is important, but it does not relate to fatigue with feedings. Options #3 and #4 will not reduce the fatigue.

13.38 ④ Low-grade fever may occur after a DTP. An antipyretic is useful prior to and after immunizations. Option #1 is not indicated. Option #2 is incorrect because the child would still receive the Pertussis which would probably cause another febrile reaction. Option #3 would be correct if there was a concern with seizures.

13.39 ③ This is a sign of placenta previa. Option #1 could be a sign of abruptio placenta. Option #2 indicates fetal distress. Option #4 is not specific of any disorder.

13.40 ② This is a factual account of exactly what happened. An incident report should be factual and objective. Option #1 is incorrect because this statement blames the physician's handwriting. Option #3, while true, does not present all of the information. It simply states a conclusion which cannot be verified without further investigation. Option #4 does not present all the facts and places blame.

13.41 ② This is an integral part of the neurological evaluation. In addition, assessments of motor activity, eyes, and pupil equality are part of the neurological work-up. Option #1 is irrelevant for a neurological assessment. Option #3 is not a correct statement. Option #4 is incorrect since signs and symptoms of increased intracranial pressure would be an increase (widening) in the pulse pressure and a complication with bradycardia. The current clinical findings in option #4 would indicate a complication of shock.

13.42 ① This indicates that osteoporosis is occurring and may lead to renal calculi. Option #2 does not respond to renal calculi. Options #3 and #4 are more likely to be seen in a client who is being treated for a chemical dependency.

13.43 ② Oxytocin is given to stimulate contraction of uterine muscle fibers. It is important to assess the contractions due to potential hypertonia and possible rupture of the uterus. Options #1 and #3 do not assess for the desired response to the medication. Option #4 is not the desired response as Pitocin does have a mild antidiuretic effect.

13.44 ② Capping the peritoneal catheter when not in use keeps the catheter sterile. Option #1 is unnecessary. Option #3 is unnecessary and probably harmful to the solution. Option #4 is incorrect because there is no arteriovenous fistula in peritoneal dialysis. This is hemodialysis access, and does not require daily cleaning with hydrogen peroxide.

13.45 ② MAO inhibitors, when combined with certain foods containing tyramine (especially aged and processed foods), cause a significant increase in blood pressure. Option #1 would be more appropriate when advising a client taking antipsychotic medications about the problem with photosensitivity. Option #3 is not relevant. Option #4 is more appropriate when advising a client taking antianxiety medications.

13.46 ③ Respirations should be counted for one full minute prior to arousing the infant with a temperature probe or stethoscope. After the infant is stimulated, the crying interferes with accurate evaluation. Option #4 is incorrect because observations should be done first.

13.47 ④ Food reduces absorption by 30–40%. Option #1 is incorrect due to the absorption reduction by food. Option #2 is incorrect because it may cause potassium toxicity. Option #3 may cause an overdose.

13.48 ③ These are major side effects of Stelazine. Extrapyramidal reactions should be reported immediately. Options #1, #2, and #4 represent possible side effects of antipsychotic medications, but do not require immediate intervention.

13.49 ① Ostomy bags should be changed at least once a week. This is a good time for the stoma to be closely inspected. Option #2 is incorrect because the bag should be changed only when the seal around the stoma is loose or leaking. Option #3 does not encourage client participation or foster independence. Option #4 is incorrect because the bag should be changed more often.

13.50 ③ This statement indicates acceptance and a readiness to participate in post-operative care. Option #1 indicates feelings of fear and helplessness. Option #2 indicates fear and lack of trust. Option #4 indicates fear that something will be missed.

13.51 ③ To prevent a post-lumbar puncture headache, the client should remain flat in bed for 8 hours after the test. Options #1 and #2 are not protocol for this test. Option #4 is inappropriate for procedure.

13.52 ④ As the client begins to escalate their anger, the nurse can be very helpful in using psychological/communication strategies. Option #1 is incorrect because it would be more useful to try option #4 first. Option #2 can become potentially dangerous to the client and property. Option #3 might further escalate frustration and anger because of ability to focus and concentrate are diminished due to an elevated anxiety level.

13.53 ④ Narcan blocks the neuroreceptors affected by opiates to reverse the effects. Option #1 is a narcotic analgesic. Option #2 is used with alcoholic clients. Option #3 is an anti-Parkinson medication.

13.54 ② Option #2 is correct as this decreases the change of atmospheric air entering the pleura, but still allows for the escape of pleural air. Option #1, chest tube insertion is a medical procedure. The old tube is contaminated. Option #3 will not be useful. Deep breathing associated with coughing can increase the amount of atmospheric air entering the pleural space. Option #4 should be reevaluated after emergency measures are instituted.

13.55 ④ Option #4 is correct: 12.5 milligrams is ¼ of a 50 mg table.

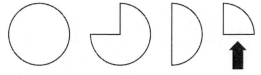

13.56 ④ Option #4 is a priority for promoting safety for this client who must get up to void during the night. Option #1 would create a safety issue for this client. Option #2 does not address the nursing concept. Option #3 is not an alternative for the client.

13.57 ② It is vitally important to complete all the penicillin. Option #1 is a true statement concerning the pregnant client not taking over-the-counter medications unless directed by a physician but is not a priority for this client. Option #3 may be unrealistic. She needs to inform others and ideally, for the present time, refrain from sexual activity. Option #4 is incorrect because communicable diseases are reportable, and partners of contacts need to be notified so they may be treated.

13.58 ③ The care of a child who has been this ill involves many disciplines, and the family will continue to need support long after discharge. Option #1 is incorrect because they should be helped to openly deal with whatever issue the child raises. Option #2 is critical at this stage. Don't limit the time; help them use it fully. Option #4 is incorrect because one of the nurse's major functions is to keep the family well informed.

13.59 ① It is very important that the geriatric client have the visual and manual skills to administer their insulin. Options #2 and #3 are important to determine; but Option #1 is a priority. Urinary tests are not commonly used to monitor diabetes.

I CAN HINT: "MAKE" will assist you in evaluating if an elderly client is competent to administer insulin to self.

Manual dexterity

Adequate vision

Kogntive (Cognitive) ability

Evaluate signs and symptoms of hyper and hypoglycemia

13.60 ③ This will prevent complications with seizures which can occur. Option #1 is incorrect because clients with meningitis are placed in droplet precautions for at least 24 hours. Option #2 is incorrect because these assessments should be done more frequently. Option #4 is incorrect because many clients will be on fluid restriction due to potential increased intracranial pressure.

13.61 ④ No blood pressure or needle sticks are done on the affected arm because of potential circulatory impairment or infection. Option #1 is unnecessary. Option #2 is avoided. Gentle exercise started early in the post-operative course helps decrease muscle tension as well as repair muscle function more quickly. Option #3 is incorrect because the appropriate support group for a post-mastectomy client is Reach to Recovery.

13.62 ③ In the selection of client assignments, it is important for the charge nurse to consider the abilities of each staff member. When a nurse is having difficulty coping with certain types of clients, the nurse needs to be reassigned until there is an ability to deal with them in a therapeutic way. Options #1 and #2 are not appropriate for the situation. Option #4 is incorrect because it would be important for the charge nurse to address the client concerns to the 3–11 nurse.

13.63 ② The client with vaso-occlusive crisis is a priority for hydration due to the physiological clumping of the RBCs. With hydration, the circulation improves, decreases discomfort, and promotes adequate oxygenation. Option #1 is incorrect because an IV may not be indicated. Option #3 may not require an IV. Option #4 will have the IV for surgery started appropriately prior to surgery.

13.64 ① Option #1 is correct. The stomach contents should be returned to the stomach so that valuable electrolytes will not be lost. In Option #2, NG tubes are ordinarily utilized for stomach decompression or nausea. The nurse would not force 350 mL of fluid on a client that has just had the tube removed. In Option #3, this distractor does not address the question. Option #4 is an unnecessary action at this point.

13.65 ③ It is important for the nurse to understand what the client expects from the rehabilitation program for future success. Options #1, #2, and #4 are important to assess, but they are not as crucial for future success as the client's goals.

13.66 ② All clients with tuberculosis are placed in standard/airborne precautions in the hospital, and the nurse should begin preparations for this immediately. Option #1 is unnecessary at this time. When indicated, the provider of care will write appropriate transfer orders. Option #3 is incorrect because the personal items do not have to be decontaminated. Option #4 is secondary.

13.67 ④ The geriatric client should be encouraged to talk about life and important things in the past. Option #1 is incorrect because he may not remember why or where he is. Option #2 is not as important as option #4. Option #3 is not priority to option #4.

13.68 ④ Indomethacin is an NSAID and is contraindicated in clients with peptic ulcer disease. It would also be contraindicated in clients with renal insufficiency. Options #1, #2, and #3 are potential orders for gout. Colchicine has an anti-inflammatory action limited to crystal-induced inflammation. Allopurinol inhibits the enzyme xanthine oxidase and blocks the formation of uric acid. Probenecid is an uriosuric drug which acts to inhibit renal tubular reabsorption of uric acid.

13.69 ③ When antacids are given 1 hour after eating, gastric acidity is minimized for another 1–2 hours, countering the food-induced stimulation of acid secretion. Options #1 and #2 are incorrect because if given with a meal, the antacid is wasted since food is an adequate buffer. Option #4 is incorrect because they interact with the medications and decrease the effectiveness.

13.70 ② Option #2 is the correct method that ensures a fresh, uncontaminated sample. Option #1 is incorrect. Urine obtained from the bag has been standing and will not give a reliable culture result. Option #3 is inappropriate and results in additional trauma to tissues. Option #4, urine collected from the bag, is not a reliable source for a culture.

13.71 ④ The client will be safest in a wheelchair. Option #1 is unsafe for an elderly client with a below-the-knee amputation. Options #2 and #3 are unmanageable without the assistance of a prosthesis.

13.72 ① Aspirin works by inhibiting prostaglandin production. As a result, a major side effect is gastric mucosal injury resulting in ulceration. Bleeding occasionally occurs from gastritis or ulceration. If PUD is already a problem, this client is predisposed to complications. Options #2, #3, and #4 would necessitate the use of aspirin.

13.73 ① This action would indicate a need for further clinical training. Securing a Foley catheter bag to the side of the bedrail can result in a reflux of urine back in the bladder. Options #2, #3, and #4 are appropriate actions.

13.74 ③ If the adult client is coughing forcefully, do not interfere with the client's attempt to expel the foreign body. Options #1, #2, and #4 are inappropriate.

13.75 ④ Option #4 is correct. This action will likely ease the breathing, so that other decisions can be made. Option #1 may not be the appropriate drug. Options #2 and #3 will likely add to the stress.

CHAPTER 14
Post-Test #2

Life is 10% what happens to you
and 90% how you react to it.
— SWINDOLL

✔ Clarification of this test …

Just keep on working on your testing practice and study. Here are more questions to help you identify your study needs.

14.1 Which of these actions is most appropriate when the nurse is documenting in the electronic medical records on the computer in a semi-private room which is located at the client's bedside?
① No nursing action is necessary following documentation since this information is fully secured.
② Following each documentation, make certain the computer is facing away from the client.
③ Pull the curtain around the computer so client and family members are unable to review.
④ Following each documentation, the nurse should log off.

14.2 What is the priority nursing action for a client who is scheduled to have a hip replacement and has signed the consent, but while completing the pre-procedure checklist, the client says, "I don't really understand what they are planning to do! I don't think I want it done"?
① Reassure the client that this is a routine surgery, and there is nothing to worry about.
② Notify the surgeon that the client has questions and concerns about the procedure.
③ Answer the client's questions, and explain the procedure.
④ Inform the client that consent for the surgery has already been done.

14.3 What personal protective equipment is necessary for the nurse to apply when providing care and assisting the health care provider with a mother with HIV and who is in the Labor and Delivery Suites actively delivering her baby? **Select all that apply.**
① Gown
② Mask
③ Goggles
④ Gloves
⑤ Sterile gown

14.4 During a rehabilitation session, a client who is four weeks post cerebrovascular accident (CVA) gets angry and yells that nobody cares about how client is feeling and starts throwing objects in the room. What would be the priority nursing action?
① Stop the session and remove client from the room.
② Communicate with client in order to gain trust.
③ Speak to client strongly and ask client to stop the behavior.
④ Administer the PRN medication that is ordered.

14.5 Which plan would the nurse review during a health promotion offering for a group of older adults in the community?
① Older adults should receive the pneumococcal immunization annually.
② The influenza immunization should not be taken if there are any known egg allergies.
③ The herpes zoster immunization should be taken if client is over age 80.
④ The meningococcal (MCV4) immunization should be taken after age 66 and repeated every 5 years if client is high-risk.

14.6 Which of these home environmental assessments would present the highest risk for injury to a client with Parkinson's Disease?
① Throw rugs on carpet in a formal living room.
② Nightlight between bedroom and bathroom.
③ Eats meals and snacks in the kitchen at the bar and uses high bar stools.
④ Uses a cane for ambulation.

14.7 Which plan(s) would the nurse include in the care for a preschool child who has been diagnosed with impetigo? **Select all that apply.**
① Apply on gloves when entering the room.
② Apply on a mask when entering the room.
③ Apply on sterile gloves prior to starting the IV.
④ Apply on a gown when entering the room.
⑤ Place in a room with another preschool child who has impetigo.

14.8 Which observation is most important during the first 48 hours after the admission of a client with severe anxiety?
① What is important to the client?
② How does the client view self?
③ In what situations does the client get anxious?
④ Who in the client's family has had mental problems?

14.9 Which clinical findings for a depressed client who has a new prescription for fluoxetine require the nurse to report immediately to the health care provider? **Select all that apply.**
① Agitation
② Hyper-reflexia
③ Vomiting
④ Hallucinations
⑤ Temperature – 103° F (39.4° C)
⑥ Lethargy

14.10 A client is ordered cefoxitin 2 gm. IV piggyback in 100 mL 5% Dextrose in water. The primary IV is 5% Dextrose in Lactated Ringers infusing by gravity. Which safety measure would be included in the administration of this medication?
① The medication should be administered slowly at 20 to 25 mL/hr.
② The primary IV solution should be changed.
③ The piggyback infusion bag should be hung higher than the primary infusion.
④ An infusion pump must be obtained prior to administration.

14.11 When exploring ways to effectively manage the budget, the nurse will most likely find that she/he will have to set goals for the unit. What would be an appropriate goal for the unit?
① Decrease overhead by limiting supplies utilized to operate the unit.
② Stabilize the total work force by utilizing only part-time employees with limited working hours.
③ Develop an incentive program that will demonstrate cost-effective measures to maintain the overall budget.
④ Participate in open-forums to discuss the issues of budget management on a consistent basis.

14.12 Which clinical findings would the nurse instruct a client who is being discharged on aripiprazole to report immediately to the health care provider? **Select all that apply.**
① Complaints of syncope
② Dry mouth
③ Feeling fatigue
④ Urinary retention
⑤ Constipation

14.13 The health care provider has just informed a client that an amputation of the leg is needed. The client is crying as the nurse enters the room. Which technique can the nurse utilize that would be most therapeutic?
① Sit with client quietly until crying stops; then inquire about feelings.
② Ask what is causing client to feel so badly.
③ Comfort by hugging and tell client not to worry.
④ Try to distract by talking about her family.

14.14 The home health nurse is assessing a 75-year-old male client who had a cerebrovascular accident (CVA) 1 month ago and is currently complaining of a terrible headache. What would be the first nursing action?
① Assess the characteristics of the headache on a pain scale of 1 to 10.
② Evaluate current medications.
③ Ask client to sit in the chair and take the blood pressure.
④ Evaluate if the client has had any caffeine.

14.15 During the newborn assessment, the nurse is evaluating the Babinski reflex. Locate where the nurse would stroke to elicit this response.

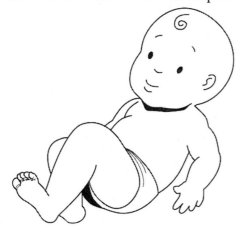

14.16 Which of these home health clients would the nurse visit and assess first?
① A student who reports experiencing severe anxiety with an exam.
② A client hearing a voice saying that it is time to accept the fact life is not worthy of living anymore.
③ A client who needs some adjustments on antipsychotic meds due to a few undesirable effects.
④ A client who refuses to come out of room and has not eaten in the last 24 hours since hearing about mother's death.

14.17 During a blood transfusion, a client presents with a hemolytic reaction. Which of these clinical findings would the nurse document in the chart? **Select all that apply.**
① Low back pain
② Urticaria
③ Chills
④ Bronchospasm
⑤ Flushing

14.18 A client is ordered to take metronidazole PO TID at home. Which client statement indicates a knowledge deficit and need for teaching?
① "I'll be sure to take this medication with meals."
② "I'll call my physician if my skin becomes itchy."
③ "I'll limit my alcohol intake to two drinks per day."
④ "I understand that my urine may become brown-colored and is normal."

14.19 Which assessment findings should be documented in the chart for a client who abuses cocaine?
① Bradycardia, miosis, hypertension
② Mydriasis, abdominal cramps, excessive salivation
③ Hypotension, bradycardia, abdominal cramps
④ Hypertension, tachycardia, tremor

14.20 Which technique would be used in the administration of heparin sodium?

① Gently massage the injection site.
② Do not aspirate after inserting the needle.
③ Use a 1-inch (2.54 cm), 18–20 gauge needle.
④ Administer the medication at the deltoid muscle.

14.21 A nursing unit is implementing a project involving changes in the way the unit is managed. The nursing manager on the unit continues to have problems with a team member that has been very disruptive regarding the implementation of the project. What is the best approach for the nurse manager in handling this situation?

① Call the unit supervisor and advise of the problems with the team member and ask how to handle the situation.
② Privately meet with the team member, review behavior, and determine if she/he is aware of the impact of her/his behavior has on the unit.
③ Involve the other members of the team in attempting to discourage the disruptive team member's behavior.
④ Counsel with the disruptive team member and ask why she/he is not happy working on this unit.

14.22 What action would the nurse implement first for a client presenting in the emergency department with a gun and is threatening to kill the nurse?

① Encourage client to discuss his anger.
② Advise the LPN on the team to notify security.
③ Firmly and calmly request client to place gun down on the floor.
④ Administer the prescribed antianxiety medication.

14.23 The nurse would teach the mother of a newborn which concept regarding umbilical cord care?

① Apply a sterile gauze dressing with petroleum jelly to cord.
② Position diaper over the umbilicus to maintain dryness.
③ Clean cord with alcohol several times a day and expose to air frequently.
④ Apply erythromycin ointment to cord several times a day to prevent infection.

14.24 What would be the priority nursing intervention for an extremely agitated client who is receiving rapid neuroleptization with haloperidol IM every 30 minutes while in the psychiatric emergency room?

① Monitor vital signs, especially blood pressure every 30 minutes.
② Remain at client's side for reassurance.
③ Tell client name and effect of medication.
④ Monitor anticholinergic effects of medication.

14.25 The nurse is caring for a client who is two days post-op abdominal surgery. Which assessment data, on the following intake and output sheet (I&O), would require further action by the nurse?

Source	7a-7p	7p-a
P.O.	0 mL	0 mL
IV	1500 mL	1500 mL
Urine	900 mL	1000 mL
Nasogastric tube	500 mL	50 mL

① P. O. intake
② Intravenous fluid balance
③ Urine output
④ Nasogastric suction drainage

14.26 What is the nurse's next action when a client states, "I am going to end it all, myself"?

① Ask the client, "Do you have a plan to kill yourself?"
② Tell the client, "Suicide is not the answer. Let's talk about what has brought you to this decision."
③ Call the health care provider and report what the client has said.
④ Ask the client, "Have you ever felt this way before?"

14.27 Which action by the nurse is most appropriate when a client requests that a nurse on a previous shift not care for him again?

① Document the issue on an incident report.
② Inform the nurse manager of the incident.
③ Explain to the client the nurse was having a bad day.
④ Address the client's concerns with the charge nurse.

14.28 Which assessment would be important to include in the history of a school-age child with glomerulonephritis?
① Strep throat 12 days ago
② Weight loss with diarrhea
③ Increase in fluid intake and voiding frequently
④ Decrease in energy with an increased need for sleep

14.29 Which vital sign recorded on a 2-month-old infant should be discussed with the pediatrician?
① Heart rate of 120 beats per minute (bpm).
② Rectal temperature of 101.5° F (38.6°C).
③ Respiratory rate of 40/min.
④ Blood pressure of 90/60.

14.30 What clinical assessment finding is a priority to report to the provider of care for a client who is taking Amphotericin B?
① Anorexia
② Muscle cramps
③ Spiked T waves
④ Skin hot and dry

14.31 What is the nurse's best response to a preschool child who asks if he is going to die?
① "Everyone dies sometime."
② "Don't be silly. You get stronger every day."
③ "You sound concerned. Tell me what made you ask that question."
④ "You are eating so much better and getting out of bed sometimes."

14.32 Which behavior indicates parental acceptance for an infant with a myelomeningocele repair?
① State the infant will outgrow this problem in time.
② Have the neighbor do bladder expression.
③ Measure the head circumference daily.
④ Discuss the expectation of child walking in one year.

14.33 Prior to administering the Measles, Mumps and Rubella (MMR) vaccine to a 15-month-old toddler, what would be most important for the nurse to assess?
① Sibling reaction to immunizations
② Allergies to eggs or neomycin
③ Allergies in family members to medications
④ Diarrhea in this client a week ago without temperature

14.34 When assessing orientation to person, place and time for an elderly hospitalized client, which principle would be understood by the nurse?
① Short-term memory is more efficient than long-term memory.
② The stress of an unfamiliar environment may cause confusion.
③ A decline in mental status is a normal part of aging.
④ Learning ability is reduced during aging.

14.35 Which nursing action is a priority for a child admitted with a positive stool culture for Salmonella?
① Change diet to clear liquids.
② Initiate intravenous fluids.
③ Place child in contact precautions.
④ Apply cloth diapers.

14.36 Which nursing care is important to include in the plan for a maternity client with preeclampsia? **Select all that apply.**
① Position client close to the nurses' station.
② Decrease fluid intake.
③ Discuss the importance of taking in a diet high in protein.
④ Encourage bed rest and place on the left lateral position.
⑤ Document the patellar reflex is +1.

14.37 Which clinical finding would be most important to report for a neonate with hyperbilirubinemia who is being treated with phototherapy?
① Bronze discoloration of the skin
② Decrease in the number of wet diapers
③ Flat anterior fontanel
④ Maculopapular skin rash

14.38 Which initial side effects from a client undergoing chemotherapy require ongoing evaluation?
① Alopecia and purpura
② Anorexia and weight loss
③ Nausea and vomiting
④ Coughing and shortness of breath

14.39 For the immobile client, which nursing assessment indicates a need for intervention?
① Drainage from the Foley catheter is clear, with a pH of 6.5.
② The client's skin blanches over the scapular areas.
③ Bilateral chest excursion is present.
④ The client drinks three glasses of orange juice every day.

14.40 Which of these clinical findings would require immediate intervention for a client who is receiving narcotics as prescribed?
① Temperature from 99.8°F to 101°F (37.7°C to 38.3°C)
② Blood Pressure from 148/86 to 150/88
③ Heart rate from 88 BPM to 56 BPM
④ Respiratory Rate from 18 to 26 per minute

14.41 What is the most appropriate action for the nurse to take after noting the sudden appearance of a fixed and dilated pupil in a neuro client?
① Reassess in five minutes.
② Check client's visual acuity.
③ Lower the head of the client's bed.
④ Call the health care provider.

14.42 In developing discharge plans with the family of the client in stage four Parkinson's disease, it is most important for the nurse to include which activities?
① Ambulate twice daily.
② ROM to all extremities four times a day.
③ Hobbies and games such as knitting and putting puzzles together.
④ Encourage and provide writing materials.

14.43 Which statement made by the client in sickle cell crisis indicates a need for further teaching?
① "My pain is from poor circulation due to sickling of the cells."
② "I will need to see a genetic counselor when I get married."
③ "I have a trip planned to snow-ski in three weeks."
④ "I need to stay away from strenuous activities."

14.44 Which statement made by a client who is prescribed Allopurinol indicates an appropriate understanding of how to safely take the medication?
① "I will take the medication 60 minutes prior to meals."
② "I will drink 2.5–3 liters of fluid per day."
③ "I will increase my intake of vitamin C."
④ "I will continue eating oatmeal and a slice of whole wheat toast for breakfast."

14.45 Which statement made by the client indicates a correct understanding of client-controlled epidural analgesia (PCA)?
① "If I start feeling drowsy, I should notify the nurse."
② "This button will give me enough to kill the pain whenever I want it."
③ "If I start itching, I need to call the nurse."
④ "This medicine will make me feel no pain."

14.46 What is the initial nursing priority for an infant admitted to the pediatric unit with possible Hemophilus influenzae meningitis?
① Encourage fluids to prevent dehydration.
② Restrain child appropriately to maintain integrity of IV site.
③ Place child in droplet precautions.
④ Encourage parents to hold and rock infant to promote comfort.

14.47 Which statement by a client indicates that the client is using the defense mechanism of conversion?
① "I love my family with all my heart, even though they don't love me."
② "I could not take my final exams because I was unable to write."
③ "I don't believe I have diabetes. I feel perfectly fine."
④ "If my wife was a better housekeeper, I wouldn't have such a problem."

14.48 Which statement indicates parental understanding about the cause of their newborn's diagnosis of cystic fibrosis?
① "The gene came from my husband's side of the family."
② "The gene came from my wife's side of the family."
③ "There is a 50 percent chance that our next child will have the disease."
④ "Both my husband and I carry a recessive trait for cystic fibrosis."

14.49 Prior to mixing different types of insulin, what would be the nursing priority?
① Rotate the vial at least 1 minute between both hands.
② Gently shake each vial for at least 1 minute.
③ Throw away all cloudy color insulin.
④ Take the vials out of the refrigerator for 30 minutes.

14.50 Which diversional activity is most appropriate for an adolescent client recovering from a sickle-cell crisis?
① Walking in the hall 20 minutes 2 times a day.
② Watching the cartoon channel all day.
③ Talking to best friend on the telephone.
④ Putting together large-pieced wooden puzzles.

14.51 Which nursing observation indicates an early complication of hypoxemia in a child with epiglottitis?
① Tachycardia
② Cyanosis
③ Circumoral pallor
④ Difficulty swallowing

14.52 Which action observed by the nurse indicates a client's ability to care for their colostomy?
① Irrigating the colostomy with 2000 mL of warm tap water.
② Changing the appliance twice a day.
③ Inserting the irrigating tube 6" into the stoma.
④ Fitting the appliance securely around the edge of the stoma.

14.53 Which nursing action is most appropriate when an infant is admitted for fever, poor feeding, irritability, and a bulging fontanel?
① Perform neuro checks every 1-2 hours.
② Place the client in droplet precautions.
③ Monitor client's urine output closely.
④ Encourage fluid intake.

14.54 Which nursing action is a priority for a newborn with a myelomeningocele?
① Elevate the head of the bed to decrease intracranial pressure.
② Immediately intubate the infant to decrease the potential for respiratory distress.
③ Position the infant supine to prevent damage to the sac.
④ Cover the sac with sterile, warm, moist compresses to maintain asepsis.

14.55 Which statement made by a client indicates a correct understanding of the side effects of phenazopyridine hydrochloride?
① "My medicine will make me urinate more frequently."
② "My medicine should be taken only at bedtime."
③ "My medicine will cause my urine to become orange."
④ "My medicine should be taken before meals."

14.56 Which recommendation by the nurse offers the greatest support to a newly diagnosed AIDS client and his family?
① Avoid all contact with anyone except immediate family.
② Speak to a representative from the local AIDS support group.
③ Stop all sexual activity immediately.
④ Begin chemotherapy as soon as possible.

14.57 Which question would best aid the nurse in assessing the orientation of a client on the psychiatric unit?
① "Who is the president of the United States?"
② "Do you remember my name?"
③ "What is your name?"
④ "What time is it?"

14.58 In performing a nursing audit, the nurse is evaluating the nursing documentation. Which would be present in the charting for a client receiving total parenteral nutrition (TPN)?
① Weight, blood glucose, I&O
② Amount of blood withdrawn for lab studies
③ Position during dressing change
④ CVP reading obtained during infusion to TPN

14.59 Which client statement indicates a need for more information regarding oral contraceptives?
① "I will need check-ups every six months."
② "I should take the pill the same time each day."
③ "If I forget a pill one day, I should take it when I remember. Then take the next pill as scheduled the next day."
④ "If I miss 2 pills, I will take them when I remember and continue the normal schedule."

14.60 Which assessments are most important regarding safety for a client receiving vincristine sulfate?
① Fatigue and nausea
② Polyphagia and polydipsia
③ Hypotension and alopecia
④ Paresthesia and difficulties in gait

14.61 During morning assignments, a nurse is assigned to several clients. Which would be first to receive morning care?
① A client with a recent appendectomy
② A client with infectious meningitis
③ An immunosuppressed client
④ A client with COPD

14.62 Which of these statements made by a RN to a GN during orientation indicates an understanding of the symptoms for an elderly client presenting with the following: a temperature of 103.4°F (39.7°C), moderate dehydration, bilateral rales in lower lobes of lungs, and disorientation to time and place?
① "The client is experiencing temporary delirium secondary to the infectious process."
② "The client is probably displaying early symptoms of Alzheimer's Disease."
③ "Elderly clients often get confused as a normal part of the aging process."
④ "A referral to a nursing home for continuing care will be necessary for this client."

14.63 A client in the ER is displaying the following symptoms:
• Elevated vital signs
• Hallucinations
• Aggressive behavior.

The client's friend says the client has been using hallucinogenic drugs. What would be the most appropriate nursing action?
① Put the client in full restraints.
② Decrease environmental stimulation.
③ Call the security guards.
④ Administer a PRN dose of chlorpromazine.

4.64 The nurse is caring for a client who is taking Disulfiram. The nurse would caution the client to avoid the intake of which of the following?
① Aged cheeses
② Liquid cough medicines
③ Chicken or beef liver
④ Yogurt or sour cream

14.65 The nurse does not know the answer to a question asked by the client. What is the most appropriate response to assist in developing a trusting relationship?
① "Why don't you ask your physician this question?"
② "Here is some written information that will answer your question."
③ "I don't know the answer, but will find out and let you know in 30 minutes."
④ "Don't worry about this issue; it should never happen to you."

14.66 The nurse is caring for a client who is extremely flirtatious, charming, and willing to manipulate others. Which measure would the nurse take?
① Set limits with the client's behavior and share plan with the nursing staff on all three shifts.
② Ask another nurse to care for this particular client.
③ Document the client's behavior, so that the health care provider will order medication to control client's behavior.
④ Listen empathetically and help meet the client's needs.

14.67 One of the goals for the nurse and client with Post Traumatic Stress Disorder (PTSD) that was mutually agreed upon was an increase in participation in "out of the apartment" activities. Which recommendation would be the most therapeutic while achieving that goal?
① Take a day trip with a friend.
② Take an 11-minute bus ride alone.
③ Join a support group and participate in a victim assistance organization.
④ Take a 10-minute walk with spouse around the block.

14.68 Which client diagnosis would be the first to receive morning care?
① Staph pneumonia
② Broken leg with skeletal traction
③ Cancer taking chemotherapy
④ COPD

14.69 A charge nurse is developing the assignment for the evening shift. In a semi-private room, Client A has neutropenia. Client B has a tracheostomy with purulent drainage and a pending C&S. Which assignment is the most appropriate?
① Assign an experienced nurse to care for both clients in the same room.
② Assign two nurses—one nurse for Client A, and another nurse for Client B—in the same room.
③ Place Client A in a private room. Assign the same nurse to care for Client A and Client B.
④ Place Client A in a private room. Assign different nurses to care for Client A and Client B.

14.70 A 6-month-old infant is on Isomil and weighs fifteen pounds. Which nursing observation on a home visit would indicate a need for further teaching?
① The infant is sucking a pacifier.
② The infant is crawling on the floor.
③ The father speaks sternly to the infant for pulling books from the bookcase.
④ The father gives the baby a bottle with whole milk.

14.71 What would be the priority assessment for an 11-month-old baby is having trouble gaining weight after discharge from the hospital?
① Observe the child at mealtime.
② Inquire regarding the child's eating pattern.
③ Weigh the baby each month.
④ Try to feed the baby for the mother.

14.72 A client has been receiving morphine sulfate 15 mg IV push for several days as pain management for severe burns. Nursing assessment reveals a decrease in bowel sounds and slight abdominal distention. Which nursing action is the most appropriate?
① Recommend morphine dose be decreased.
② Withhold pain medication.
③ Administer medication by another route.
④ Explore alternative pain management techniques.

14.73 Which assessment would be a priority for evaluating the status of a pleurevac connected to a right middle lobe chest tube?
① Incentive spirometry
② Breath sounds
③ Chest tube drainage
④ Chest x-ray

14.74 Following hip replacement surgery, an elderly client is ordered to begin ambulation with a walker. In planning nursing care, which statement by the nurse will best help this client?
① "Sit in a low chair for ease in getting up to the walker."
② "Make sure rubber caps are present on all four legs of the walker."
③ "Begin weight-bearing on the affected hip as soon as possible."
④ "Practice tying your own shoes before using the walker."

14.75 An elderly client with mild osteoarthritis needs instruction on exercising. In planning nursing care, which instruction would best help this client?
① Swimming is the only helpful exercise for osteoarthritis.
② Warm-up exercises should be done prior to exercising.
③ Exercises should be done routinely even if joint pain occurs.
④ Isometric exercises are most helpful to prevent contractures.

Category Analysis—Post-Test #2

1. Management of Care
2. Management of Care
3. Safety and Infection Control
4. Psychosocial
5. Health Promotion
6. Reduction of Risk Potential
7. Safety and Infection Control
8. Psychosocial
9. Pharmacology
10. Pharmacology
11. Management of Care
12. Pharmacology
13. Psychosocial
14. Reduction of Risk Potential
15. Health Promotion
16. Psychosocial
17. Safety and Infection Control
18. Pharmacology
19. Safety and Infection Control
20. Pharmacology
21. Management of Care
22. Psychosocial
23. Health Promotion
24. Pharmacology
25. Physiological Adaptation
26. Psychosocial
27. Safety and Infection Control
28. Health Promotion
29. Health Promotion
30. Pharmacology
31. Psychosocial
32. Health Promotion
33. Health Promotion
34. Health Promotion
35. Safety and Infection Control
36. Health Promotion
37. Basic Care and Comfort
38. Basic Care and Comfort
39. Reduction of Risk Potential
40. Pharmacology
41. Reduction of Risk Potential
42. Reduction of Risk Potential
43. Physiological Adaptation
44. Pharmacology
45. Pharmacology
46. Reduction of Risk Potential
47. Psychosocial
48. Health Promotion
49. Basic Care and Comfort
50. Health Promotion
51. Health Promotion
52. Basic Care and Comfort
53. Health Promotion
54. Health Promotion
55. Pharmacology
56. Psychosocial
57. Psychosocial
58. Management of Care
59. Health Promotion
60. Pharmacology
61. Management of Care
62. Physiological Adaptation
63. Psychosocial
64. Pharmacology
65. Psychosocial
66. Psychosocial
67. Psychosocial
68. Safety and Infection Control
69. Safety and Infection Control
70. Health Promotion
71. Health Promotion
72. Basic Care and Comfort
73. Physiological Adaptation
74. Health Promotion
75. Health Promotion

Chapter 14: POST-TEST #2

Directions

1. Determine questions missed by checking answers.
2. Write the number of the questions missed across the top line marked "item missed."
3. Check category analysis page to determine category of question.
4. Put a check mark under item missed and beside content.
5. Count check marks in each row and write the number in totals column.
6. Use this information to:
   - identify areas for further study.
   - determine which content test to take next.

We recommend studying content where most items are missed—then taking that content test.

Number of the Questions Incorrectly Answered

Post-Test	Items Missed																				Totals
C Management of Care																					
O Safety and Infection Control																					
N Health Promotion and Maintenance																					
T Psychosocial Integrity																					
E Physiological Adaptation: Fluid Gas																					
N Reduction of Risk Potential																					
T Basic Care and Comfort																					
Pharmacology and Parenteral Therapies																					

Answers & Rationales

Chapter 14: ANSWERS & RATIONALES   321

14.1 ④ Option #4 is correct. The Health Insurance Portability and Accountability Act (HIPAA) requires client confidentiality. It is required that after each use of the computer and when exiting the room of the client, the nurse log off from the computer. It is important that the others do not see the information on the screen. Option #1 is an incorrect statement. Options #2 and #3 do not address the need to log off of the computer. Just because the computer is not facing the client or the curtain is around the computer does not assure someone will not review the information on the screen.

14.2 ② Option #2 is correct. It is the physician's responsibility to explain the procedure and to obtain the consent. The nurse can answer client's questions, but it is ultimately the surgeon's responsibility. Option #1 is minimizing the client's concerns, and option #4 is incorrect. Consent can always be withdrawn.

14.3 ① Options #1, #2, #3, #4 are correct. This is
       ② based on the CDC standards of care for a
       ③ client in labor and delivery and who has been
       ④ diagnosed with HIV. These same precautions should be followed even with no diagnosis of HIV in order to protect the nurse. CDC has outlined the Standard Precautions based on the nursing care being provided. If there is a risk for the nurse to come in contact with the client's blood and/or body fluids during delivery, then the first four options must be applied. Option #5 is not necessary for this client.

14.4 ① Option #1 is the correct answer. It is the standard of care to remove the combative client from a setting where the client may harm self and/or others. Option #2 is important, but if client is yelling, it would not be the top priority for this situation. Option #3 is setting limits, and is an appropriate second action, but not a priority over option #1 which has a focus on client "SAFETY." Option #4 would be last if all else fails.

14.5 ② Option #2 is correct. The immunization would be contraindicated for clients with known egg allergies. Options #1, #3, and #4 are incorrect. Option #1 is incorrect. If the client was not previously vaccinated or has no evidence of disease then one dose should be given at age 65. Option #3 is incorrect. The guidelines recommend this immunization for all adults over 60 year. Option #4 is incorrect. The meningococcal (MCV4) immunization is recommended for adults greater than age 56. Revaccination may be recommended after 5 years for adults at high risk for infection.

14.6 ③ The bar stools present the highest risk factor for falls to this client. Option #1 is a concern but not a priority over option #3. Options #2 and #4 may assist client versus being a risk factor.

14.7 ① This child will require contact precautions.
       ④ Staphylococcus causes impetigo. These preca-
       ⑤ utions require both a gown and gloves when entering the room. If no private rooms are available, then assign client to a room with another child close to the same developmental age and who has the same infection. Options #2 and #3 are not required for this organism.

14.8 ③ This will provide necessary information in the baseline assessment of the client's anxiety. Options #1, #2, and #4 are helpful data which can be collected during treatment, but do not take priority during the first 48 hours.

14.9 ① Fluoxetine is a selective serotonin reuptake
       ② inhibitor (SSRI). This classification
       ③ of medication can result in a possible lethal
       ④ condition known as serotonin syndrome. It
       ⑤ can occur within 2 to 72 hours after beginning the SSRIs. The only incorrect option is #6. Agitation, insomnia, and nervousness may occur, but not lethargy. The other options reflect serotonin syndrome.

14.10 ③ When using a gravity drip, the piggyback fluid level should be higher than the primary infusion. Option #1 is incorrect because the antibiotic should be administered within one hour. Options #2 and #4 are not necessary for safe infusion.

14.11 ③ Developing an incentive program to maintain revenue will involve the whole unit. This will also give accountability and responsibility back to the staff on the unit. Option #1 may be counter-productive. Option #2 may decrease quality of care. Option #4 may be useful and secondary to option #3.

14.12 ①
③ Options #1 and #3 are correct. Aripiprazole is a 3rd generation antipsychotic medication. The syncope may be a result of the orthostatic hypotension that my occur from the undesirable effects of cardiac changes. Option #3 may occur from the undesirable effect of bleeding. These two findings need to be immediately reported. Options #2, #4, and #5 are anticholinergic effects, and do not present an immediate threat to the client.

14.13 ① "Being with" the client as acknowledgement and dealing with impending loss demonstrates the nurse's acceptance of the client's need to grieve. Allowing the client time to cry and then asking to describe feelings demonstrates the nurse is willing to listen and validate the client's feelings. Option #2 is not acknowledging the situation requiring an amputation. Option #3 might be somewhat premature and uncomfortable unless both participants in the relationship find touching acceptable. It is inappropriate to tell her not to worry. Option #4 is avoidance of the situation.

14.14 ③ The major risk for a CVA is arterial hypertension. A symptom of hypertension is a headache. If BP is elevated, client needs to be evaluated in the emergency department. Option #1 would not affect the care the home health nurse provides in the home. It is important to initiate option #2, but the nurse must first attempt to identify the cause. Option #4 is incorrect for this question.

14.15

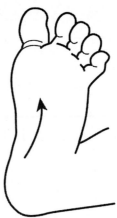

14.16 ② Option #2 is correct. This client may consider suicide and SAFETY becomes an immediate concern. Option #1 is not correct. While it is important for intervention so the anxiety does not escalate to a state of panic, it would not be a priority over option #2 who may be suicidal. Option #3 is not correct. This client needs intervention, but not a priority over #2. Option #4 is indeed important to assess, but client does not have energy to perform suicide. There is no increase in energy, no plan, etc. The client is very depressed and needs help, but option #2 needs immediate assessment due to the voices being heard about not being worthy to live.

14.17 ①
③
⑤ These are correct. Hemolytic transfusion reaction clinical findings include: low back pain, hypotension, tachycardia, tachypnea, apprehension, sense of impending doom, fever, chills, flushing, chest pain, dyspnea, and onset is immediate. Options #2 and #4 are allergic reactions. Allergic reactions include: urticaria, pruritus, facial flushing, severe shortness of breath, bronchospasm.

I CAN HINT: The key word is "*hemolytic versus allergic*" in the stem of the question. An allergic reaction would result in a release of histamines. This would be the same clinical presentation that would occur if the client had an allergic reaction from penicillin, pollen, chocolate, etc.

14.18 ③ Metronidazole will produce a disulfiram-like (Antabuse) reaction if any form of alcohol is used. Options #1, #2, and #4 indicate an understanding of the concepts related to taking this medication.

Chapter 14: ANSWERS & RATIONALES

14.19 ④ Cocaine elevates the blood pressure and pulse along with causing a fine tremor. Cardiac dysrhythmias can occur, especially with the use of crack cocaine. Excessive salivation and bradycardia are not found with cocaine abuse.

14.20 ② Aspirating the syringe with a subcutaneous heparin solution can cause bruising. Option #1 is incorrect because the heparin injection site should not be rubbed. Option #3 is incorrect because the needle is too long. Option #4 is incorrect because the medication should be given subcutaneously.

14.21 ② It is important to determine what the problem is with the disruptive team member. The best way to do that is in private. Review with him/her the disruptive behavior and attempt to determine the source of the problem. If this does not solve the situation, then the supervisor should be notified. Option #2 better describes the solution than does option #4. Other team members should not be brought into the situation

14.22 ③ The first action is to calmy attempt to diffuse the hostile situation. Option #1 is incorrect. This may result with the client killing an innocent person. Option #2 in addition to notifying the local police department are important for safety for the man, other clients, and staff. The first action is to diffuse the hostile situation. Option #4 is not correct for this situation.

14.23 ③ This will encourage drying and assist in preventing infection. Option #1 is appropriate for circumcision care. Option #2 will keep the area moist. Diaper should be placed below the umbilicus. Option #4 is incorrect because the antibiotic ointment is not necessary.

14.24 ① While all of these nursing interventions are necessary during rapid neuroleptization, monitoring vital signs is of utmost importance to assure client safety and physiological integrity. Rapid neuroleptization is a pharmacological intervention used to rapidly diminish severe symptoms which accompany acute psychosis. The alpha-adrenergic blockade of peripheral vascular system lowers blood pressure and causes postural hypotension. Options #2 and #4 are secondary. Option #3 may be done later.

14.25 ④ Option #4 is correct. Sudden cessation or drastic decrease of nasogastric drainage indicates blockage or disruption of the drainage system. Normal gastric production is 1-1.5 L daily. 500 mL per twelve-hour shift is expected. Option #1 is incorrect because the client has a draining nasogastric tube. P.O. intake is not expected. Option #2 demonstrates that the I.V. fluid balance is appropriate. Option #3 is incorrect because the urine output is slightly more than intake and is not a cause of concern.

14.26 ① Option #1 is priority to identify if the client has a plan for suicide before proceeding to intervention. Options #2, #3, and #4 do not assess if the client has a plan which is priority if a client mentions suicide intent.

14.27 ④ As a client advocate, the nurse needs to intervene to assure the client's request is met. The issue needs to be discussed with the charge nurse, so that accurate communication occurs between the shifts and personnel involved. Option #1 is inappropriate. Option #2 should occur, but after the charge nurse is advised of the situation. Option #3 is making excuses and not addressing the issue.

14.28 ① There is a 10–14 day latent period between group A beta hemolytic streptococcal infection and the onset of signs of glomerulonephritis. Option #2 includes signs of hypovolemia. Option #3 includes signs of diabetes mellitus. Option #4 is not specific to a particular diagnosis.

14.29 ② Option #2 is correct because a temperature above 101.3°F (38.5°C) rectally in a child less than 3 months old is abnormal and can signify a serious infection. Options #1, #3, and #4 are normal in a 2-month-old infant.

14.30 ② Option #2 is correct since a complication that may occur with a client who is taking amphotericin may experience an undesirable effect of hypokalemia. Hypokalemia may present with muscle cramps or a flattened or inverted T wave. Other complications that may occur include weakness of the skeletal muscles, hyporeflexia, irritability, and decreased bowel sounds. Option #1 is incorrect. Option #3 would be appropriate for hyperkalemia. Option #4 is incorrect.

Chapter 14: ANSWERS & RATIONALES

14.31 ③ Exploring what happened to cause the client to ask the question would assist the nurse in answering questions. Options #1, #2, and #4 do not explore the client's feelings.

14.32 ③ Parents' participation in care may be the first sign of acceptance. Measuring the head circumference is important due to the risk of hydrocephalus following surgery, but even simple care like bathing the child, could bring acceptance. Option #1 is incorrect because the child has a chronic problem. Option #2 indicates parents' lack of interest and inability to care for child. Option #4 shows a lack of understanding about myelomeningocele.

14.33 ② Allergies to MMR come from egg, fowl, and neomycin due to the growth of the live virus in egg embryo. Option #1 is incorrect because there is no absolute relationship between the siblings' allergic responses. Option #3 is not relevant to this vaccination. Option #4 is more significant for oral polio administration.

14.34 ② The stress of an unfamiliar situation or environment may lead to confusion among the elderly. Option #1 is incorrect because long-term memory is more efficient than short-term. Options #3 and #4 are not affected by aging. The elderly client may be slower at doing things.

14.35 ③ Contact precautions prevent the transmission of Salmonella to other individuals. Options #1, #2, and #4 may be appropriate but are not a priority over option #3 which will prevent transmission.

14.36 ③ A diet high in protein to replace the lost protein in the urine is important for the plan. Placing client on the left lateral position will optimize uteroplacental blood flow. Option #5 only needs to be documented since it is a normal finding. Option #1 is incorrect. Too much stimuli can cause a seizure. Client should drink 6-8 glasses of water daily.

14.37 ② Option #2 is the correct answer. A potential risk with the treatment of hyperbilirubinemia with phototherapy is alteration in fluid and electrolytes from the numerous stools. One way to evaluate the hydration of a neonate is the number of wet diapers in addition to the weight and characteristics of the fontanels. Option #1 is incorrect since this is an expected finding for a neonate with hyperbilirubinemia. Option #3 is incorrect. If the neonate was dehydrated, the fontanels would be sunken. Option #4 is incorrect for this clinical situation.

14.38 ③ The most common initial side effects of chemotherapy are nausea and vomiting. Options #1 and #4 are typically later findings. Option #2 can be a result of option #3.

14.39 ② Blanching or hyperemia that does not disappear in a short time is a warning sign of pressure ulcers. Option #1 is normal urine. Option #3 is a normal respiratory assessment finding. Option #4 is irrelevant.

14.40 ③ Narcotics can cause a decrease in heart rate. Option #1 is irrelevant. Option #2 is incorrect because hypotension will result. Option #4 is incorrect because respiratory depression will result.

14.41 ④ A fixed and dilated pupil represents a neurological emergency. Option #1 does not take-action necessary for the immediate situation. Option #2 cannot accurately be evaluated with increased ICP. Option #3 would increase the intracranial pressure.

14.42 ② In stage four Parkinson's disease, the client is immobile. Option #1 is incorrect because the client would be unable to ambulate. Options #3 and #4 are incorrect because the client cannot perform activities which require small muscle dexterity.

14.43 ③ The mountains are low in oxygen concentration which, along with increased activity, would contribute to sickling of the cells. Options #1, #2, and #4 indicate a correct understanding.

14.44 ② Fluids are imperative to decrease the side effects of a gout attack or renal stones. Option #1 is incorrect because the drug should be taken following meals due to nausea and vomiting. Option #3 will increase the likelihood of renal calculi formation. Option #4 is high in purine which is a precursor to uric acid. This counteracts the purpose of administering the medication.

14.45 ③ A common side effect of narcotics used in epidural pain management is itching. Options #2 and #4 are incorrect. Option #1 is secondary.

14.46 ③ To prevent the spread of the infection, the client is placed in droplet precautions for at least 24 hours after implementation of antibiotic therapy. Option #1 is incorrect because the fluids are determined by client status. Fluids are usually limited to prevent cerebral edema. Option #2 is appropriate but is not a priority to option #3. Option #4 would cause discomfort to the client's head.

14.47 ② The client has converted his anxiety over school performance into a physical symptom that interferes with his ability to perform. Option #1 may be reaction formation. Option #3 is denial. Option #4 is projection.

14.48 ④ Cystic fibrosis is inherited by an autosomal recessive trait. Both parents are carriers of the abnormal gene. There is a 25 percent chance of passing the gene on to any of their offspring. Options #1, #2, and #3 are inaccurate.

14.49 ① Rotating resuspends the modified insulin preparations and helps to warm the medication. Option #2 causes bubbles and foam which can alter the dose. Option #3 is incorrect because longer acting insulins are supposed to be cloudy. Option #4 is incorrect because insulin does not have to be refrigerated as long as it is at normal room temperature.

14.50 ③ This will conserve energy and still meet psychosocial needs of peer involvement. Option #1 will not conserve much needed energy. Option #2 is an isolating activity and is not age appropriate. Option #4 is appropriate for preschool children.

14.51 ① Option #1 is correct. The heart rate correlates with hypoxemia and is an early finding along with restlessness. Options #2 and #3 would be late signs. Option #4 is a sign of epiglottitis.

14.52 ④ The appliance should fit easily around the stoma and protect the skin. Option #1 is incorrect because no more than 1000 mL of irrigation fluid should ever be used. Option #2 is incorrect because the appliance should only be changed when it begins to leak or becomes dislodged. Option #3 is incorrect because the catheter should not be inserted over 4" into the stoma.

14.53 ② These are classic signs of meningitis, and the client should be isolated from other clients. Options #1 and #3 are appropriate but are not a priority over option #2 when the client is first admitted. Option #4 is inappropriate for this situation.

14.54 ④ Prevention of infection is critical for this infant. The head of the infant's bed should remain flat unless otherwise ordered. Option #2 is irrelevant to this situation. Option #3 is of utmost importance, but to do this, the infant must be prone or on his side.

14.55 ③ The drug may change the urine to an orange color. Option #1 is not accurate because this drug is not a diuretic. It has a local anesthetic action on the urinary tract mucosa. Options #2 and #4 are incorrect because the drug should be taken after meals.

14.56 ② The establishment of a support system from the beginning is very important to any terminally ill client, especially with a disease like AIDS that is associated with a social stigma. Option #1 is incorrect because general isolation is not necessary. The client does need education regarding exposure to infectious agents. Option #3 is not necessary as long as precautions are taken to prevent spreading the disease. Option #4 is inappropriate to the situation.

14.57 ③ This is a specific question related to the orientation of the person. Option #1 is incorrect because some well-oriented people do not know the answer to this question depending upon their age, educational level, etc. Option #2 is irrelevant. Option #4 is incorrect because without consulting a watch or clock, most well-oriented people cannot answer this question.

14.58 ① Daily weights, blood glucose, and I&O evaluate the effectiveness of TPN. Option #2 is unnecessary. Option #3 may be charted but is secondary to #1. Option #4 is incorrect. The CVP should not be determined with TPN infusing.

14.59 ④ If 2 pills are missed, they should be taken. However, another form of contraception for the remainder of the month should be used. Options #1, #2, and #3 are correct and do not require more information.

14.60 ④ These assessments indicate a problem with peripheral neuropathy. These can result in difficulties with safety and will mandate a change in the plan of care. Option #1 does occur but is not a priority over option #4. Option #2 includes signs of diabetes. Option #3 is not a priority over option #4.

14.61 ③ WBCs are usually decreased in the immuno-suppressed client which predisposes to infection. AM care should be completed on this client first, especially before the client with meningitis. Option #1: the nurse may find it useful to provide time for a PRN for pain to work before beginning AM care on this client. Option #4: this client would need care done slowly so as not to fatigue client.

14.62 ① Delirium, accompanied by some disorientation, is often caused by a systemic infection such as pneumonia, especially in an older person who may be more vulnerable to illness. Options #2, #3, and #4 are premature assumptions and are not based on the data presented.

14.63 ② The symptoms may subside with time and decreased stimulation. Options #1 and #3 are not necessary at this time. Option #4 is inappropriate.

14.64 ② Many liquid cough medicines have an alcohol base which will interact with the Antabuse to produce nausea and vomiting. Options #1, #3, and #4 are foods which interact with MAO inhibitor medications.

14.65 ③ Option #3 is most appropriate in developing a trusting relationship. Option #1 is practicing nurse avoidance. Option #2 is only providing information. Option #4 provides false reassurance.

14.66 ① A manipulative client needs firm limits, and those limits must be known and followed by all the nursing staff. If not, client will be able to split the staff into opposing forces. Options #2, #3, and #4 are inappropriate nursing actions with this client.

14.67 ③ Support groups of people who have suffered similar acts of violence can be helpful and supportive in teaching clients how to deal with the traumatizing situation and the emotional aftermath. Options #1, #2, and #4 are all reasonable recommendations to begin utilizing in a systematic desensitization program after the crisis period is alleviated.

14.68 ③ In an immuno-suppressed client, the WBC's are usually decreased which predisposes the client to infections. It would be important to do this client's AM care first, especially before all clients with a probable infection as the clients in options #1, #2, and #4.

14.69 ④ Infection in a neutropenic individual may cause morbidity and fatality if untreated. Place neutropenic client in a private room. Limit and screen visitors and hospital staff with potentially communicable illnesses. Options #1, #2, and #3 may be harmful to client A.

14.70 ④ A 6-month-old on a soy-based formula is probably allergic to cow milk products. Many children who are sensitive to cow's milk cannot tolerate it until the age of 2. Options #1, #2, and #3 are acceptable activities in caring for this age child.

14.71 ① Direct observation of a typical mealtime will give the most information. Option #2 may or may not secure an accurate picture. The weight should be obtained more often or on each visit as opposed to option #3. Option #4 circumvents the routine patterns of behavior surrounding feeding times.

14.72 ④ Morphine is the drug of choice for burn pain management. When a side effect becomes apparent, exploration of alternative techniques such as visualization become important. Option #1 might be used, but with a possible impending ileus suspected, this option is not ideal. Options #2 and #3 are inappropriate.

14.73 ④ The chest x-ray will be able to visualize fluid and air in the pleural space. Options #1, #2, and #3 would be beneficial to evaluate but are not as inclusive as option #4.

14.74 ② Intact rubber caps should be present on walker legs to prevent accidents. Options #1, #3, and #4 should be avoided for 4-6 weeks.

14.75 ② Warm-up or stretching exercises should always be done prior to and after exercising. Option #1 is one helpful exercise. It is not the only one. Option #3 is incorrect because painful joints should not be exercised. Option #4 does not involve joint movements.

CHAPTER 15
Post-Test #3

Your vision of where or what you want to be is the greatest asset you have. Without having a goal it's difficult to score.
— PAUL ARDEN

✔ Clarification of this test …

Just keep working on your testing practice and studying. Here are more questions to help you identify your study needs.

15.1 Which of these actions by the unlicensed assistive personnel (UAP) caring for a client with infective endocarditis requires immediate intervention from the nurse?
① The UAP reminds the client to take rest periods throughout the day.
② The UAP helps the client with his/her activities of daily living.
③ The UAP encourages frequent ambulation in the hall during the day.
④ The UAP reports to the nurse the client's HR has increased from 68 bpm to 88 bpm.

15.2 What would be the first action by the nurse on evening shift who smells alcohol on the breath of the charge nurse?
① Give her one more chance since she has never done this before.
② Discuss this with the nurse practitioner who is working on the unit.
③ Make an appointment with the evening supervisor and discuss concerns.
④ Document and report to the Vice President of Nursing.

15.3 What would be the initial action for the charge nurse who observes two LPN/VNs having an argument in the hallway?
① Write up a disciplinary action regarding their behavior.
② Advise the LPN/VNs to go to the office to discuss their differences.
③ Notify the charge nurse to break up the dispute and discuss the argument.
④ Request they stop arguing in the hallway.

15.4 Which action by the unlicensed assistive personnel (UAP) would require intervention from the charge nurse for a client with end-stage renal disease?
① Performs oral hygiene routinely.
② Encourages client to drink fluids hourly.
③ Refuses to give client the fruit salad with oranges for a snack.
④ Takes the weight daily and records it.

15.5 What task can be delegated to the unlicensed assistive personnel (UAP) in the intensive care unit?
① Take the serum specimen to the laboratory.
② Assess and monitor the vital signs following a cardiac catheterization.
③ Assist the health care provider during an endotracheal intubation.
④ Assist with a bath for a client with asthma and COPD.

15.6 Which of these pediatric clients would be a priority to assess first on the pediatric unit?
① A toddler with a temperature of 102.4°F (39.11°C) and is drooling
② A preschool child who fell at school and is presenting with pain in the right arm
③ A school age child who is admitted with headaches of unknown origin
④ An adolescent who is experiencing polyphagia, polydipsia, with a weight loss

15.7 A woman at 34 weeks gestation has been admitted to the ER following a car accident. Which of these clinical assessment findings require immediate intervention?
① BP 150/88, periorbital edema, +3 protein in urinalysis.
② Painless bright red vaginal bleeding with variability; BP—110/80, HR—88 bpm, FHR—140.
③ Contractions periodically occurring in the lower abdominal area.
④ Dark red vaginal bleeding and a hard, painful uterus; BP—98/62, HR—102 bpm, with pale and clammy skin.

15.8 Which client is a priority to assess immediately following shift report?
① A laboring client at 7 cm dilated with a temp of 100°F (37.78°C), FHR—170 bpm.
② A laboring client presenting with early decelerations.
③ A laboring client presenting with an increase in variability.
④ A laboring client presenting with one variable deceleration.

15.9 The Pediatric ICU nurse is requesting to transfer a client from the PICU to the Pediatric Unit to make room for a new client. Which client would be most appropriate to transfer?
① The client with Kawasaki Disease who is presenting with new symptoms of edema and oliguria.
② The client with cystic fibrosis and is coughing and expectorating small amounts of yellow secretions and decrease breath.
③ The client who is one day post-operative for cast application on the left arm.
④ The client who is two hours post-operative for an appendectomy and requiring pain medication.

15.10 What clinical finding would cause the nurse to suspect the prescribed dwelling time is not being followed when the client is receiving peritoneal dialysis?
① WBC—18,000 mm³ (18 x 10⁹/L).
② Serum glucose—200 mg/dL (11.1 mmol/L).
③ Serum phosphorus level—3.8 mEq/L (3.8 mmol/L).
④ Complaints of headache, nausea and vomiting.

15.11 What is the priority plan of care for a client with Raynaud's Phenomenon?
① Report swelling of the joints and fingers.
② Put gloves on client when out in cold weather.
③ Evaluate oxygen saturation by placing the probe on the finger.
④ Inform client that there will be a feeling of intense heat in the fingers.

15.12 What is priority to include in the health promotion plan for the parents of a newborn regarding car seat safety who is being discharged from the hospital?
① Position car seat in the back seat, forward facing.
② Position car seat in the front seat, forward facing.
③ Position the newborn in the rear-facing car seat until 1 year old.
④ Use an approved rear-facing car seat in the middle of the back seat.

15.13 Which action would be most appropriate for the nurse manger to implement first for a nurse on the pediatric unit who has four medication errors in the last 4 months?
① Enroll nurse in a medication course.
② Review the errors with the nurse to evaluate if there is a problem with the medication system.
③ Continue to evaluate nurse for any additional medication errors in the future.
④ Engage in the formal counseling protocol for the medication errors.

15.14 What plan would be priority for an elderly client who informs the nurse, "I am unsteady with getting in and out of my bathtub"?
① Discuss the possibility of taking a shower instead of a bath.
② Recommend a physical therapist consult.
③ Review the importance of taking voltaren prior to taking a bath.
④ Determine if the bathroom has grab bars for client to hold.

15.15 Which of these clients would be priority to assess immediately following shift report?
① A client with chronic renal failure who is preparing for hemodialysis in one hour and is presenting with HR—100 bpm and BP—160/92 with weight increase of 2 kg/48 hours.
② A newly diagnosed client with chronic renal failure who has begun hemodialysis and is presenting with nausea and vomiting, a change in LOC, and agitated.
③ A client who is receiving an initial round of peritoneal dialysis and is draining straw colored dialysis return.
④ A client who is receiving peritoneal dialysis with an order to infuse in 500 mL of dialysate and only drains out 450 mL.

15.16 What is the priority assessment for an older adult client who is presenting with delirium?
① Agitation and confusion
② Frequent hand washing
③ A gradual decline in memory
④ A recent change in medication

15.17 What is the priority care for a maternity client presenting with painless bright red blood in the last trimester of pregnancy?
① Assess cervix to determine how many cm dilated client is.
② Place client in bed and on the fetal heart monitor.
③ Prepare client for an emergency cesarean section.
④ Explain the bleeding is from premature separation of the placenta.

15.18 Two days after admission to the hospital, an elderly client reports that her hands are shaking, she cannot relax, and she feels "things moving around in her bed." The nurse assesses her pain level to be a 4 on a 10 scale. Which would be the best follow-up response from the nurse?
① "This hospitalization is causing you to be anxious."
② "What pain medication do you normally take at home?"
③ "Can you attribute your hands shaking to a particular event?"
④ "I'd like to review your drug and alcohol history with you."

15.19 Which statement by a client with gastroexophageal reflux disease (GERD) suggests an understanding of the teaching?
① "I usually drink a small glass of water before bed."
② "I avoid food such as celery and bran cereal."
③ "I changed from butter to margarine."
④ "I quit drinking coffee and cola drinks."

15.20 A terrorist attack on a public building has resulted in several injured clients arriving at the ER simultaneously for treatment. Which victim is highest priority for immediate treatment?
① A toddler with his forehead wound bleeding profusely.
② A pregnant woman with a fetal heart rate of 120 bpm.
③ An adolescent with a painful rigid abdomen.
④ A client with bilateral fractures of the forearms.

15.21 Which question is most appropriate for the nurse to ask clients before a blood sample is drawn for a middle-aged male client who is offered a psotrate-specific antigen test?
① "Are you allergic to iodine or radiopaque dyes?"
② "Have you had rectal penetration in the last 48 hours?"
③ "Do you strain when you void or have a bowel movement?"
④ "Have you eaten red meat within 24 hours?"

15.22 A client with Parkinsonism is having problems with ambulation and is experiencing wavering and stumbling. Which client teaching would be most beneficial in preventing the client from falling?
① Keep the arms as still as possible when walking.
② Walk with the feet spaced at hip width.
③ Maintain a slightly forward-leaning position.
④ Focus eyes on the level of the horizon.

15.23 A client's thrombocyte count is 510,000/mm³. Which nursing intervention is the highest priority?
① Observe for nosebleeds.
② Use a manual sphygmomanometer.
③ Encourage fluid intake.
④ Minimize physical activity.

15.24 Which behavior by the client indicates a need for further teaching when changing the dressing on the left deltoid following an incision and drainage of an abscess?
① Using clean gloves to remove the dressing
② Removing the tape by pulling away from the wound
③ Cleansing the wound with saline
④ Measuring the wound's length and width

15.25 Which information would be included in the incident report for a client who received the wrong medicine?
① The nurse's opinion of why the incident occurred.
② The name of the staff member who was to blame for the incident.
③ A statement that a copy of the report was filed in the client's chart.
④ An objective account of the incident and when it occurred.

15.26 A client diagnosed with a lower GI bleed has an order for 1 unit of packed red blood cells. What information is most important to be documented during this procedure?
① Vital signs prior to procedure
② Confirmation that the nurse alone verified the blood label information
③ The total volume that is to be infused
④ Vital signs before, during, and after procedure, date and time started and completed

15.27 Which plan is the most appropriate for a 34-week-pregnant woman who is being treated with magnesium sulfate and bed rest for preeclampsia?
① Assessing the equality of the pedal pulse
② Assessing the abdominal circumference
③ Assessing for an increase in the urine output
④ Obtaining the client's daily weight

15.28 What plan is the highest priority for a client who is 24 hours post-operative following a renal transplantation and begins presenting with hematuria?
① Reporting discomfort at the transplant site and T—102.1°F (38.9°C).
② Advising the provider that fluid intake should be increased.
③ Continuing to monitor the urine's volume and appearance.
④ Using a urine dipstick to check for proteinuria.

15.29 Which client would be delegated to the RN?
① A client who started her menses within the last 24 hours.
② A client whose family insists she get the "best care available."
③ A client who is arriving as a transfer from a skilled nursing facility.
④ A client who has a diagnosis of Type I diabetes with a blood sugar of 180 mg/dL (9.99 mmol/L).

15.30 Which behavior by the client demonstrates an understanding of how to take cyclosporine?
① Client mixes it in a citrus juice and stirs it well.
② Client waits at least 30 minutes to take the drug after mixing it in a solution.
③ After taking the medication, client adds water to the container and drinks that, too.
④ Client uses a plastic or styrofoam cup to mix the medication solution.

15.31 Six months after her vaginal hysterectomy, a client tells the nurse, "Sex with my husband is painful." Which is the most appropriate response from the nurse?

① "Are you using a water-soluble lubricant during intercourse?"
② "Tell me what aspect of sex is painful to you."
③ "It may be too early after surgery to be having sex."
④ "I will advise your surgeon to talk to you about this."

15.32 What is the priority of care for a client who is one day post-operative following an abdominal hysterectomy and is presenting with edema in the left leg?

① Instruct the client to increase the frequency of post-op leg exercises.
② Consult the client's chart for a history of renal or heart failure.
③ Elevate the foot of the client's bed at least thirty degrees.
④ Measure both legs at mid-thigh and mid-calf.

15.33 Which client can be discharged to make room for an emergency admission?

① A young-adult client, post-op bowel obstruction with nasogastric tube in place.
② The client admitted today in heart failure.
③ An older-adult client with bronchial asthma and oxygen saturation on room air of 95%.
④ A client with a fractured femur and possible fat embolus.

15.34 What is the priority plan for a licensed practical nurse (LPN) who documented one hour prior to turning client there was "No skin breakdown"; and when turning the client, the registered nurse notices a stage 1 pressure injury on the client's coccyx area?

① Talk to the practical nurse about the assessment when client returns to the unit.
② Correct the practical nurse's charting to address the pressure injury.
③ Document that there has been a change in the client's skin assessment.
④ Ask the client to state a time when the practical nurse did the skin assessment.

15.35 What is the priority of care for a client who has a right radius and ulna fractures with an external fixator and develops loss of two-point discrimination in the fingers on right hand?

① Elevate the right arm on pillows.
② Place the right arm at heart level.
③ Put the right arm in a dependent position.
④ Vary the right arm position every 15 minutes.

15.36 What is the priority of care for a client who sustained a closed-head injury, is being monitored for increased intracranial pressure, and has a $PaCO_2$ of 33 mm Hg?

① Encourage the client to slow his breathing rate.
② Auscultate the client's lungs and suction if indicated.
③ Advise the health care provider (HCP) that the client needs supplemental oxygen.
④ Report the results and continue to monitor for signs of increasing intracranial pressure.

15.37 What is the priority plan for a client who presents with a positive Brudzinski sign and has a recent history of sinusitis?

① Control intracranial pressure.
② Administer prescribed antibiotics.
③ Add pads to the side rails of the bed.
④ Hydrate the client with 0.45% saline.

15.38 Which of these nursing actions by the LPN for a newborn with a congenital heart defect require immediate intervention by the charge nurse?

① Encourages family to ventilate their concerns and anxiety about the diagnosis.
② Encourages family to touch and have physical contact with the newborn.
③ Encourages stimulation and crying to assist prevention of pneumonia.
④ Evaluates pulses for presence and quality.

15.39 The nurse observes that a fire has started in the nursery. Which action would the nurse take first?

① Confine the fire to the nursery.
② Extinguish the fire.
③ Pull the fire alarm.
④ Rescue the babies.

15.40 A city council person is admitted to the hospital after experiencing chest pain at a ribbon-cutting ceremony. A journalist from the newspaper contacts the hospital's nursing supervisor and asks her for a report on the client's status. What would be the next nursing action?
① Advise the journalist of HIPAA guidelines.
② Contact the hospital's chief executive officer.
③ Ensure the journalist is authorized to receive such information.
④ Obtain signed authorization from the client.

15.41 Which assignment would be appropriate for the Labor and Delivery (L&D) nurse who will be working for one shift on the Medical Surgical unit?
① A toddler with croup
② A young adult client with malignant hypertension
③ A middle-aged client with unstable angina
④ An older adult client with heart failure

15.42 After establishing IV access, what would be the best for the nurse to document immediately after procedure?
① The type of catheter used and number of venipuncture attempts.
② The type of IV fluid hung and equipment used.
③ The date, time, venipuncture site, type and gauge of catheter, and IV fluid hung.
④ Type, amount, and flow rate of IV fluid, condition of IV site.

15.43 What question would be most important to ask a male client who is in for a digital rectal examination?
① "Have you noticed a change in the force of the urinary stream?"
② "Have you noticed a change in tolerance of certain foods in your diet?"
③ "Do you notice polyuria in the AM?"
④ "Do you notice any burning with urination or any odor to the urine?"

15.44 Which statement made by the new mother indicates an understanding of screening for PKU for her newborn son who she is breastfeeding?
① "I will have him tested 24 hours after birth."
② "I will return to the clinic in 48 hours for the screening."
③ "I will return in 1 week to obtain blood samples."
④ "I will return in 1 month for the screening."

15.45 Which of these schedules would be the most appropriate to recommend to a pre-menopausal woman regarding her self breast exam?
① One week prior to the monthly period
② One week after the menstrual period
③ During every shower
④ The same day monthly

15.46 During the history, which information from a young adult client would indicate a risk for development of testicular cancer?
① Genital Herpes
② Hydrocele
③ Measles
④ Undescended testicle

15.47 Which plan is least appropriate for meeting the needs of a family after a loved one has died?
① Allow the family to wash the body.
② Allow the minister to touch the body.
③ Allow chanting to be done during the "last rites."
④ Call the funeral home immediately to remove the bad spirit.

15.48 What is the priority clinical assessment finding indicating a common side effect for a client who receives a positive end expiratory pressure (PEEP) at the end of the ventilator respiration cycle?
① Increased blood pressure
② Decreased cardiac output
③ Decreased lung compliance
④ Increased venous return to heart

15.49 Organize the following steps to suctioning in chronological order (with 1 being the first step in this procedure).

① Put on sterile glove.
② Lubricate catheter with normal saline.
③ Apply suction for 5–10 seconds.
④ Explain procedure to client.
⑤ Wash hands thoroughly.

15.50 Which findings would indicate that a client with Adult Respiratory Distress Syndrome (ARDS) is deteriorating?
① PaO_2—88%; R—24
② PaO_2—87%; HR—80
③ PaO_2—58%; HR—108
④ PCO_2—47 mm Hg; R—32

15.51 Which of the clinical assessment findings requires further evaluation due to risk of a potential complication with appendicitis?
① Sharp pain with extreme gastric distention
② Rebound tenderness in the right lower abdominal quadrant, with decreased bowel sounds
③ Growing pain, radiating to the lower back
④ Pain on light palpation in epigastric area with diarrhea

15.52 Which clinical assessment finding indicates a complication resulting in a low volume alarm on a volume-cycled positive pressure ventilator?
① Client is biting on the tubing.
② Excessive fluid is in the ventilator tubing.
③ A leak is in the client's endotracheal tube cuff.
④ Client is lying on the tubing.

15.53 Which of these documentations indicate the nurse understands how to accurately evaluate the client's stool for occult blood?
① Collect stool placed in a clean container to examine for pathological organisms.
② Remained on regular diet prior to test being done.
③ Stool sample obtained from one area of the stool.
④ Guaiac testing positive for occult blood. Paper turned blue.

15.54 What is the priority of care after the urinary catheter is removed?
① Encourage client to eliminate fluid intake.
② Document size of catheter and client's tolerance of procedure.
③ Evaluate client for normal voiding.
④ Documentation of client teaching.

15.55 The client is admitted to ER with severe discomfort and an inability to urinate after today's A&P repair. The nurse inserts the Foley catheter all the way up to the collecting tube without urine return. Which nursing action would be next?
① Leave the catheter in place and wait for an hour to determine if it is in the correct position.
② Change the position of the catheter in an attempt to get urine flow.
③ Acquire a new catheter and attempt to place in the appropriate orifice.
④ Try an alternate method to get the client to urinate.

15.56 Which of these statements made by a female client who has been abused by her spouse indicates the counseling has been effective?
① "I know my husband will never hurt me again."
② "I know it is my fault that he hits me."
③ "I promise I will get him to promise that he will not do it again."
④ "I have made arrangements to go to the battered women's shelter the next time he hits me."

15.57 Which clinical findings indicate a complication from diabetes insipidus?
① Urine specific gravity—1.001
② Serum sodium—135 mEq/L (135 mmol/L)
③ Urine output greater than 200 mL/hr
④ Weight loss of 2 lbs. (0.9 kg)

15.58 Which nursing action is most appropriate for a client receiving a tube feeding around the clock?
① Rinse the bag and change the formula every 4 hours.
② Rinse the bag and change the formula every shift.
③ Change the bag and formula every shift.
④ Rinse the bag and change the formula every 2 hours.

15.59 An adolescent is beginning chemotherapy for her malignancy. Which statement indicates she has a realistic perception of her health status?
① "I will be cured after my therapy is completed."
② "I may lose my hair during chemotherapy."
③ "I will be able to continue my current school schedule."
④ "I must have done something to cause this illness."

15.60 What nursing action is most appropriate when inserting a vaginal suppository?
① Remove the suppository from the wrapper and lubricate it with Vaseline.
② Instruct client to place in tampon after inserting the vaginal medication.
③ With an applicator on the forefinger of your free hand, insert the suppository about 2" (5 cm) into the vagina.
④ Direct the applicator up initially and then down and forward.

15.61 Which statement made by the client with a cast on his right leg indicates he understands how to safely walk up stairs with his crutches?
① "I will put my right leg up first."
② "I will put my left leg up first."
③ "I will put both of my crutches up first."
④ "I will put both of my legs up first."

15.62 Which statement made by the nurse while teaching the client about the purpose of a continuous bladder irrigation (CBI) for the first-day post-operative TURP indicates an understanding of the procedure?
① Prevents urinary stasis and infection.
② Maintains urinary dilution to prevent irritation.
③ Keeps urine flowing by preventing clot formation.
④ Delivers medication directly to operative area.

15.63 What would the nurse ask the client to do when evaluating the cranial nerve 1?
① Ask client to smell and identify different odors.
② Ask client to shrug the shoulders.
③ Ask client to read a Snellen chart.
④ Ask client to stick out tongue and move from side to side.

15.64 Which plan is most appropriate for a client in septic shock?
① Position client with head down and feet up.
② Place in Sims position.
③ Restrict dietary protein.
④ Increase flow rate of IV fluids.

15.65 A client with a closed-head injury has a nasogastric tube in place and begins to vomit. What is the highest priority?
① Check the nasogastric tube for appropriate placement.
② Reposition client in bed to a side-lying position.
③ Notify the health care provider (HCP).
④ Remove the tube immediately.

15.66 The client has had an acute myocardial infarction and is on a cardiac monitor. She is beginning to have premature ventricular contractions (PVCs) at 10/minute. The nurse will administer which of these ordered drugs?
① Atropine
② Nitroglycerin
③ Propanolol
④ Lidocaine

15.67 Organize these steps in chronological order with #1 being the first step for a client who is having a nasogastric tube removed.

① Assist client into semi-Fowler's position.
② Ask client to hold her breath.
③ Assess bowel function by auscultation for peristalsis.
④ Flush tube with 10 mL of normal saline.
⑤ Withdraw the tube gently and steadily.
⑥ Monitor client for nausea and vomiting.

15.68 Prior to administering atenolol and digoxin, which assessment is most important to report and document?
① HR—56 bpm
② HR—92 bpm
③ BP—140/92
④ Serum potassium—3.8 mEq/L (3.8 mmol/L)

15.69 A psychiatric client with the diagnosis of schizophrenia tells the nurse that he is Elvis Presley. What would be the priority action for the nurse?
① Confront the client regarding this delusion and bring him back to reality.
② Reflect this statement back to the client to encourage therapeutic communication.
③ Respond with an open-ended response to get client to further discuss his thoughts.
④ Verify identify of the client prior to administering his medication.

15.70 A client is experiencing septic shock and the provider wants dosing of medications to be regulated so that a mean arterial pressure (MAP) between 65 and 75 mm Hg is maintained. Which of the client's blood pressure readings meet this goal?
① 135/90
② 125/80
③ 115/70
④ 105/60

15.71 What would be most important to monitor on a client who is taking Lisinopril?
① Serum potassium
② Serum pH
③ Serum calcium
④ Heart rate

15.72 Following an automobile accident, a client is admitted to the hospital with a head injury. Which clinical finding would indicate the cerebral edema is increasing and the client is deteriorating?
① Increase in pain
② Irregular respiratory pattern
③ Narrowing of the pulse pressure
④ Increase in heart rate

15.73 The physician orders heparin 7,000 U S.C. q8h for a client with deep vein thrombosis. The heparin available is 20,000 units per 1 mL. How many milliliters of heparin should the nurse administer?
① 0.2 mL
② 0.3 mL
③ 0.35 mL
④ 3.5 mL

15.74 Which interventions would be most appropriate for an infant in a right hip spica cast?
① Palpate the left radial artery and compare it to the right.
② Check cast for tightness by inserting fingers between skin and cast.
③ Blanch the skin of areas proximal to the casted right leg.
④ Medicate frequently for pain.

15.75 The nurse is caring for a female client in the ER who was attacked and raped 6 hours ago. What initial nursing action would be most important?
① Clean wounds immediately.
② Obtain written informed consent for examination.
③ Determine if the woman has bathed or douched.
④ Obtain laboratory specimens.

Category Analysis—Post-Test #3

1. Management of Care
2. Management of Care
3. Management of Care
4. Management of Care
5. Management of Care
6. Management of Care
7. Health Promotion
8. Health Promotion
9. Safety and Infection Control
10. Reduction of Risk Potential
11. Reduction of Risk Potential
12. Health Promotion
13. Safety and Infection Control
14. Safety and Infection Control
15. Physiological Adaptation
16. Psychosocial
17. Management of Care
18. Pharmacology
19. Basic Care and Comfort
20. Management of Care
21. Physiological Adaptation
22. Reduction of Risk Potential
23. Basic Care & Comfort
24. Basic Care & Comfort
25. Management of Care
26. Pharmacology
27. Basic Care & Comfort
28. Basic Care & Comfort
29. Management of Care
30. Pharmacology
31. Health Promotion
32. Basic Care and Comfort
33. Management of Care
34. Management of Care
35. Basic Care and Comfort
36. Reduction of Risk Potential
37. Reduction of Risk Potential
38. Management of Care
39. Safety and Infection Control
40. Management of Care
41. Management of Care
42. Pharmacology
43. Health Promotion
44. Health Promotion
45. Health Promotion
46. Health Promotion
47. Psychosocial
48. Physiological Adaptation
49. Physiological Adaptation
50. Physiological Adaptation
51. Basic Care and Comfort
52. Physiological Adaptation
53. Reduction of Risk Potential
54. Basic Care and Comfort
55. Basic Care and Comfort
56. Psychosocial
57. Basic Care & Comfort
58. Basic Care & Comfort
59. Psychosocial
60. Pharmacology
61. Reduction of Risk Potential
62. Basic Care and Comfort
63. Reduction of Risk Potential
64. Physiological Adaptation
65. Basic Care and Comfort
66. Pharmacology
67. Basic Care and Comfort
68. Pharmacology
69. Psychosocial
70. Physiological Adaptation
71. Pharmacology
72. Reduction of Risk Potential
73. Pharmacology
74. Reduction of Risk Potential
75. Management of Care

Chapter 15: POST-TEST #3

Directions

1. Determine questions missed by checking answers.
2. Write the number of the questions missed across the top line marked "item missed."
3. Check category analysis page to determine category of question.
4. Put a check mark under item missed and beside content.
5. Count check marks in each row and write the number in totals column.
6. Use this information to:
   - identify areas for further study.
   - determine which content test to take next.

We recommend studying content where most items are missed—then taking that content test.

Number of the Questions Incorrectly Answered

Post-Test	Items Missed																Totals
C Management of Care																	
O Safety and Infection Control																	
N Health Promotion and Maintenance																	
T Psychosocial Integrity																	
E Physiological Adaptation:Fluid Gas																	
N Reduction of Risk Potential																	
T Basic Care and Comfort																	
Pharmacology and Parenteral Therapies																	

Answers & Rationales

15.1 ③ Option #3 is correct. Clients with endocarditis should be on bed rest to decrease cardiac demands during the infection and inflammation. This does require immediate intervention from the nurse, since it is not within the standard of care for these clients. Options #1, #2, and #4 are not correct. None of these require immediate intervention from the nurse.

15.2 ③ Option #3 is correct. The evening supervisor or the manager of the unit has the authority to mandate the charge nurse to submit to drug screening. With this situation, the supervisor on the evening shift should handle the situation. Option #1 is not correct. This does not follow the ethical responsibility that nurses have to uphold the safety and quality care for all clients. Alcohol will diminish the ability to make safe decisions. Option #2 is not correct. The nurse practitioner does not have the authority necessary to mandate the drug screening. Option #4 is not correct, since this would not be communicating within the appropriate levels of management in a systemic manner.

15.3 ④ Option #4 is correct. The initial action is to stop the argument occurring in public. The charge nurse should not discuss the behavior in public. Option #1 is not correct. The charge nurse can discuss the behavior with the LPNs and evaluate whether the manager needs to be involved. Option #2 would be the second action. They need a private place to discuss their differences. Option #3 is not the first action. The charge nurse may need to mediate the argument; however, this is not the initial action.

15.4 ② Option #2 is correct. A client in end-stage renal disease should not be encouraged to drink fluids hourly. In fact, they should limit their fluid intake. The UAP is not following the standard of practice for this medical condition. Option #1 is not correct. This is appropriate care and does not require intervention by the charge nurse. Option #3 is not a correct answer because oranges are high in potassium, and renal clients should not take in foods high in potassium. Option #4 is also not correct, since it is within the standard of care for these clients to be weighed daily and monitor the trends.

15.5 ① Option #1 is correct. The UAP can take specimens to the laboratory. Option #2 is not correct because these have to be compared to previous readings, analyzed, and there are risks involved following this procedure. Option #3 is not correct. The UAP is not able to assist the HCP with an invasive procedure at the bedside. Option #4 is not correct. Bathing can increase the metabolic rate of the client and require more oxygen. The UAP does not have the knowledge to understand if there is a need to stop the bath due to clinical findings of hypoxia.

15.6 ① Drooling with a high temperature are the signs of epiglottitis, that can be life threatening. This is the child that needs to be assessed first. The nurse should not attempt to assess the throat area due to risk of a laryngospasm. The health care provider will need to do this and be prepared for an emergency tracheostomy if necessary. Options #2, #3, and #4 are not correct. While each of these children need further evaluation, they are not a priority to option #1.

15.7 ④ The vital signs in option #4 indicate a complication with bleeding and the assessment findings may indicate an abruptio placenta. Option #1 presents with preeclampsia but is not priority to bleeding. There are no assessments in option #1 indicating headache, blurred vision or epigastric pain that may result in a seizure from sodium imbalance. Option #2, vital signs and FHR are within the defined range. Option #3 is not priority in contrast to option #4.

15.8 ① Option #1 is the priority to assess. This client has a temperature and the FHR is fast. The FHR should be 120 to 160. Options #2, #3, and #4 do not require immediate assessment. Option #2 indicates head compression and is not a complication. Option #3 indicates increase in oxygenation that is a good assessment. Option #4 is not a priority over #1. This clinical finding may be from cord compression, but is only one and not consistent.

15.9 ③ Option #3 is the correct answer. This client is the most stable to transfer to the Pediatric Unit. There is no indication of any complications with compartmental syndrome, drainage, temperature, etc. Option #1 may indicate child is developing heart failure and needs further assessment and intervention. Option #2 may have an infection occurring. Option #4 is not stable enough to be transferred.

15.10 ② Option #2 is correct. With the serum glucose being elevated, this can result from the hyperosmolarity of the dialysis. Glucose may be absorbed from the dialysate. The longer the fluid dwells the higher the risk for hyperglycemia. Options #1, #3, and #4 are not related to the dwelling time. Option #1 may occur from an infection which can occur from the micro-organisms in the peritoneum (Peritonitis). Option #3 is not from dwelling time. This elevation in serum phosphorus is from the renal failure. Option #4 is not correct. This is not from dwelling time; this is from a rapid decrease in the BUN ad volume.

I CAN HINT: The strategy for answering this question correctly is to focus on what it is asking which is the "dwelling time". The correct pathophysiology needs to be connected to the clinical findings as outlined in the rationale above.

15.11 ② Option #2 is correct. Raynaud's Phenomenon consists of intermittent episodic spasms of the arterioles, most frequently in the fingers, toes, ear, and tip of the nose. When the client experiences a feeling of coldness, vasoconstriction occurs then client will have an increase in achiness, tingling, and numbness. Hands, feet, nose, and ears need to be protected when exposed to cold weather. Client should wear gloves/socks when in contact with objects from the refrigerator or freezer. Option #1 is incorrect. Swelling does not occur, but pallor, achiness, tingling, throbbing, and numbness may occur. Option #3 is not correct. The reading will not be accurate due to the vasoconstriction that occurs with this medical condition. Option #4 is not correct.

15.12 ④ Option #4 is correct. Option #1 is incorrect due to safety issues. It should read, in the backseat, rear-facing. Option #2 is unsafe as well. Option #3 should read 2 years of age versus 1 year old.

15.13 ② Option #2 is correct. The first action by the manager is to assess if the system is contributing to the errors (i.e., pharmacy sends up incorrect dose or not available at correct time). Option #1 is not correct. The manager should first talk with the nurse to determine if there is a system problem. Option #3 is not correct. Four medication errors in this short period of time require the manager to further analyze the situation. Option #4 is not correct. This is not the first action, but may be necessary if the manager determines the nurse needs additional education regarding safe medication administration.

15.14 ④ Option #4 is correct. The priority concern is environmental safety. This assessment is making this determination. Option #1 is not correct. While it may be safer to take a shower, the priority is for the nurse to determine if the bathroom is safe for either a shower or bath by having the bars in place. Option #2 is not the first priority. Safety is priority. While the physical therapist would be an excellent professional to include on the team, it is not the priority first over safety. Option #3 may be used for pain. This plan would not address the safety issues regarding bath and shower safety.

15.15 ② Option #2 is correct. This client is presenting with disequilibrium syndrome which may be caused by too rapid a decrease of BUN and circulating fluid volume. It may result in cerebral edema and increased ICP. Early recognition of disequilibrium syndrome is essential. Signs include nausea, vomiting, change in level of consciousness, seizures and agitation. Option #1 is not correct. This is the reason the client is preparing from hemodialysis in one hour due to the renal failure and with an increase in fluid there would be an increase in the HR, BP and weight. Option #4 does require some repositioning of the client in order to facilitate the drainage, but it is not a priority to option #2 which is a complication. Option #3 is expected.

I CAN HINT: In addition to disequilibrium syndrome, other complications that may occur from dialysis could include sepsis, and hepatitis B and C.

15.16 ④ Option #4 is correct. Alcohol and drug use are common unrecognized problems in the elderly in the United States. This client may be exhibiting manifestation of substance withdrawal; and in recognizing this should gather more data from the client. Option #1 is incorrect because it makes an unfounded assumption and ignores the client's symptoms, Option #2 is incorrect as it is a symptom of Obsessive Compulsive Disorder, not delirium. Option #3 is incorrect as there is a difference in suspected delirium and slow onset memory loss as in Alzheimer's.

15.17 ② There is also a fetus that needs to be evaluated. Prior to any intervention, the fetus needs to be evaluated due to risk of hypoxia from the bleeding. If there was a complication with hypoxia, the fetus would present with late decelerations and decrease in variability. Option #1 is contraindicated due to risk of bleeding. Options #3 and #4 are incorrect. Placent previa is when the placenta is abnormally implanted in the lower segment of the uterus, near or over the cervical os rather than attaching to the fundus.

15.18 ④ Option #4 is correct. Alcohol and drug use is a common unrecognized problem in the elderly in the United States. The client may be exhibiting manifestation of substance withdrawal; and in recognizing this, the nurse should gather more data from the client.

15.19 ④ Option #4 is correct. Coffee and cola drinks are discouraged in GERD because the increased gastric motility and the likelihood of reflux. Drinking before bed is discouraged because it is preferred that the stomach be empty when reclining. High fiber and low fat diets are recommended in cases of GERD.

15.20 ③ Option #3 likely has a severe injury that is causing hemorrhaging internally. Option #1 should be seen next as children lose volume rapidly. Option #2 should be seen as soon as possible to assess for fetal distress. Option #4 may be the last one to be seen. There are no good options; they are all terrible as is the terrorist attack that caused this situation.

15.21 ② Option #2 is correct. Rectal penetration such as a digital exam or rectal intercourse can cause a false high PSA result. If this has occurred, 48 hours must pass before the test can be done. Allergies to iodine or radiopaque dye, straining with voiding or defecation, and eating red meat are not contraindications for testing.

15.22 ④ Option #4 is correct. Focusing on the horizon level helps maintain the balance of a client with Parkinsonism who is having ambulation difficulties. The client should be taught to swing the arms when walking, not to keep them still. The feet should be widely spaced at shoulder width or greater. The client should try to maintain an erect posture, not a forward-leaning one.

15.23 ③ Option #3 is correct. The client has thrombocytosis, which predisposes him to thrombus formation. Fluid intake reduces the risk of thrombus by maintaining an adequate amount of water in the serum. The other measures identified are associated with thrombocytopenia.

15.24 ② Option #2 is correct. When removing a dressing, the tape should be removed toward the wound, not away from it, as pulling away from the wound may disrupt healing. Home care of an abscess wound requires medical asepsis so clean gloves are acceptable during the procedure. It is standard practice to clean wounds with saline. Measuring the wound can give the provider information regarding the progress of the healing.

15.25 ④ Option #4 is correct. Just the facts ma'am. Other options are incorrect.

15.26 ④ Option #4 is correct. Option #1 is not as inclusive as #4. In Option #2, blood should be verified with another nurse. Option #3 should be actual volume versus projected amount since the infusion may need to be discontinued prior to total amount being infused.

15.27 ④ Option #4 is correct. This is a primary concern since it provides a baseline and an ongoing record of potential increase in the weight. Options #1, #2, and #3 are incorrect. Option #1 should read the patellar reflexes since they are more indicative of neurological problems with PIH or magnesium sulfate toxicity. Option #2 is not routinely done. Option #3 would be a decrease in urine output if assessing magnesium sulfate toxicity.

15.28 ① Option #1 correct. The highest priority is to report evidence of transplant rejection such as hyperacute which occurs within 48 hours after surgery and would include symptoms such as: fever, hypertension, and pain at the transplant site. The acute rejecton occurs 1 week to 2 years after surgery and would include symptoms such as oliguria, anuria, low-grade temperature, hypertension, tenderness over the transplanted kidney, lethargy, azotemia, and fluid retention. This question is asking about the hyperacute rejection since it is within 24 hours following the renal transplantation. Option #2 is incorrect since fluids should only be administered as prescribed and not increased. While option #3 is important, the assessment of the urine appearance and odor hourly (initially pink and bloody, gradually returning to normal in a few days to several weeks, is not a priority over option #1. This hematuria is an expected finding following this surgery. Option #4 is incorrect. While the daily urine tests are important, they would not be a priority over option #1 since signs or rejection must be reported immediately.

15.29 ③ Option #3 is correct. Of the four clients described, the only one that must receive an assessment from the RN is the newly arriving client. An RN must perform the initial assessment of a client.

15.30 ③ Option #3 is correct. To ensure getting the full dose of the drug, after the dose has been taken, water should be added to the container, swished around to mix with the residue of the drug, and the water should then be drunk. Option #1 is incorrect because not all citrus juices should be mixed with the drug. Grapefruit juice is contraindicated. Option #2 is incorrect because the drug should be taken immediately after mixing. Option #4 is incorrect because the drug will adhere to the sides of a plastic or styrofoam cup. Only a glass container should be used.

15.31 ② Option #2 is correct. The nurse needs more information, more assessment, before optimal help can be given to the client. Therefore, it is ideal for the nurse to ask for clarification of the client's statement. Options #1, #3, and #4 are all incorrect because these responses bypass the necessary assessment. The client did not state that intercourse is painful so #1 is making an assumption. Option #3 is incorrect because in most cases, intercourse after a vaginal hysterectomy does not need to be postponed for 6 weeks. Option #4 is incorrect because it undervalues the nursing role and overlooks the opportunity to help the client in her dilemma.

15.32 ④ Option #4 is correct. One of the most reliable physical findings of a deep vein thrombosis, a post-op complication, is edema of the affected leg. When discovered, a nurse should measure both legs at mid-thigh and mid-calf so that the nurse's report to the provider is complete and accurate. Option #1 is incorrect because increased activity of the leg without concurrent treatment for deep vein thrombosis may actually dislodge the clot. Talk to the provider before instituting this strategy. Option #2 is incorrect because it does not address the immediate need of the client, and in renal failure and heart failure, edema is bilateral. Option #3 is incorrect because it does not address the immediate need of the client and will not help to resolve the problem of a deep vein thrombosis.

15.33 ③ The client in option #3 is in the least distress and should be discharged. We would like to see the N/G removed before going home, but option #1 could be the second to go if an emergency and appropriate discharge instructions were given. Options #2 and #4 could have life threatening emergencies and should remain hospitalized if possible.

15.34 ① Option #1 is correct. There is a significant difference in the skin assessment of the practical nurse and the registered nurse. The registered nurse is obligated to discuss the matter with the practical nurse. Option #2 is incorrect. One nurse should not alter the charting of another nurse. Option #3 is incorrect. The nurse should not make this assumption without talking to the practical nurse first. Option #4 is incorrect. As a matter of professional respect, it is preferred that the registered nurse speak to the practical nurse before involving the client in the matter.

15.35 ② The client has a symptom of compartment syndrome which is a complication of trauma and fractures. In this case, the best position for the arm is neutral or at heart level. Option #1 is incorrect because it reduces arterial flow to the arm and increases tissue ischemia. Option #3 is incorrect because it can increase swelling and further impair circulation to the extremity. Option #4 is incorrect because it both reduces arterial flow and increases swelling of the extremity.

15.36 ④ Option #4 is correct. A lower-than-normal $PaCO_2$ can actually benefit the client because it reduces intracranial pressure by preventing cerebral vasodilation. The results should be reported to the physician, and monitoring for signs of increased intracranial pressure should continue. Option #1 is incorrect. Instructing the client to slow his breathing rate is inappropriate because it could elevate the $PaCO_2$ which could increase intracranial pressure. Option #2 is incorrect. There is no evidence that suction is indicated. Suctioning elevates intracranial pressure and therefore should be avoided. Option #3 is incorrect. There is no evidence that supplemental oxygen is needed. An abnormal $PaCO_2$ does not indicate the need for supplemental oxygen.

15.37 ② Option #2 is correct. The Brudzinski sign indicates bacterial meningitis, a complication of sinusitis. The client's greatest need is a regimen of antibiotics to which the causative agent is sensitive. Option #1 is incorrect. Bacterial meningitis causes increased intracranial pressure, and it is important for the nurse to monitor for manifestation of increased intracranial pressure. However, in this circumstance, it is not the highest priority. Option #3 is incorrect. Because of the risk for seizures in bacterial meningitis, padded side rails are an important nursing intervention. However, this intervention does not have priority over instituting the client's antibiotic therapy. Option #4 data does not indicate the use of a hypotonic solution for hydrating the client

15.38 ③ Option #3 is correct. Stimulation and crying need to be kept at a minimum for this newborn with a cardiac defect. Oxygen and energy need to be conserved. Options #1 and #2 do not require immediate intervention since they would be included in the care. Option #4 is an appropriate plan for any newborn who has an alteration in perfusion due to a congenital cardiac defect.

15.39 ④ Option #4 is correct. Just remember, "RACE." (Rescue, Alarm, Confine, and Extinguish).

15.40 ④ Option #4 is correct. Maintaining client confidentiality/privacy is most important to this situation. Options #1, #2, and #3 do not address this concern with privacy. These answers focus on the journalist and hospital. The correct answer is the answer that is client-focused.

15.41 ② Option #2 is correct. The L&D nurse provides care for clients with pregnancy induced hypertension. These assessments and plans of care would correlate with the nurse's skills. Options #1, #3, and #4 would not be appropriate for this nurse. L&D nurses do not routinely provide care for children. Options #3 and #4 require an understanding of cardiology.

15.42 ③ Option #3 is the most correct answer. Options #1 and #2 are appropriate but not as inclusive as option #3. Option #4 should be included in the once-per-shift documentation. This question states "after establishing IV access."

15.43 ① Option #1 is correct. This change would be most indicative of a potential complication with (BPH) benign prostate hypertrophy. Options #2, #3, and #4 are incorrect. Option #4 would be indicative of an infection.

Chapter 15: ANSWERS & RATIONALES

15.44 ③ Option #3 is correct since the newborn is only getting colostrum for the first few days. This screening may have a possible false negative result with the initial screening. Options #1, #2, and #4 are inaccurate and would not provide valid information.

15.45 ② Option #2 is correct because this is when the breasts are least congested. Option #1 is when the breasts are most congested. Option #3 is unnecessary. The recommended frequency is monthly. Option #4 is for post-menopausal women.

15.46 ④ Undescended testicles make the client high risk for testicular cancer. Mumps, inguinal hernia in childhood, orchitis, and testicular cancer in the contra lateral testis are other predisposing factors. Options #1, #2, and #3 are not factors that contribute to testicular cancer.

15.47 ④ Families of most cultures choose to "say goodbye in their own ways."

15.48 ② Option #2 is correct. As a result of the PEEP, the cardiac output may decrease. Options #1, #3, and #4 are incorrect for PEEP.

15.49

| ④Explain procedure to client. |
| ⑤Wash hands thoroughly. |
| ①Put on sterile glove. |
| ②Lubricate catheter with normal saline. |
| ③Apply suction for 5 to 10 seconds. |

15.50 ③ Option #3 is correct. ARDS is a form of pulmonary edema that is characterized by dyspnea, labored respiration, and low PaO_2. Option #3 indicates client's deterioration. Options #1 and #2 are incorrect. In Option #4, increasing levels of CO_2 are generally not a problem.

15.51 ② Option #2 is correct. Rebound pain is manifested by pressing firmly over the area known as McBurney's point. The rebound pain, decreased bowel sounds, tender abdomen, and fever, are all characteristic of appendicitis. Options #1, #3, and #4 are incorrect.

15.52 ③ Option #3 is correct. When the low alarm sounds, this usually indicates a leak. Options #1, #2, and #4 would result in a high volume alarm.

15.53 ④ Option #4 is correct. Options #1, #2, and #3 are incorrect. Option #1 should be in a sterile container. In Option #2, client may be on a specific type of diet prior to test being done to minimize false results. Option #3 should be collected from various areas of stool.

15.54 ③ Option #3 is a priority. Within 24 hours client should be voiding normally. Options #1, #2, and #4 are incorrect. Option #1 should be increased. Option #2 is not totally correct. The size of the catheter should be documented when it is placed. Option #4 is important but is not a priority for this question.

15.55 ③ Option #3 is correct. The bladder is not as deep in the body cavity as the full length of a Foley. The catheter is obviously in the wrong orifice. Option #1 will leave the client in pain for another hour and is not acceptable. Option #2 can be dangerous if the old catheter is pulled from the vagina and placed into the urethra. Option #4 is too late as client is in pain.

15.56 ④ Option #4 is correct. Most abused women eventually leave the situation. Interventions may not produce quick outcomes, but they can begin to facilitate the process of healing. Options #1, #2, and #3 are incorrect. In option #1, the husband will not change without identifying cause of anxiety and altering the manner he deals with it. Options #2 and #3 do not indicate counseling was effective.

15.57 ④ Option #4 is correct. Clinical manifestations from diabetes may result in severe dehydration. These manifestations may include: dry skin and mucous membranes; weight loss; decrease in blood pressure; decrease in central venous pressure; weakness; confusion; or speech difficulty in elderly. Options #1 and #3 are clinical manifestations of diabetes insipidus but not complications. Option #2 is within the normal reference range.

15.58　① Research indicates there is an increased growth of organisms after four hours. Options #2 and #3 are inappropriate due to increased organism growth. Option #4 is not a necessary action to maintain asepsis.

15.59　② This statement reflects the client's understanding of the side effects of chemotherapy. Option #1 may or may not occur. Option #3 is not realistic. It may be possible at times, but the question requests a "realistic perception." Option #4 is inaccurate and may reflect blame and guilt.

15.60　③ Option #3 is correct. Option #1 is incorrect. It should be lubricated with a water-soluble lubricant. Option #2 should not be done because the tampon would absorb the medication and decrease its effectiveness. Option #4 should read to direct the applicator down initially (toward the spine), and then up and back (toward) the cervix.

15.61　② Option #2 is correct. The unaffected leg moves up first, followed by the crutches, and the affected leg. Options #1, #3, and #4 are incorrect. When going downstairs, affected leg and crutches move down first.

15.62　③ Continuous bladder irrigation prevents the formation of clots which can lead to obstruction and spasm in the post-operative TURP client. Option #1 refers to a possible preoperative complication of infection due to the enlarged prostate. Option #2 will be ineffective. Option #4 is incorrect because medicine is not routinely administered via CBI in a first-day post-op TURP.

15.63　① Option #1 is correct for the CN1 (olfactory). Option #2 would be correct for CN11 (spinal accessory). Option #3 is evaluates CN2 (optic). Option #4 evaluates for CN12 (hypoglossal).

15.64　④ Option #4 is correct. Due to dilation of blood vessels from the overwhelming infection, the client experiences a decrease in venous return. To maintain adequate circulation, IV fluid replacement is essential. Position should be supine with legs elevated.

15.65　② Option #2 is correct. It is done to decrease risk of aspiration. Options #1, #3, and #4 are incorrect. While the nurse may implement option #1, it is not a priority to option #2.

15.66　④ Lidocaine decreases cardiac irritability and is the first line drug for treatment of PVCs. Option #1, atropine, is used to treat bradycardia and heart block effect. Option #2, nitroglycerin, is primarily given for anginal pain. Option #3, Inderal, is used (primarily) to treat supraventricular dysrhythmias.

15.67

| ③ Assess bowel function by auscultation for peristalsis. |
| ① Assist client into semi-Fowler's position. |
| ④ Flush tube with 10 mL of normal saline. *Flushing will ensure that the tube doesn't contain stomach contents that could irritate tissues during tube removal.* |
| ② Ask client to hold her breath. *This is to close epiglottis.* |
| ⑤ Withdraw the tube gently and steadily. |
| ⑥ Monitor client for nausea, vomiting. *For 48 hours, monitor client for GI dysfunction including nausea, vomiting, abdominal distention, and food intolerance.* |

15.68　① Option #1 is correct. When clients take beta blockers concurrently with cardiac glycoside and/or calcium channel blockers, there is an increased risk for bradycardia. Options #2, #3, and #4 are not correct for this situation. Option #4 is within the normal reference range.

15.69　④ Option #4 is correct. Safety is a priority in the clinical situation. Client identification is imperative since he is delusional. Option #1 is not a priority to #4. Options #2 and #3 include strategies for "therapeutic communication" versus "out of touch with reality."

15.70　④ Option #4 is correct. The formula for mean arterial pressure (MAP) is SBP + 2 DBP divided by 3. The blood pressure with mean arterial pressure between 65 and 75 is 105/60 (MAP = 75).

15.71 ① Option #1 is priority. This medication may cause retention of potassium. Options #2, #3, and #4 are incorrect.

15.72 ② Clients with increased intracranial pressure have bradycardia, an irregular respiratory rate, and a widening of the pulse pressure. Option #1 is not a sign that a client with a head injury is deteriorating. The earliest sign of a change in the client's neurological status is an alteration in the level of consciousness. In Option #3 there is a widening of pulse pressure with increased intracranial pressure. Narrowing of the pulse pressure indicates hypovolemic shock. Option #4, bradycardia, is a sign of increasing intracranial pressure, not increase in heart rate.

15.73 ③ Option #3 is correct.

$$\frac{20{,}000\ U}{1\ mL} = \frac{7{,}000\ U}{X}$$

$$20{,}000\ X = 7{,}000\ U$$

$$X = \frac{7{,}000\ U}{20{,}000\ U}$$

15.74 ② Option #2 is correct. Check the cast to make sure it is not constricting circulation. The child is not in traction; the arms are not part of the treatment; and the circulation is checked distal to the cast, not proximal. Medicating frequently is inappropriate.

15.75 ② Option #2 is correct. Consent must be a priority action before obtaining laboratory specimens and completing a specific interview or calling the police.

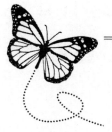

Notes

CHAPTER 16
Practice Exam

Every accomplishment starts with the decision to try.
— UNKNOWN

✔ **Clarification of this test …**

The Practice Exam has been designed to be comparable to NCLEX® with items represented according to these categories:

➢ **Safe and Effective Care Environment**
- Management of Care — 15–21%
- Safety and Infection Control — 10–16%

➢ **Health Promotion and Maintenance** — 6–12%

➢ **Psychosocial Integrity** — 6–12%

➢ **Physiological Integrity**
- Basic Care and Comfort — 6–12%
- Pharmacological and Parenteral Therapies — 13–19%
- Reduction of Risk Potential — 9–15%
- Physiological Adaption — 11–17%

The majority of the items are decision-making questions. When you master the top NCLEX® standards and concepts listed at the beginning of the chapters, you are on the path to NCLEX® success!

16.1 A client with a new onset of increased intracranial pressure (ICP) has an order to administer morphine for severe headache. What is the priority nursing care?

① Assess respiratory rate prior to administering.
② Have naloxone at the bedside.
③ Notify the primary health care provider and verify appropriateness for this order.
④ Recommend client to cough and deep breathe on a regular schedule.

16.2 After report, which of these clients would be the priority for the nurse to evaluate?

① An immobilized client with peripheral edema who suddenly becomes anxious and very short of breath (SOB).
② A client with pneumonia with a WBC count of 20,000 mm³ and presenting with lymphadenopathy, temperature of 102.8°F (39.3°C) and O_2 stat of 92%.
③ A client with bronchitis with an O_2 sat of 90% expectorating thick, pale-yellow secretions and temperature of 101.2°F (38.4°C).
④ An older adult client who is ambulating and suddenly stops and complains of pain in the calf in the right leg.

16.3 After a client had a renal transplant, which nursing actions indicate an understanding of how to safely provide care for this client? **Select all that apply.**
① Apply goggles.
② Place client in a room with negative-pressure air flow.
③ Wear gloves and gown/mask when in contact with client.
④ Do not allow fresh flowers in the room.
⑤ Double glove.

16.4 What is the expected outcome for a maternity client who is in preterm labor at 31 weeks of gestation, and receiving betamethasone?
① Contractions are regular and increasing in intensity.
② LS ratio is 2:1.
③ Temperature is 99.1° F.
④ WBC—8, 000 mm³.

16.5 Which of these nursing actions should be included in the rehabilitation plan for a client with a left cerebral hemisphere CVA? **Select all that apply.**
① Complete sentences that the client is unable to complete.
② Only use a communication board for all communication to prevent stress.
③ Look at client directly while communicating.
④ Speak slowly.
⑤ Give instructions one step at a time.

16.6 During hospital rounds, a nursing supervisor smells smoke coming from a client's bathroom. She/he opens the bathroom door and finds the client unresponsive on the floor and the waste can on fire. Which is the most appropriate response?
① Drag the client from the bathroom and close the door.
② Activate the fire alarm located outside the client's room.
③ Move the waste can to the shower and turn the shower on.
④ Call for help from other staff members.

16.7 During a cardiac assessment, where would the nurse place the stethoscope to accurately evaluate the aortic heart sound?
① The second intercostal space right of the sternum
② The second intercostal space left of the sternum
③ The fifth intercostal space at the left mid-clavicular line
④ The third intercostal space right of the sternum

16.8 What is the most appropriate nursing action after a nurse observes another nurse contaminating a chest tube?
① Report the incident to the supervisor.
② Clean the catheter with betadine and continue with procedure.
③ Ignore the incident.
④ Offer to assist and get another sterile chest tube.

16.9 The client is returning from surgery with a chest tube after a lobectomy. Select the equipment that would be at the bedside for this client. **Select all that apply.**
① Clamp
② Sterile gauze
③ Sterile gloves
④ IV cut-down tray
⑤ Suction equipment

16.10 While performing an electrocardiogram (ECG), which of the interventions is most appropriate to implement?
① Use alcohol or acetone pads on the client's fleshy areas and secure electrodes.
② Have the client lie in the Semi-Fowler's position for the procedure.
③ Encourage client to breathe deeply during procedure.
④ If client has excess hair on his chest, shave the area, rub area with alcohol, and dry it before placing the electrodes.

16.11 During suctioning of a client with an endotracheal tube, the heart rate decreases from 100 to 50 beats per minute. What is the priority nursing action?
① Continue suctioning client.
② Administer epinephrine to increase the HR.
③ Stop procedure and evaluate the breath sounds.
④ Discontinue the procedure and reconnect client to the ventilator.

16.12 What is the priority nursing action for a client at home who has diabetes mellitus and is presenting with diaphoresis, lethargy, but is still arousable?
① Administer Glucagon subcutaneous (SC).
② Check HbA1c.
③ Give an 8 oz. (237 mL) glass of milk.
④ Notify the health care provider.

16.13 In preparing for a traumatic wound debridement, what intervention is most appropriate?
① Pack the wound with betadine soaks prior to debridement.
② Prior to procedure, clean wound with alcohol.
③ Irrigate wound in preparation for debridement with 10 psi.
④ Pack the wound with gauze pads soaked in normal saline solution until debridement.

16.14 The nurse indicates an appropriate understanding of prioritizing the workload when implementing which client's plan of care first?
① A school-age child in a sickle cell crisis
② A school-age child admitted for shunt revision
③ An adolescent with a fractured femur
④ A young adult client with pelvic inflammatory disease

16.15 Which of these would be included in the plan of care for a client who has chronic kidney disease? **Select all that apply.**
① Assess for a flat T wave on the ECG monitor.
② Discuss the importance of using salt substitutes.
③ Encourage taking an NSAID for discomfort.
④ Review the importance of taking aluminum hydroxide gel with meals.
⑤ Review the importance of monitoring and reporting trends in weight gain.

16.16 Which of these plans is appropriate while monitoring the care of a client on a ventilator and troubleshooting ventilator alarms? **Select all that apply.**
① Suction for high alarms.
② Silence alarms while at bedside during night hours.
③ Assess for leak or disconnection for low pressure alarms.
④ Manually ventilate if alarms sound without apparent cause.
⑤ Check for kinking or compression of endotracheal tube for high alarms.

16.17 A client in a long-term care facility with heart failure has an order to receive a daily dose of enalapril 10 mg and is scheduled for hemodialysis this morning. When would the nurse plan to administer this medication to the client?
① The morning of dialysis
② The day after dialysis
③ 2 hours into dialysis
④ Upon return from dialysis

16.18 Which of these assessments is a priority for the nurse to report to the physician 6 hours after a cast has been applied to the left leg?
① The pedal pulse is stronger on the left foot.
② The left foot is cool to touch.
③ There is an alteration in the sensation to the left foot.
④ The capillary refill to the toes is less than 2 seconds.

16.19 On the fourth post-operative day after GI surgery, the nurse assesses a client shaking, diaphoretic, with a temperature of 103.6°F (39.8°C). What would be the priority assessment after the health care provider (HCP) is called for antibiotic orders?
① Client's weight
② Vital signs
③ Blood and urine cultures
④ Neurological evaluation

16.20 After evaluating the circulation in an arm in a cast, which assessment requires health care provider notification?
① Apical pulse of 88
② Tingling, cold fingers
③ Lack of cooperativeness by the client
④ Warm fingers with an alteration in capillary refill

16.21 While evaluating a quality indicator of client room placement, which of the following client transfers from the medical/surgical units to the maternity unit indicates the nurses know how to safely manage room placement for clients?
① A client with rubella
② A client with chronic hepatitis B
③ A client with RSV
④ A client with systemic lupus erythematosus

16.22 A client is to undergo an emergency appendectomy. Which assessment would be a priority before the anesthesia is administered?
① Location, intensity, and duration of the pain
② Last time client ate any solid food
③ Evaluation of vital signs
④ History of previous surgeries

16.23 What would be the priority nursing evaluation for a 30-hour-old newborn who begins to exhibit a high pitched cry, irritability, diarrhea, sneezing, and frequent tremors?
① History of maternal drug abuse
② Newborn sepsis
③ Cardiac dysrhythmias
④ Maternal sepsis

16.24 Which nursing plan is the highest priority for a client after a grand mal seizure?
① Elevate the head of the bed.
② Place an oxygen mask on the client.
③ Report the characteristics and the length of the seizure.
④ Administer Valium IV push.

16.25 Select the correct procedures when following standard precautions. **Select all that apply.**
① Wear gloves when coming in contact with any body fluid.
② Place the client in a private room that has negative air pressure in relation to surrounding area.
③ Discard used needles immediately in the trash can.
④ Wear gloves when entering the room.
⑤ Avoid contact with client if nurse has an exudative lesion.

16.26 Which technique is appropriate to promote chest physiotherapy in an active preschool child with cystic fibrosis?
① Perform percussion while having child sitting playing video games.
② Facilitate bronchial drainage by allowing child to hang upside down on monkey bars.
③ Encourage child to participate by beginning first with a healthy snack.
④ Provide a heavy blanket to provide warmth, comfort and to protect the skin.

16.27 A radium implant is found in the bed of a client who is being treated for cervical cancer. What is the most appropriate plan for the nurse to include in the care for this client?
① Reposition the implant immediately in the cervix with the physician's assistance.
② Remove it from the bed and discard in the unit's biohazardous materials container.
③ Remove it from the bed using tongs, discard in the biohazardous materials container in the room, and notify Radiology.
④ Remove it from the room after notifying the physician.

16.28 The nurse has administered sublingual nitroglycerin to a client complaining of chest pain. Which observation is most important for the nurse to report to the next shift?
① The client indicates a need to urinate frequently.
② Blood pressure has decreased from 140/80 to 98/62.
③ Respiratory rate has increased from 16 to 24.
④ The client indicates the chest pain has subsided.

16.29 A client was admitted for regulation of insulin. Client takes 15 units of Humulin N insulin at 8:00 AM every day. At 4:00 PM, which nursing observation indicates a complication due to the insulin?

① Acetone odor to breath, polyuria, and flushed skin
② Irritability, tachycardia, and diaphoresis
③ Headache, nervousness, and polydipsia
④ Tenseness, tachycardia, and anorexia

16.30 After abdominal surgery, a client is admitted from the recovery room with intravenous fluid infusing wide open. He receives 850 mL in less than 60 minutes. Which observation would indicate a problem?

① CVP reading of 8 mm Hg and bradycardia
② Tachycardia and hypotension
③ Dyspnea and oliguria
④ Rales and tachycardia

16.31 During the initial assessment of a client with myxedema, the nurse would carefully observe for which symptoms?

① Tachycardia, fatigue, and intolerance to heat
② Polyphagia, nervousness, and dry hair
③ Lethargy, weight gain, and intolerance to cold
④ Tachycardia, hypertension, and tachypnea

16.32 An elderly client is admitted with a possible fractured right hip. During the initial nursing assessment, which of the following observations of the right leg would validate or support this diagnosis?

① The leg appears shortened, is abducted, and externally rotated.
② Plantar flexion is observed with sciatic pain occurring down the leg.
③ From the hip, the leg appears longer and is externally rotated.
④ There is evidence of paresis with decreased sensation and limited mobility.

16.33 Which of the following instructions given to the client taking warfarin sodium indicates the nurse is negligent?

① Notify provider of care if stool becomes tarry.
② Eat a diet high in green leafy vegetables.
③ Return to the clinic for periodic blood tests.
④ Discontinue taking ginseng while taking coumadin.

16.34 A client develops acute renal failure and is on continuous peritoneal dialysis. Which assessment finding indicates the most common complication associated with this procedure?

① Hypotension
② Hypertension
③ Pruitis
④ Bradycardia

16.35 Which of these tasks is most appropriate for the nurse to delegate to an experienced UAP?

① Observe a newly diagnosed client with diabetes mellitus practice injection techniques using an orange.
② Obtain a clean catch urine specimen from a client suspected of having a urinary tract infection.
③ Obtain a 24-hour diet recall from a client recently admitted with anorexia nervosa.
④ Observe the amount and characteristics of the returns from a continuous bladder irrigation for a client after a transuretheral prostate resection.

16.36 Which reflex would be abnormal to observe in a 6-month-old child?

① Presence of a positive Babinski reflex.
② Extrusion reflex occurs when feeding.
③ Able to voluntarily grasp objects.
④ Rolls from abdomen to back at will.

16.37 A client is admitted to the emergency room with a gunshot wound in the chest and in severe respiratory distress. Which nursing action has the highest priority when managing the emergency?

① Establish and maintain an open airway.
② Start cardiopulmonary resuscitation.
③ Initiate oxygen therapy.
④ Obtain an arterial blood gas.

16.38 A toddler admitted with an elevated blood lead level is to be treated with intramuscular injections of calcium disodium edentate and dimercaprol. Which nursing action would have the highest priority?

① Keep a tongue blade at the bedside.
② Encourage the child to participate in play therapy.
③ Apply cool soaks to the injection site.
④ Rotate the injection site.

16.39 Which assessment finding indicates gentamycin toxicity?

① Decreased hearing
② Blurred vision
③ Nausea and vomiting
④ Macular rash

16.40 Which assessment documents an allergic blood transfusion reaction?

① Hypotension
② Chills
③ Respiratory wheezing
④ Lower back discomfort

16.41 Prior to administering atenolol and digoxin, which assessment is most important to report and document?

① Bradycardia
② Tachycardia
③ Hypertension
④ Serum potassium—3.8 mEq/L (3.8 mmol/L)

16.42 What would be the priority assessment for a client who is admitted to the outpatient oncology unit for routine chemotherapy transfusion with the current lab reports: WBC—2,500 mm³; RBC—5,100 mm³; and calcium 5 mg/dL (1.25 mmol/L)?

① Fatigue related to decrease in red cells.
② Infection related to low white cell count.
③ Anxiety secondary to hyperparathyroid disease.
④ Fluid volume deficit due to decreased fluid intake.

16.43 A urinalysis has been done on a client who has been complaining of dysuria, urinary frequency, and discomfort in the suprapubic area. After evaluation of the results, the nurse would order a repeat urinalysis based on:

① Negative glucose
② RBCs present
③ No WBCs or RBCs reported
④ Specific gravity 1.018

16.44 What is the priority care for a client in Buck's traction?

① Turn the client every two hours to the unaffected side.
② Maintain client in a supine position.
③ Encourage client to use a bedside commode.
④ Prevent foot drop by placing a foot board to the bed.

16.45 Which assignment is most appropriate for the UAP?

① Doing a sterile dressing change on a client admitted for skin grafts.
② Obtaining a temperature on a client receiving the final 40 minutes of a blood transfusion.
③ Assisting a client newly diagnosed with a CVA to eat his dinner.
④ Completing the initial vital signs on a client who has just returned to her room after having abdominal surgery.

16.46 What would be the primary goal of nursing interventions for a client who has Multiple Sclerosis with a progressive disability?

① Maintain a cheerful, positive outlook.
② Remain physically active and independent.
③ Maintain good personal hygiene.
④ Remain in a quiet environment to decrease stimuli.

16.47 A client is admitted to the emergency room after an acute asthmatic attack. Vital signs on admission include:
- Pulse 98 bpm
- Respiratory rate 40 with substernal retracting

Immediate care would include placing the client in which position?
① High Fowler's
② Supine position
③ Trendelenburg
④ Sim's position

16.48 A young adult client is seen in the emergency room for an overdose of acetylsalicylic acid. Which plan represents correct care in the Emergency Room?
① If aspirin was ingested within the last two hours, administer activated charcoal powder.
② Initiate an intravenous infusion and administer protamine sulfate.
③ Since aspirin overdose will cause bleeding, AquaMephyton should be given.
④ Obtain an arterial blood gas and request respiratory therapy to begin respiratory support.

16.49 Which client condition could precipitate a toxic reaction to Phenytoin?
① Impaired liver function
② Decreased hemoglobin and hematocrit
③ White blood count of 10,000/mm^3 and serum sodium of 140 mEq/L (140 mmol/L)
④ Depressed neurological functioning

16.50 An infant is admitted for vomiting and diarrhea. The anterior fontanelle is depressed and a fever of 103.2°F (39.6°C) is noted. What would be the initial plan to assist with rehydration?
① Determine daily weights and evaluate weight loss.
② Evaluate child's ability to take in oral fluids.
③ Place a full bottle of Pedialyte at bedside.
④ Document I & O.

16.51 What is the priority nursing action while assisting the physician with the spinal tap on a 4-month-old?
① Restrain the child appropriately.
② Instruct parents about procedure.
③ Provide support to the child.
④ Elevate the head of the bed.

16.52 Which of these nursing actions by the licensed practical nurse (LPN), when working with a client with a nasogastric tube, requires intervention by the charge nurse?
① The tube is flushed after an enteral feeding is given.
② The tube is secured by taping the tube to the client's cheek with a short length of tubing looped on the nose.
③ When the gastric residual was 150 mL, the feeding was held and rechecked residual in 1 hour.
④ The client is positioned in the semi-Fowler's position when residuals are high.

16.53 Which teaching is appropriate regarding wearing anti-embolism stockings following surgery?
① Wear them when legs are cramping.
② Wear them the entire time client is in the hospital.
③ Put stockings on in the evening prior to going to bed.
④ Put stockings on after client has been out of bed and walked around.

16.54 An infant is in Bryant's traction. During the neurovascular assessment, the nurse notes that the foot of the uninjured leg feels warmer to touch than that of the broken leg. What action would the nurse implement now?
① Recognize that as long as the foot of the injured leg is warm to touch, circulation is doing well.
② Encourage child to move his foot by playing a toe-moving game with him.
③ Cover the colder foot with a sock and check its temperature in one hour.
④ Recognize that the strapping may be too snug and notify the health care provider.

16.55 Which nursing action indicates an understanding of how to administer AquaMephyton to a neonate?
① Administers an injection into the vastus lateralis.
② Mixes it in the formula.
③ Applies drops into the inner canthus.
④ Administers a subcutaneous injection into the anterior thigh.

16.56 Which plan is a priority in an emergency wound evisceration?
① Maintain moisture to the wound.
② Start an IV and begin antibiotics.
③ Keep a sterile dressing over the wound.
④ Irrigate the wound with normal saline.

16.57 During chemotherapy of an outpatient who is lethargic, weak, and pale, which intervention is most important for the nurse to implement?
① Establish emotional support.
② Position for physical comfort.
③ Maintain respiratory isolation.
④ Hand washing prior to care.

16.58 Which response to mannitol is desired for decreasing the intracranial pressure of a client with a closed head injury?
① The blood pressure increases to 150/90.
② Urinary output increases to 175 mL/hour.
③ Decrease in the level of activity.
④ Absence of fine tremors of the fingers.

16.59 A young adult client, gravida 2, para 1, in her third trimester of pregnancy has had diabetes since age 14. Which statement made by the client indicates an understanding regarding the insulin requirements during the third trimester?
① "I cannot continue to exercise as this will increase my insulin needs."
② "I understand my insulin requirements will increase as my pregnancy progresses."
③ "Since the baby has a normal pancreas, my insulin needs will not change."
④ "The more weight I gain, the more insulin I will need to take."

16.60 Which observation indicates the client has an understanding of appropriate crutch walking?
① Weight bearing is under the arm on the axillary area.
② The crutches are placed about 18–20 inches (46–50.8 cm) in front of him with each step.
③ The weight of the body is being transferred to the hands and the arms.
④ Leather sole shoes are worn to increase the smooth motion across the floor.

16.61 Which of these instructions is most important to include with the discharge teaching for a client who is going to be discharged on simvastatin?
① "Return to the office in 7 days to determine if the lipids have decreased."
② "Take the medication on an empty stomach to assist with absorption."
③ "Review the importance of taking with food and at bedtime."
④ "Discuss the importance of decreasing the fiber in diet when taking this medication."

16.62 A client is currently hospitalized with renal failure and has 3+ pitting edema of the lower extremities. Which nursing observation indicates a therapeutic response to therapy for the edema?
① Potassium level of 4.0 mEq/L (4.0 mmol/L)
② Serum glucose of 140 mg/dL (7.77 mmol/L)
③ Increased specific gravity of the urine
④ Weight loss of 5 lbs. (2.3 kg) over last 2 days

16.63 Several days after a myocardial infarction, a client was placed on a 2 Gm sodium diet. Which selection indicates compliance with the diet?
① Scrambled egg, orange slices and milk
② Instant oatmeal, toast, and orange juice
③ Poached egg, bacon, and milk
④ Biscuit, fruit cup, and sausage

16.64 Which actions would be implemented for a client admitted with left ventricular heart failure who is presenting with a sudden onset of dyspnea, breathlessness, moist cough, and a rapid and weak heart rate while lying in the bed? **Select all that apply.**
① Administer morphine sulfate 4 mg intravenously (IV) as prescribed.
② Prepare to administer cyclophosphamide as prescribed.
③ Prepare to administer furosemide IV as prescribed.
④ Initiate oxygen via a high-flow rebreather mask per protocol.
⑤ Reposition client to the left side to facilitate cardiac contractility.

16.65 Which would be most responsible for prolonging wound healing in the older client?
① Depression
② Increased social contacts
③ An increase in the adipose tissue
④ An intake of 20 to 35 g. of fiber per day

16.66 In the immediate post-operative period, which nursing assessment is a priority in a client with a pneumonectomy?
① Presence of breath sounds bilaterally
② Position of trachea in sternal notch
③ Amount and consistency of sputum
④ An increase in the pulse pressure

16.67 What is the priority nursing assessment for a client who is a primipara in early labor with newly ruptured membranes?
① Determine the pH of the amniotic fluid.
② Evaluate the mother's blood pressure.
③ Check the monitor for an early deceleration with the next contraction.
④ Observe the perineal area for evidence of a prolapsed cord.

16.68 Which diet selections would be included in the teaching plan of the client with osteoporosis?
① Steak and baked potato
② A glass of skim milk and a toasted cheese sandwich
③ Chicken and salad
④ French fries and fish

16.69 A client is in labor and is receiving magnesium sulfate IV. Which assessment is most important to report to the nurse on the next shift?
① Respiratory rate change from 13/minute to 15/minute
② Increase in anxiety and hyperactivity
③ Presence of nausea and refusal to take clear liquids
④ Urine output change from 60 mL/hr to 40 mL/hr

16.70 Which of these statements made by the nurse indicates an understanding of the reason a client with chronic renal failure is receiving calcium carbonate?
① "This medication will minimize the complications with constipation."
② "This medication will prevent the development of osteoporosis."
③ "Calcium carbonate will prevent the development of ulcers."
④ "Calcium carbonate will bind with phosphorus to decrease concentrations."

16.71 Which of these clinical assessment findings would be reported to the provider of care for an older adult who has been vomiting and had diarrhea for the last 32 hours? **Select all that apply.**
① Heart Rate—68 bpm
② Blood Pressure—156/88
③ Furrowed dry tongue
④ Confusion
⑤ Increase thirst

16.72 What is the priority nursing assessment(s) after a client returns from having a liver biopsy?
① Urine output—50 mL/hr
② HR—105 bpm; RR—32 breaths/min; BP—100/68
③ Evaluate pretest prothrombin time and INR
④ Evaluate peripheral pulses

16.73 In the crowded hospital cafeteria, a nurse overhears an unlicensed assistive personnel (UAP) openly discussing a client with her peers. Which nursing action has the highest priority?
① Report the UAP's behavior to the Director of Nursing.
② Complete an incident report regarding the behavior.
③ Discuss the importance and implications of client confidentiality with the UAP.
④ Report the incident to the evening charge nurse.

16.74 The charge nurse is making the morning assignment for a group of clients including several who are HIV positive, or who have AIDS. There are three unlicensed assistive personnel (UAPs) to assist with morning care. One of the UAPs states: "I am not going to take care of anyone who has AIDS." What is the best nursing action for the charge nurse to take regarding the assignment of the morning?
① Tell the UAP that when she was hired she was advised about HIV-positive clients, and she does not have a choice in the type of assignments she receives.
② Respect the UAP's request and assign all of the HIV-positive clients to the other two UAPs.
③ Determine what type of education the UAP received regarding standard precautions, and evaluate her ability to follow the precautions.
④ Discuss with the UAP in private that it is necessary for her to provide care to these clients and attempt to determine the source of fear.

16.75 What information is important for the nurse to explain to the mother whose child has been discharged on Tylenol?
① Acetaminophen is the generic name for Tylenol; any acetaminophen product in the children's strength is okay for her to use.
② The mother may purchase Tylenol in the children's or infant's strength for her child.
③ Determine if the mother has any acetaminophen at home either in the adult strength or in the children's strength for her child.
④ Tylenol is the generic name for the brand names of Advil or Motrin. Either of these in the children's strength may be used.

16.76 What would be most important to have at the bedside of a 36-month-old client with a fever of 103.4°F (39.7°C), respirations at 49/minute with suprasternal retractions present, drooling, and an enlarged epiglottis?
① Defibrillator
② Tracheostomy set-up
③ Tongue blade
④ IVAC pump

16.77 A client is given Aminophylline capsule 4 hours too early. This incident is discovered 30 minutes after administration. Which plan would be the most appropriate?
① Document the event on an incident report, and notify the health care provider (HCP).
② Change time for next medication administration.
③ Assess for bradycardia and lethargy, and notify physician.
④ Skip the next dose of medication.

16.78 A client at 38 weeks gestation is admitted in active labor. The nursing assessment reveals a decreased blood pressure to 90/50 and the FHR is 130 and regular. Which nursing action is the most important?
① Call the physician and advise of the decrease in blood pressure.
② Elevate the head of the bed to facilitate respirations.
③ Check the client's blood pressure and FHT every 30 minutes for the next 2 hours.
④ Place the client on her left side and reevaluate the blood pressure.

16.79 The client has an order for IV fluid of D5.2 Normal Saline, 1000 mL to run from 9 AM to 9 PM. The drip factor on the delivery tubing is 15 gtts/mL. The nurse would adjust the IV to infuse at what rate?
① 21 gtt/min
② 12 gtt/min
③ 25 gtt/min
④ 31 gtt/min

16.80 After a right radical mastectomy, which position is the most appropriate for a client?
① Left side with right arm protected in a sling
② Right side with right arm elevated
③ Semi-Fowler's position with right arm elevated
④ Prone position with right arm elevated

16.81 Which nursing assessment is a priority for an elderly client who is very confused and disoriented when admitted from a long-term care facility?
① Determine level of mobility regarding safe walking.
② Evaluate teeth and determine appropriate diet.
③ Determine if a family member can remain at bedside.
④ Assess the respiratory status and evaluate for hypoxia.

16.82 A client is admitted to the Emergency Room with second and third-degree burns to the anterior chest, both arms, and right leg. What would be the priority information to determine at the time of admission?
① Percentage of burned surface area.
② Amount of IV fluid necessary for fluid resuscitation.
③ Any evidence of heat inhalation or airway problems.
④ Circumstances surrounding the burn and contamination of the area.

16.83 Which nursing action is correct regarding the initial infusion of oxytocin?
① Mix oxytocin in D_5W, begin at 5 mg/mL as primary IV to gravity flow.
② Decrease the rate/flow of oxytocin if fetal heart rate is below 150.
③ Piggyback the oxytocin into mainline IV and maintain flow by gravity.
④ Start an IV line and piggyback the oxytocin with an infusion pump.

16.84 The nurse is caring for a client who vigorously follows several rituals daily, including frequent hand washing. The client's hands are now reddened and sensitive to touch. Which nursing action would be least helpful initially?
① Provide special skin care.
② Give positive reinforcement for nonritualistic behavior.
③ Limit the amount of time the client may use to wash hands.
④ Protect the client from ridicule by other clients on the unit.

16.85 A client is admitted for a total abdominal hysterectomy. When the nurse gives the client the operative consent, client refuses to sign it. Which documentation in the chart is appropriate?
① The surgeon was notified and stated he/she would return to speak with the client.
② The client was informed about the importance of signing the consent, and advised to call the physician.
③ The husband was notified and gave a telephone consent.
④ The operating room was notified and surgery was canceled.

16.86 During a well-baby check-up on a 6-month-old, what would the nurse expect on assessment?
① Pincer grasp
② Sit with support
③ Birth weight tripled
④ Presence of the posterior fontanelle

16.87 Which nursing assessment is indicative of a positive tuberculin skin test reaction?
① Induration of 10 mm at the site
② A pruitic rash of 5 mm at the site
③ High fever and congested cough
④ Erythema and inflammation at the site

16.88 To assess the right middle lobe (RML) of the lung, the nurse would auscultate at which location?
① Posterior and anterior base of right side
② Right anterior chest between the fourth and sixth intercostal
③ Left of the sternum, midclavicular at fifth intercostal space
④ Posterior chest wall, midaxillary right side

16.89 1000 mL 5% dextrose in 0.45 saline is to be administered IV over 8 hours using an infusion pump for an adult client. What is the correct rate setting on the IV infusion pump?

_____ mL/hr

16.90 The parents of a newborn with a meningocele have been grieving the loss of their perfect child. After 3 days of grieving, progress in their emotional status would be indicated by which comment made by the parents?
① "When will it be safe for us to hold our baby?"
② "We would rather you feed our baby."
③ "What did we do to cause this problem?"
④ "When do you anticipate our baby going home?"

16.91 The nurse is assigned to work with the parents of a mentally and physically delayed child. With regard to the parents, which nursing action should be included in the care plan?
① Need to interpret the grieving process for the parents.
② Discuss the reality of institutional placement.
③ Assist the parents in making decisions and long-term plans for the child.
④ Perform a family assessment.

16.92 The provider of care prescribes Lactated Ringer's 50 mL IV to be infused over 20 min. What should the nurse set the IV flow rate to deliver how many mL/hr?
_____ mL/hr

16.93 A woman being evaluated for infertility is given clomiphene citrate 50 mg daily to take for 5 days. The client asks the nurse the purpose of the medicine. What would the nurse instruct the client about regarding the action of clomiphene citrate?
① Clomiphene citrate will induce ovulation by changing the hormone effects on the ovary.
② Clomiphene citrate will change the uterine lining to be more conducive to implantation.
③ Clomiphene citrate will alter the vaginal pH to increase sperm motility.
④ Clomiphene citrate will produce multiple pregnancies for those who desire twins.

16.94 During the initial prenatal visit, the physician orders an iron supplement to be taken throughout the client's pregnancy. What information is important for the nurse to tell the client regarding the iron?
① The medication should be taken with orange juice.
② Take the medication with antacids to decrease gastric distress.
③ Drinking 8 ounces of water will enhance absorption of the medication.
④ Notify the physician if stools become dark or loose.

16.95 A client with Addison's disease has been placed on prednisone. Which comment by the client indicates an understanding of how to take the medication?
① "I should take the medication one hour before meals."
② "It is important to take the medication with my meals."
③ "I will take the medication on an empty stomach."
④ "I will not drink milk right after I take my medicine."

16.96 A client has an order for a low-sodium, low-cholesterol diet. Which selection reflects the client's compliance?
① Vegetable soup, applesauce, and hot chocolate
② Cheeseburger, French fries, and milk
③ Tomato and lettuce salad, and roasted chicken
④ Tuna fish sandwich, cottage cheese, and a Coke

16.97 What is the priority of care for an elderly client who is taking amitriptyline?
① Monitor urine output every 12 hours.
② Stand up slowly from sitting or lying positions.
③ Provide oral care every 12 hours.
④ Review foods that are low in fiber.

16.98 Which evaluation indicates a therapeutic response to volume replacement in hypovolemic shock?
① Urine output increased to 50 mL per hour
② Blood glucose of 180 mg/dL (9.99 mmol/L), serum potassium of 4.0 mEq/L (4.0 mmol/L)
③ CVP of 2 mm Hg, pupils equal and reactive
④ Pulse rate of 110 with no dysrhythmias

16.99 A post-operative client has returned to the room from the surgical recovery area. The client is sleeping and is disoriented when aroused. What is a nursing action to promote the client's safety?
① Placing the call bell within the client's reach.
② Staying with the client until totally oriented.
③ Restraining all four extremities until client is oriented.
④ Placing the side rails up until the client is fully awake.

16.100 Which nursing action is most appropriate for an infant who is post operative for cleft lip and palate repair and is presenting with upper airway congestion and slightly labored respirations?
① Elevate the head of the bed.
② Suction the infant's nose.
③ Position the infant on his side.
④ Administer oxygen until breathing is easier.

16.101 An American Indian client is scheduled for a joint replacement. Upon admission for surgery, the client says to the nurse, "I need to have the tissues that are removed, so they can be buried with me when I die. Without them, I will not be whole in my afterlife." What action would the nurse take?
① Inform the client this request violates protocol.
② Inform the client this request does not make sense.
③ Inform the surgeon of the client's request.
④ Inform the operating room staff to save the tissue removed.

16.102 An unaccompanied client, who is six months pregnant, is admitted to the nursing unit with vaginal bleeding. Which comment made by the client indicates a need for the nurse to assess the adequacy of the client's emotional support?
① "My husband will be so angry with me if I lose this baby."
② "I'm afraid I am going to lose my baby."
③ "I can't stay here. I don't have any insurance."
④ "I feel so guilty. I didn't want to get pregnant."

16.103 On a home health visit, an elderly client states, "This neighborhood has really gone down. I feel like a prisoner in my own home with all the trouble out there." Which nursing response would be priority?
① "Have you and your neighbors formed a Neighborhood Watch?"
② "It must be very difficult for you to live in this neighborhood."
③ "I see a lot of police cars. You should be pretty safe."
④ "Tell me what has happened to make you feel that you are not safe."

16.104 A client is experiencing septic shock and the provider wants dosing of medications to be regulated so that a mean arterial pressure (MAP) between 65 and 75 mm Hg is maintained. Which of the client's blood pressure readings meet this goal?
① 135/90
② 125/80
③ 115/70
④ 105/60

16.105 A client on the psychiatric unit was observed crying in her room following a visit from the health care provider (HCP). Which nursing docmentation is the most appropriate regarding this observation?
① Depressed following visit with health care provider (HCP).
② Appeared depressed after the visit from health care provider (HCP).
③ Crying in her room following visit by health care provider (HCP).
④ Upset with the health care provider (HCP) after his visit.

16.106 Which of these clients would the nurse question the new prescription for sildenafil citrate?
① A client with a history of headaches
② A history of shingles
③ A history of bronchitis
④ Heart failure and hypotension

16.107 A recently widowed elderly client has been hospitalized following a suicide attempt. Which behavior most clearly indicates the client remains a suicide risk?
① He admits having vague suicidal ideas in the past.
② His history indicates difficulty forming relationships with caregivers.
③ He becomes emotional and cries when talking about his late wife.
④ He begins to give away some of his most prized possessions.

16.108 Which of these clinical assessment findings would be reported to the health care provider for a client who has a nasogastric tube with suctioning? **Select all that apply.**
① Spiked T waves
② Hyperactive bowel sounds
③ Positive Chvostek's sign
④ Muscle cramping
⑤ Syncope when getting up out of bed

16.109 The nurse is administering Desmopressin Acetate (DDAVP) to a client diagnosed with diabetes insipidus. Which of the following assessments indicates the desired outcome of treatment?
① BP was 189/101 and is now 160/90.
② Blood glucose was 140 mg/dL (7.77 mmol/L) and is now 110 mg/dL (6.11 mmol/L).
③ Client intake of meal increased from 50% to 75%.
④ Urine output was 300 mL hr and is now 65 mL hr.

16.110 Which of the following actions is appropriate for the nurse to delegate to the UAP for a client who is one day post-operative choleycystectomy?
① Empty the T-tube drainage bag and report the amount of drainage noted.
② Instruct the client to avoid broccoli, fried chicken, and cheese.
③ Obtain vital signs and monitor for changes.
④ Assist the client to ambulate in the hall.

16.111 An LPN is caring for a client who has acquired third-degree full thickness burns, and is experiencing an excessive fluid loss. Which nursing action indicates the LPN understands how to provide appropriate care?
① The LPN is administering PO pain medications.
② The LPN assists the client to elevate extremities.
③ The LPN is administering hypotonic IV fluids.
④ The LPN assists the client to dangle his legs.

16.112 After a client is started on haloperidol 5 mg TID, which would be a priority for the nurse to discuss with the client?
① Stay away from foods high in tyramine.
② Move slowly to a standing position.
③ May experience a dry mouth.
④ Limit salt intake.

16.113 An elderly client in the Rehabilitation Department was evaluated to determine at what risk the client was for developing a pressure ulcer. How would the charge nurse intervene with a score of 21 points on the Braden Scale?
① A multidisciplinary client care meeting would be held to develop a plan for prevention, since the client is high risk.
② Since this client is high risk, review with staff that a Stage II ulcer involves the partial thickness skin loss involving epidermis and/or dermis. This ulcer may present clinically as an abrasion, blister, or shallow crater.
③ Interpret this score as an excellent one, and continue with protocol for skin care to prevent any complications.
④ Review with the UAPs how to move client up in bed since a major cause of pressure sores are secondary from friction and shear.

16.114 A home care nurse is caring for an older adult client that is taking docusate sodium. Which of these clinical assessment findings indicates an undesirable effect from this medication?
① Orange urine
② Abdominal distention with absent bowel sounds
③ HR of 72 bpm
④ Abdominal cramps

16.115 A client with chronic bronchitis is receiving supplemental oxygen via nasal cannula and orders state that the SpO_2 would be maintained at 90 percent or higher. During the nursing assessment, the nurse notices that the oxygen delivery is set at 7 liters per minute with an SpO_2 of 88 percent. What would be the priority nursing action?
① Reduce the oxygen delivery to the client no more than 2 liters per minute and stay with the client.
② Change the method of oxygen delivery to a simple mask or face tent.
③ Validate the SpO_2 value and further assess the client for possible causes of hypoxemia.
④ Investigate if the client, a significant other or a staff member set the oxygen at 7 liters.

16.116 After a client has returned to the floor from thyroidectomy surgery, which nursing intervention has the highest priority?
① Monitor vital signs every four hours.
② Monitor for hemorrhaging by observing frequent swallowing.
③ Monitor signs of respiratory distress frequently.
④ Position client in supine position.

16.117 The nurse is preparing a client to be discharged and who will be going home with crutches. The following are instructions for going down the stairs. Put the steps in order. Use all of the options.

| ①Shift weight to the unaffected leg. |
| ②Transfer weight to the crutches and move the unaffected leg to that step. |
| ③Assume tripod position at the top of the stairs. |
| ④Move crutches and the affected leg down onto the next step. |

| |
| |
| |
| |

16.118 Which of these nursing actions by the LPN when performing nasopharyngeal suctioning requires intervention by the charge nurse due to the standard of practice not being followed?
① Applying suction only when withdrawing the catheter and rotating it with the thumb and forefinger.
② Allowing the client 10 to 15 seconds for recovery between suctioning sessions.
③ Advancing the catheter the approximate distance from the tip of the nose to the base of the earlobe.
④ Suctioning client for 10 to 15 seconds.

16.119 Which of these documentations by the RN indicates an understanding of how to safely provide care for a peripherally inserted central catheter?
① Flushed port with 10 mL 0.9% sodium chloride as per facility protocol for intermittent medication administration.
② Applied a gauze dressing over site and changed gauze dressing every 24 hours.
③ Cleansed the insertion port with betadine for 10 seconds and allowing it to dry completely prior to accessing it.
④ Informed client that after 24 hours a shower can be taken with no precautions to site.

16.120 The nurse is caring for a client in labor. The nurse palpates a firm round form in the uterine fundus. On the client's right side, small parts are palpated, and on the left side, a long, smooth curved section is palpated. Which location would the nurse auscultate the fetal heart?

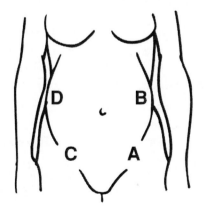

Category Analysis—Practice Exam

1. Management of Care
2. Physiological Adaptation
3. Safety and Infection Control
4. Pharmacology
5. Basic Care and Comfort
6. Management of Care
7. Physiological Adaptation
8. Safety and Infection Control
9. Management of Care
10. Physiological Adaptation
11. Physiological Adaptation
12. Physiological Adaptation
13. Basic Care and Comfort
14. Management of Care
15. Physiological Adaptation
16. Physiological Adaptation
17. Pharmacology
18. Reduction of Risk Potential
19. Pharmacology
20. Reduction of Risk Potential
21. Management of Care
22. Basic Care and Comfort
23. Reduction of Risk Potential
24. Reduction of Risk Potential
25. Safety and Infection Control
26. Safety and Infection Control
27. Safety and Infection Control
28. Pharmacology
29. Pharmacology
30. Physiological Adaptation
31. Reduction of Risk Potential
32. Reduction of Risk Potential
33. Pharmacology
34. Basic Care and Comfort
35. Reduction of Risk Potential
36. Health Promotion
37. Physiological Adaptation
38. Pharmacology
39. Pharmacology
40. Pharmacology
41. Pharmacology
42. Safety and Infection Control
43. Basic Care and Comfort
44. Reduction of Risk Potential
45. Management of Care
46. Reduction of Risk Potential
47. Physiological Adaptation
48. Pharmacology
49. Pharmacology
50. Basic Care & Comfort
51. Reduction of Risk Potential
52. Basic Care and Comfort
53. Basic Care & Comfort
54. Reduction of Risk Potential
55. Pharmacology
56. Basic Care & Comfort
57. Safety and Infection Control
58. Pharmacology
59. Health Promotion
60. Basic Care & Comfort
61. Pharmacology
62. Physiological Adaptation
63. Basic Care and Comfort
64. Physiological Adaptation
65. Psychosocial
66. Physiological Adaptation
67. Health Promotion
68. Basic Care and Comfort
69. Pharmacology
70. Pharmacology
71. Physiological Adaptation
72. Reduction of Risk Potential
73. Management of Care
74. Management of Care
75. Pharmacology
76. Physiological Adaptation
77. Pharmacology
78. Health Promotion
79. Pharmacology
80. Reduction of Risk Potential
81. Psychosocial

82.	Physiological Adaptation	95.	Pharmacology	108.	Physiological Adaptation
83.	Pharmacology	96.	Basic Care and Comfort	109.	Physiological Adaptation
84.	Psychosocial	97.	Basic Care and Comfort	110.	Management of Care
85.	Management of Care	98.	Physiological Adaptation	111.	Basic Care and Comfort
86.	Health Promotion	99.	Safety and Infection Control	112.	Pharmacology
87.	Safety and Infection Control	100.	Physiological Adaptation	113.	Basic Care and Comfort
88.	Physiological Adaptation	101.	Psychosocial	114.	Pharmacology
89.	Physiological Adaptation	102.	Psychosocial	115.	Physiological Adaptation
90.	Psychosocial	103.	Health Promotion	116.	Physiological Adaptationl
91.	Psychosocial	104.	Physiological Adaptation	117.	Safety and Infection Control
92.	Pharmacology	105.	Psychosocial	118.	Physiological Adaptation
93.	Pharmacology	106.	Pharmacology	119.	Pharmacology
94.	Basic Care and Comfort	107.	Psychosocial	120.	Reduction of Risk

Directions

1. Determine questions missed by checking answers.
2. Write the number of the questions missed across the top line marked "item missed."
3. Check category analysis page to determine category of question.
4. Put a check mark under item missed and beside content.
5. Count check marks in each row and write the number in totals column.
6. Use this information to:
   - identify areas for further study.
   - determine which content test to take next.

We recommend studying content where most items are missed—then taking that content test.

Number of the Questions Incorrectly Answered

Post-Test	Items Missed																											Totals
C Management of Care																												
O Safety and Infection Control																												
N Health Promotion and Maintenance																												
T Psychosocial Integrity																												
E Physiological Adaptation:Fluid Gas																												
N Reduction of Risk Potential																												
T Basic Care and Comfort																												
Pharmacology and Parenteral Therapies																												

Answers & Rationales

16.1 ③ Option #3 is correct. Morphine should be contraindicated since this will mask the neurological assessment for this client. Option #1 is incorrect since the medication should be contraindicated for this client and should not be administered. Option #2 is incorrect due to the same rationale as #1. The client should not be receiving this medication, so there would be no need for the antidote at the bedside. Option #4 is not consistent with the standard of care for clients with increased intracranial pressure. Coughing will increase the ICP.

16.2 ① Option #1 is correct. Based on the clinical findings, the client is presenting with an acute episode of hypoxia. The key statement is *"suddenly becomes anxious and very SOB."* This may be from heart failure, but with the current clinical data provided the nurse must make a clinical decision based on this limited information. There is a need for further assessments and an immediate intervention. Of course, part of this clinical decision making strategy is to compare and contrast the options in order to make a clinical judgment. Option #2 is not a priority over #1. The client in option #2 is septic and the body is responding physiologically like it should with a WBC count of 20,000 mm³ and a diagnosis of pneumonia. In contrast, however, option #1 has a client presenting with a *"sudden onset of hypoxia."* Option #3 is a concern due to the saturation and temperature, but is not a priority over option #1. A key to answering this question would be to review the similarity between options #2 and #3. Remember, this is not a question evaluating *"select all that apply."* Option #4 is also a concern. This client is presenting with intermittent claudication which is secondary to arterial insufficiency. Yes, the nurse needs to see this client, but this client still is not as acute as the client in option #1.

16.3 ③ Options #3 and #4 are correct. Protective
    ④ isolation is used to protect clients who have an increased susceptibility to infection such as if they are receiving chemotherapy or are immuno-suppressed or neutropenic. Clients who have had a renal transplant are immuno-suppressed. Option #3 is included in the standard of care for these isolation guidelines. Option #4 is reinforced to minimize exposure to microorganisms found on the outer layers of fresh flowers. This also applies to fruits and vegetables. Option #1 is incorrect. The nurse is not concerned with protecting self from the client's secretions as a result of being splattered. The goal is to prevent the client from getting infected. If the question, however, did indicate that the nurse was going to engage in nursing care that would require the nurse to come in contact with the client's body secretions such as with entubation, suctioning, etc., then the goggles would be required based on the standard/universal precautions outlined by CDC. Option #2 is incorrect. The client should be placed in a ventilated positive pressure room for maximum protection. Negative-pressure airflow would be appropriate for a client with tuberculosis. Option #5 is not within the standard of care for this type of infection prevention precaution.

16.4 ② Betamethasone is a glucocorticoid agent that produces and releases lung surfactant to stimulate fetal lung maturity. This value indicates sufficient surfactant is present. Option #1 would be an outcome form oxytocin. Options #3 and #4 do not address the question that is the expected outcome from the medication, betamethasone.

16.5 ③ Options #3, #4, #5 are correct. This question
    ④ is evaluating *"How to communicate with*
    ⑤ *the client with sensory deficits."* Looking at the client directly while communicating, speaking slowly, and giving instructions one at a time will result in effective communication. Additional nursing actions may also include: remaining in the client's field of vision if possible; using a warm, pleasant voice and not speaking loudly; explaining procedures prior to starting them; and keeping background noise to a minimum. When a subject is changed, it is imperative to slow down or to use key words to indicate the change. Option #1 is incorrect since this may have an effect on the self-esteem of the client,

and does not assist in a development of independence. Option #2 is incorrect since the communication board is another devise to assist with communication, but is not the ONLY method. The entire distractor must be correct for it to be a correct answer.

16.6 ① Option #1 is correct. When confronted with a fire, the most important response from a nurse is to rescue the client. In order of priority, the proper responses are: 1) rescue; 2) alarm; 3) confine the fire; and 4) evacuate or extinguish.

16.7 ① Option #1 is correct. Option #2 would be appropriate position to auscultate the pulmonic heart sound. Option #3 would be the appropriate location to auscultate the PMI. Option #4 is incorrect.

16.8 ④ This is being a client advocate. The observed nurse may need some assistance, and this would be an excellent opportunity to provide education regarding this procedure. Options #1 and #3 do not address the problem. Option #2 is unsafe practice and can lead to infection.

16.9 ① Options #1, #2, and #3 are correct.
      ② Options #4 and #5 are not necessary for
      ③ this procedure.

16.10 ④ Option #4 is correct. Option #1, alcohol or healer acetone pads in place of the electrode paste or gel may impair electrode contact with the skin and diminish the transmission quality of electrical impulses. Option #2, the client should be instructed to lie in a supine position. Option #3 is incorrect. Client should breathe normally.

16.11 ④ Option #4 is correct. The client is getting hypoxic and needs oxygen. Options #1 and #2 are incorrect. Option #1 is unsafe. Option #3 is partially correct. Stopping procedure is correct, but evaluating breath sounds is not a priority in this clinical situation over option #4.

16.12 ③ Option #3 is the correct answer. The client is experiencing hypoglycemia, but is still arousable. Diaphoresis and lethargy are symptoms of hypoglycemia. Additional symptoms of hypoglycemia may be shakiness, anxiety, nervousness, nausea, chills, headache, weakness, and confusion. The guidelines for this hypoglycemic client would be to treat with 15 to 20 Gm carbohydrates. Examples of this amount of carbohydrates may include: 4 oz. (118.3 mL) orange juice, 2 oz. (59 mL) grape juice, 8 oz. (237 mL) milk, glucose tables per manufacturer's suggestion to equal 15 GM. Option #2 is incorrect. Option #2 is part of the standard of care for the diabetic client, but is not the priority for this clinical situation. The HbA1c is the best indicator of the average blood glucose level for the past 120 days. This lab assists in evaluating treatment effectiveness and compliance. This option does not answer the question which requires immediate intervention. Option #4 should be done after an intervention, based upon the outcomes from the nursing action. It is, however, not the priority over treating the hypoglycemia.

I CAN HINT: One of the key words in this question is "arousable". If, however, the client was unconscious or unable to swallow, the home health nurse would need to administer (Option #1) glucagon SC or IM (repeat in 10 min if still unconscious), and notify the health care provider. Since the client is arousable, option #3 is the priority.

16.13 ④ Option #4 is correct. Option #1 is incorrect. Betadine is an inappropriate option. Option #2 is incorrect. Avoid using alcohol because it causes pain and tissue dehydration. Hydrogen peroxide may be used. The foaming action facilitates debris removal. However, peroxide should never be instilled into a deep wound because of the risk of embolism from evolving gases. Option #3 is incorrect when irrigating a traumatic wound, avoid using more than 8 psi of pressure. High-pressure irrigation can seriously interfere with healing, kill healthy cells, and allow bacteria to infiltrate the tissue.

16.14 ① The sickle cell crisis would be a priority due to the need to start IV fluids for hydration purposes. The hypoxia must be corrected immediately with IV fluids and oxygen. Option #2 would only be a preparation prior to surgery. Options #3 and #4 are important but not priorities to option #1.

16.15 ④ Options #4 and 5 are correct. Option #4 will bind with phosphates to decrease phosphates and assist with increasing calcium level. Option #5 is correct due to the problem with fluid excess secondary to the chronic renal disease. Option #1 is incorrect due to the complication that can occur is hyperkalemia which would result with a peaked T wave. Option #2 is incorrect because these are high in potassium. Option #3 is incorrect due to NSAIDs requiring normal renal function.

16.16 ①
③
④
⑤
All are appropriate interventions for trouble shooting ventilator alarms with the exception of option #2, silencing alarms. Alarms should never be turned off for the protection of the client. When in doubt of the cause of the alarm, the nurse should manually ventilate the client with an ambule bag while another nurse or respiratory therapist determines the functioning of the ventilator. High pressure alarms frequently indicate a need for suctioning or a kinked/compressed ET tube. Low pressure alarms indicate a leak or possible disconnection.

16.17 ④ Correct answer is option #4. Enalapril (Vasotec) is an ace inhibitor used to treat hypertension. If given upon return from dialysis, this will prevent a hypotensive effect. Vasotec should not be given before dialysis because the client could experience a hypotensive episode. If given the day after dialysis, this would disrupt the way that the medication is to be administered to the client.

16.18 ③ Option #3 is the priority due to potential risk of compartmental syndrome. This is a sign of potential nerve involvement which can result in permanent damage. Option #1 presents no problem. Option #2 makes no comparison to the right foot. Option #4 is no problem.

16.19 ③ The client is presenting with signs of an infection. The cultures should be completed prior to antibiotic therapy in order to determine what organism the client is growing. If the antibiotic is started prior to getting the cultures, then the report will not be valid. This will not assist the health care provider in determining if the antibiotic is effective. While option #1 is important to have to assist the HCP in calculating the antibiotic dose, the question reads "*after the HCP has been called for the order.*" Option #2 has already been evaluated based on the stem of the question. Option #4 is not specific to this case.

16.20 ② This is indicative of an alteration in the circulation from the cast being too tight causing an unsafe evaluation that could result with the client losing part of his extremity. Option #1 is irrelevant. Option #3 is important, but is not the priority as option #2. Option #4 is partially acceptable. The capillary refill can lead to option #2. Therefore, option #2 is the priority of concern with alteration in perfusion.

16.21 ④ Option #4 is correct. Options #1, #2, and #3 are dangerous for a maternity client since these diseases are communicable. Infection prevention is the priority concern here.

16.22 ② This is a priority due to the possibility of aspiration. While it is important to complete options #1, #3, and #4, they are not a priority over option #2.

16.23 ① This is the priority evaluation since the signs of drug withdrawal are more frequently associated with central nervous system alterations, gastrointestinal disturbances, and tachypnea. Options #2, #3, and #4 are secondary.

16.24 ③ It is important to monitor the beginning, the behaviors during the seizure, and the duration of the seizure. This will assist the neurologist in determining a more specific location and cause of the seizures. Option #1 is incorrect because the client should be positioned on side to facilitate the draining of oral secretions and minimize aspiration. Option #2 is incorrect since this is not an automatic protocol, and there is not enough data to substantiate this action. Option #4 is incorrect after the seizure is over.

16.25 ①
⑤
Options #1 and #5 are correct. Standard precautions are to prevent any contact with any blood or body secretions. Option #2 would be appropriate if the client had tuberculosis. Option #3 is never appropriate. Options #4 is not necessary unless the nurse is going to come in contact with client's blood

or body secretions, and this would need to be indicated in the stem of the question.

16.26 ② Option #2 is the only appropriate option for this active preschool child. Playground activities that are fun and promote bronchial drainage will engage the child in the intervention as well as meet his developmental needs. Option #1 is wrong. The best position to target the lung bases for cystic fibrosis is reverse Trendelenburg not sitting. Option #3 is incorrect. Avoid performing CPT immediately after eating to prevent vomiting and aspiration. Option #4 is incorrect. Client should have a lightweight layer covering their skin to get the most of the percussion effects.

16.27 ③ This is the safest plan for the radioactive material. Safety is a priority when dealing with implants—the client's, the nurse's, and the visitor's. Option #1 is inappropriate. Option #2 does not clarify how to remove it from the bed. Option #4 is incomplete and is unsafe for any radioactive material.

16.28 ② Hypotension is a significant side effect of nitroglycerin. While the effect may be transient, the client's blood pressure needs to be closely observed to assure that it does not continue to fall. Options #1 and #3 are not relevant to this medication. Option #4 is an expected outcome.

16.29 ② Humulin N insulin is an intermediate insulin that peaks from 8-12 hours after onset. This is when signs and symptoms of hypoglycemia occur. Options #1, #3, and #4 are signs of hyperglycemia.

16.30 ④ Rales and tachycardia would indicate a cardiovascular fluid overload. Option #1 is a normal CVP reading. Options #2 and #3 do not contain information relevant to fluid overload.

16.31 ③ These are signs and symptoms of hypofunction of the thyroid. Some other assessments would include dry hair, facial expression mask-like, thickened skin, enlarged tongue, and drooling. Options #1 and #4 contains signs of hyperfunction of the thyroid. Option #2 contains signs of hyperthyroidism.

16.32 ① These are accurate assessments of the position of a fractured hip prior to repair. Option #2 occurs with foot drop. Option #3 is incorrect because the leg will not appear longer. Option #4 occurs with injury to the lumbar disc area.

16.33 ② Option #2 is correct. Green, leafy vegetables are high in vitamin K, and this is the antidote for coumadin. Options #1, #3, and #4 are correct instructions. Option #1 would be indicative of bleeding. Option #3—client will need to have pT and/or INR evaluated. Option #4—Ginseng and Coumadin will increase the risk for bleeding.

16.34 ① As with hemodialysis, hypotension is most likely to result from rapid removal of fluid from the intravascular space. Options #2, #3, and #4 are not complications associated with this procedure.

16.35 ② Option #2 is correct. The scope of practice for the UAP is if the activity delegated is performed according to an established routine sequence of steps (*that do not require clinical decision making*), then this is most likely within the scope of practice for the UAP. Other aspects of care that may be delegated to the UAP include: tasks that frequently recurs in the daily care of a client or group of clients; tasks that involve little to no modification from one client care situation to another; task may be performed with a predictable outcome; task does not inherently involve ongoing assessment, interpretation, or decision making which cannot be logically separated from the procedure(s) itself; and the task does not endanger the client's life or well-being. Option #1 is incorrect since this involves assessment of the injection technique, and this is not within the scope of practice for the UAP. Option #3 is incorrect since this is not a routine task, and will require some teaching regarding the process for the task of obtaining the 24-hour diet recall. Option #4 requires evaluation which is not within the scope of practice for the UAP.

16.36 ② The extrusion reflex disappears between 3–4 months of age. Option #1 disappears at approximately 1–2 years of age. Options #3 and #4 are normal occurrences at this age level.

Chapter 16: ANSWERS & RATIONALES

16.37 ① The first action is to establish an airway. If there is no airway, any other resuscitation will not be helpful. Since the client hasn't had a cardiac arrest, option #2 is inappropriate. Option #3 does not deal with the problem of the severe dyspnea. Option #4 is not a priority.

16.38 ④ The highest priority is to prevent tissue damage and promote tissue absorption of the medicine which is accomplished through rotation of the injection sites. Option #1 is incorrect. It is important to have appropriate seizure precautions and emergency respiratory equipment available. Option #2 is important to implement but is not a priority. Option #3 contains incorrect information.

16.39 ① Decreased hearing and vertigo can occur as a result of involvement of the 8th cranial nerve which is caused from gentamycin (Garamycin) toxicity. Options #2, #3, and #4 are not toxic effects of this antibiotic.

16.40 ③ Allergic reaction is characterized by wheezing, urticaria (hives), facial flushing, and epiglottal edema. Options #1, #2, and #4 are indicative of a hemolytic transfusion reaction.

16.41 ① Option #1 is correct. When clients take beta blockers concurrently with cardiac glycoside and/or calcium channel blockers, there is an increased risk for bradycardia. Options #2, #3, and #4 are not correct for this situation. Option #4 is a therapeutic lab value.

16.42 ② Clients with a low WBC count are susceptible to infection. Option #1 contains incorrect information. The RBC's are not decreased. Option #3 is not correct. The calcium level is low versus high. Option #4 is a potential, but not a priority. In reality, this option is not addressed in the stem of the question. For this to be correct, it would be important to have labs indicating a complication with fluid volume deficit such as the urine specific gravity, BUN, Hct or even clinical findings indicting dehydration such as weight loss, decrease in the skin turgor, dry lips and mucous membranes, dry skin, vomiting etc.

I CAN HINT: If the stem of the question gives you lab reports, assessments, vital signs, etc., PAY ATTENTION. The key here is to know the normal values for the following: WBC's: 5,000–10,000 mm^3; RBC: 4,200–5,400 mm^3; and Calcium: 9.0–10.5 mg/dL (2.25–2.62 mmol/L).

16.43 ③ With the client complaints, WBCs and RBCs should be present. WBCs are a response to the inflammation process and irritation of the urethra. RBCs are increased when the bladder mucosa is irritated and bleeding. Option #1 is not a primary component in determining urinary tract infections. Option #2 is not as complete a response as option #3. Option #4 indicates the concentration of the urine for this specimen and is not specifically associated with a urinary tract infection.

16.44 ① Immobility is a leading cause of problems with Buck's traction. It is important to turn client to the unaffected side. Option #2 is incorrect because the head of the bed can be elevated 15 to 20 degrees, since the supine position can increase problems with immobility. Option #3 is incorrect because the client is on strict bed rest. Option #4 would interfere with the traction.

16.45 ② Option #2 is correct since it is in final time of transfusion. Option #1 is not appropriate. Option #3 is newly diagnosed. Option #4 is initial and would be inappropriate.

16.46 ② The goal of care for this disease is to maintain independence as long as client is able. Options #1 and #3 are not primary goals, but are included in the care plan. Option #4 is inappropriate for this client.

16.47 ① This will facilitate maximum expansion of the lungs and will decrease the pulmonary workload. Options #2, #3, and #4 would not improve the quality of respirations and would increase client anxiety.

16.48 ① The charcoal, if given within two hours, will absorb the particles of salicylate. Option #2 is an antidote for Heparin. Option #3 is an antidote for warfarin (Coumadin). Option #4 may be necessary later after evaluating the response to charcoal.

16.49 ① Phenytoin (Dilantin) is metabolized by the liver. Elderly clients frequently have some degree of liver impairment and are a high risk for the toxic reaction. Options #2 and #3 are not affected by Dilantin. Option #4 is incorrect.

16.50 ② This will assist in determining if hydration can be done through oral fluids alone. Option #1 is done, but is not to assist with rehydration. It evaluates rehydration. Option #3 does not solve the problem, since it doesn't guarantee the child is taking fluids. Option #4 evaluates the amount of fluid taken in, but does not actually assist with rehydration.

16.51 ① The safest objective is to prevent trauma to the child during the procedure, so the child must be restrained. Option #2 would be done prior to obtaining consent and performing the procedure. Option #3 should be done before and/or after the procedure. Option #4 will not expose the spinal column of a 4-month-old necessary for this procedure to be performed safely.

16.52 ② Option #2 is correct. This action needs intervention since this is not the standard of care for this procedure. The tape should be secured from the client's nose to the nasogastric tube in order to secure placement. The tube is too bulky for the nurse to create a loop. Options #1, #3, and #4 are all correct and safe nursing care for this client.

16.53 ② The stockings should be worn the entire time the client is in the hospital. They should be removed with the bath and replaced after the skin is dry and prior to the client getting out of bed. Option #1 is incorrect because the stockings should be worn to prevent any discomfort and to increase the blood flow. Option #3 is incorrect because the stockings should be worn during the day and when the client is non-ambulatory. Option #4 is incorrect because the stockings should be applied prior to getting out of bed.

16.54 ④ The assessment indicates that the ace is too tight and it needs readjusting. Option #1 ignores the possibility of the ace being too tight. Options #2 and #3 do not relieve the circulation problem.

16.55 ① AquaMephyton is given in the vastus lateralis. Options #2, #3, and #4 are not correct routes of administration of this medication.

16.56 ① The priority is to maintain moisture to prevent the wound from drying out and becoming necrotic prior to returning to surgery. Option #2 is inappropriate. Option #3 needs to be moist in order to be correct. Option #4 needs to be continuous to be correct.

16.57 ④ Chemotherapy can lead to immuno-suppression which predisposes the client to infection. Hand washing is one of the most effective means of decreasing the infection transmission. Options #1 and #2 are appropriate but not a priority. Option #3 is not the correct precaution during chemotherapy.

16.58 ② Mannitol (Osmitrol) is an osmotic diuretic, thus increasing the urinary output. The diuresing effects facilitate the decrease in the intracranial pressure. Options #1, #3, and #4 are not indications of desired effects of the medication.

16.59 ② During both the second and third trimester, the need for insulin will increase due to insulin antagonism by the placental hormones. Option #1 is incorrect because the client is encouraged to continue to exercise. Option #3 is incorrect because the baby's pancreas is normal. However, the mother's insulin needs will increase. Option #4 is incorrect because weight gain in pregnancy and insulin needs do not correlate.

16.60 ③ The arms should be bent at 35 degree angle and weight should be placed on the hands and arms. Option #1 is incorrect because pressure placed on the axillae can damage the brachial plexus. Option #2 is incorrect because crutches should be placed 8-10 inches in front with each step. Option #4 is unsafe. Shoes should be non-slip soles.

16.61 ③ "Statins" should be taken at bedtime and with food. Option #1 is incorrect since it will take several weeks before the lipids decrease. Option #2 is incorrect. Option #4, clients should be instructed to increase fiber in their diet (whole grain cereals, fruits, and vegetables).

16.62 ④ Edema is a result of sodium and fluid retention. Weight loss should occur if therapy is effective. Options #1 and #2 do not relate to edema. Option #3 is inappropriate for this client.

16.63 ① All are low in sodium, and milk is allowed on a salt-restricted diet. Option #2 is incorrect because instant oatmeal is high in sodium. Option #3 is incorrect because bacon is high in sodium. Option #4 is incorrect because all baked breads are high in sodium along with the sausage.

16.64 ①③④ Options #1, 3, and 4 are correct. Option #1 will reduce peripheral resistance and venous return. This will result in a redistribution from the pulmonary circulation to other body systems. It will cause a pooling of blood in the peripheral blood vessels, resulting in a reduction of the amount of blood returning to the heart which will decrease the work of the heart. Option #3 is correct because furosemide (Lasix) will facilitate the excretion of water and sodium and decrease the amount of blood returning to the heart. Option #4 is correct because a high-flow rebreather mask should be used for oxygen therapy in pulmonary edema to relieve the feeling of breathlessness and support the signs of hypoxemia the client is experiencing. Option #2 is incorrect. This is an alkylating agent used for chemotherapy. There is no need for this agent with this client's clinical assessment findings. Option #5 is incorrect. The client should be positioned upright, preferable with the legs dangling over the side of the bed, to reduce venous return to the heart.

16.65 ① Depression is a frequent cause of malnutrition in the older client. Psychological, sociological, and economic factors, chronic disease, and polypharmacy all contribute to the potential or actual problem of malnutrition which will prolong wound healing. Option #2 could be a contributing factor if said decrease in social contacts. Option #3 is a normal process with aging and is not responsible for prolonging wound healing unless it is an extreme increase. Option #4 is the recommendation from the American Cancer Association for dietary fiber. This may improve the intake of vitamins and minerals as well as being beneficial for glucose tolerance.

16.66 ② The position of the trachea should be evaluated. With a tracheal shift, an increase in pressure could occur in the operative side and cause pressure against the mediastinal area. Option #1 is incorrect because on the surgical side, breath sounds will be absent. Option #3 is important to observe, but not as high a priority as option #2. Option #4 does not relate to the situation.

16.67 ④ The initial assessment is to check for a prolapsed cord. Option #1 is a useful assessment, but not the priority assessment over option #4 due to safety. It will determine if the fluid is urine (acidic) rather than amniotic fluid, but this can be assessed later. Option #2 is incorrect because the mother's blood pressure is not affected by rupture of the membranes. Option #3 would read variable decelerations for a cord compression or prolapse versus early deceleration.

I CAN HINT: The book *Nursing Made Insanely Easy*, has great images to simplify these decelerations. Just remember, *Early decelerations = Head compression; Variable decelerations = Cord compression; Late decelerations = Uteroplacental insufficiency.*

16.68 ② The calcium intake is important in minimizing the development of osteoporosis. Both of these contain calcium. The other options are not focused on calcium intake.

16.69 ④ Magnesium sulfate is a central nervous system depressant. A side effect is oliguria. Option #1 is not a concern because the respirations are increasing. Options #2 and #3 are not relevant for the medication.

16.70 ④ Option #4 is correct. Clients with chronic renal failure have hyperphosphatemia. Calcium carbonate will bind with the phosphorus to assist with the phosphorus excretion. Some examples of these calcium-based phosphate binders include calcium acetate, calcium carbonate, or aluminum hydroxide gel. The other options are not correct for this client with chronic renal failure.

I CAN HINT: Remember it is important to focus on what information is in the stem of the question. The key here is the diagnosis with the medication.

16.71 ③ Options #3 and #4 are correct. Older
④ clients are at greater risk than young people for dehydration and hypovolemia. If hypovolemia is present which is a risk from vomiting and diarrhea, they may present with tachycardia, hypotension, tachypnea, a furrowed dry tongue, and sunken eyeballs, and confusion. Option #1 is a normal rate and Option #2 would typically be decreased with this clinical presentation. Option #5 is not a reliable assessment in the older client, since this is typically decreased with age.

16.72 ② Option #2 is the priority since the client is at high risk for hemorrhaging or shock due to the liver being a vascular organ. Option #1 is WNL. Option #3 is pretest, and Option #4 would become an issue if the bleeding continued and client was to progress into shock.

16.73 ③ The unlicensed assistive personnel (UAP) needs to be re-educated about the importance of maintaining client confidentiality. Options #1, #2, and #4 are avoiding the current situation. If the behavior continues, then this must be communicated to a different level of authority.

16.74 ④ The charge nurse should discuss standard precautions (universal precautions) with the unlicensed assistive personnel (UAP) and determine the nature of her problem. It may be easily solved with education, or the UAP may need to be transferred to another unit. Option #1 may cause the UAP to resign when she may be retrained. Option #2 does not show respect for other UAPs. Option #3 is not an issue.

16.75 ① The generic children's strength acetaminophen is less expensive than the brand names (Tylenol) and may be used. Options #2 and #3, the mother should be instructed to use only the children's strength. The infant's strength of Tylenol is more concentrated. Option #4, acetaminophen is not the generic name for Advil or Motrin. These are Ibuprofen.

16.76 ② An airway is a priority. Epiglottitis can cause a sudden total airway obstruction. Option #1 is not appropriate to this situation. Option #3 is incorrect because this client has airway problems, not a seizure problem, plus a padded tongue blade is no longer recommended. Option #4 is not specific for the potential emergency of airway obstruction.

16.77 ① Document the error on an incident report, assess for side effects, and notify the health care provider (HCP). Options #2 and #4 are unsafe, incorrect nursing interventions. Option #3 is incorrect information. Tachycardia and hyperactivity are signs of aminophylline overdose.

16.78 ④ The decrease in blood pressure is most likely due to pressure on the inferior vena cava which occurs in the supine position (vena-caval syndrome). By positioning the client on her side, the pressure is relieved and the blood pressure will increase. Option #1 may be necessary, but option #4 should be done first. Option #2 does not address the problem of low blood pressure. Option #3 is incorrect because the problem needs to be addressed immediately.

16.79 ① The IV is to run in 12 hours, or 720 minutes. The formula is: volume to be infused is divided by 720 times 15. Another calculation may be used to determine the number of mL's per hour, then per minute and multiplied by the drip factor. Options #2, #3, and #4 are incorrect calculations.

16.80 ③ This position will facilitate the removal of fluid from the venous pathways and lymphatic system through gravity. The arm is elevated to enhance circulation and prevent edema. Option #1 is incorrect because a sling is not necessary; the arm needs to be elevated. Option #2 is incorrect because the right arm cannot be elevated from this position. Option #4 is incorrect because the prone position is inappropriate.

16.81 ④ The presence of hypoxia needs to be addressed immediately. The hypoxia also contributes to the confusion. Once hypoxia is ruled out, then the confusion could be from being in a new environment. Always start with assessing physiological issues! Options #1, #2, and #3 are important to consider but are secondary to Option #4.

Chapter 16: ANSWERS & RATIONALES

16.82 ③ The priority of care is to determine if any heat inhalation has occurred that would cause airway problems. Option #1 is secondary. Option #2 will be done as soon as option #1 is completed. Option #4 will also be done, but option #3 remains the priority.

16.83 ④ The Pitocin should always be a secondary infusion and the infusion controlled by an IV pump. Option #1 is incorrect because Pitocin should be a secondary infusion. Option #2 contains incorrect information. Normal range for fetal heart tones is 120 to 160 per minute. Option #3 is incorrect because the rate should be maintained by an infusion pump.

16.84 ③ Placing a limit on the ritual initially will only increase the client's anxiety and need for the rituals. Limits must be gradually instituted. Options #1, #2, and #4 are appropriate nursing actions.

16.85 ① The client and/or family must be informed about questions or concerns about the surgery prior to signing the consent. After notifying the physician, the physician's response should be documented. Options #2, #3, and #4 do not protect the client's rights.

16.86 ② A 6-month-old should sit with help. Option #1 is present at 9 months of age. Option #3 is present at 1 year. Option #4 is closed by 2–3 months.

16.87 ① A positive skin test is determined by the area of induration (raised) rather than the area of inflammation. This correctly describes a positive reaction to the skin test. Options #2 and #4 describe other types of inflammatory responses. Option #3 does not have anything to do with reading the skin test.

16.88 ② The RML is found right anterior between the fourth and sixth intercostal spaces. Options #1 and #4 are incorrect because the RML cannot be auscultated from the posterior. Option #3 is the point of maximum impulse or apical pulse.

16.89 125 mL/hr

Pump rates are always set in mL's per hour. 1000 mL divided by 8 hours equals 125 mL/hour.

16.90 ① This comment indicates a desire to begin stroking and cuddling this baby. This must happen before parents can actually provide physical care. Option #2 indicates a fear or a sense of insecurity with the feedings. Option #3 indicates some feeling of guilt. Option #4 is a request for information and does not address the question.

16.91 ④ This will help the nurse know where the family is in regards to grieving, coping, etc. Options #1, #2, and #3 are inappropriate before the assessment. Actions can be taken only when the circumstances are known.

16.92 150 mL/hr

Step One: What is the volume to be infused? 50 mL

Step Two: What is the time for the infusion? 20 min.

Step Three: Set up the equation and calculate:

$$\frac{\text{Volume (mL)}}{\text{Time (min)}} = \frac{x \text{ mL}}{60 \text{ min}}$$

$$\frac{50}{20} = \frac{x \text{ mL}}{60 \text{ min}}$$

$$20x = 3{,}000$$

$$x = 150 \text{ mL/hr}$$

150 mL IV pump to deliver 150 mL/hr

I CAN HINT: Reassess to review if the answer makes any sense. It does make sense to infuse 50 mL over 20 min to administer 150 mL/hour.

16.93 ① Clomiphene Citrate (Clomid) induces ovulation by altering the estrogen and stimulating follicular growth to produce a mature ovum. Options #2 and #3 are infertility problems, but Clomid does not affect them. Option #4 is not an appropriate use of the medication.

16.94 ① Vitamin C facilitates the absorption of iron. Option #2 is incorrect because antacids will decrease the absorption of the iron. Option #3 is incorrect because although the client needs increased fluids, fluids will not affect absorption. Option #4 is incorrect because dark stools are characteristic of iron therapy, and there is no need to notify the physician.

16.95 ② Prednisone (Deltasone) can cause ulcers. Administering it with meals or with milk will assist in protecting the GI mucosa. Options #1 and #3 do not protect the stomach. Option #4 is incorrect because the drug is recommended to be given with milk.

16.96 ③ Fresh fruits and vegetables are low sodium, and roasted chicken is low cholesterol. Option #1 is incorrect because canned foods contain increased salt, and milk contains cholesterol. Option #2 is incorrect because breads contain sodium, and frying increases the cholesterol. Option #4 is incorrect because bread and carbonated beverages contain sodium.

16.97 ② Option #2 is correct due to the risk for falling from orthostatic hypotension. This is a safety issue, and the number one injury to older adults is falls. Options #1 and #3 are correct, but not frequent enough, so would not be a priority over "*safety with the risk for falling.*" Option #4 is incorrect, since the foods should be high in fiber.
I CAN HINT: Amitriptyline (Elavil) has anticholinergic effects and can result in a few complications such as with low blood pressure, constipation, urinary retention, and dry mouth.

16.98 ① The primary objective of fluid replacement is to perfuse the vital organs. The increase in urine output to a normal range indicates that the kidneys are adequately perfused. Therefore, other major organs are being perfused also. Option #2 does not give any indication of adequate fluid replacement. Option #3 is incorrect because although the CVP is an indicator of fluid balance, a CVP at 2 mm Hg is in the low range and does not indicate tissue perfusion. Option #4 is incorrect because the client is tachycardiac, and the absence of dysrhythmias does not indicate tissue perfusion.

16.99 ④ Side rails should be up for any disoriented client. Option #1 is appropriate, but is not the safety priority. Option #2 is incorrect because it is not necessary to stay with the client, especially while sleeping. Option #3 is incorrect because restraints are not necessary at this time.

16.100 ② Suctioning the nose will help open the airway. Option #1 will not promote adequate drainage from the upper airway. Option #3 will facilitate drainage of mucous from the upper airway and will assist the adjustment to breathing through the nose, but is secondary to option #2. Option #4 does not relieve the congestion.

16.101 ③ Option #3 is the correct answer. It is imperative the nurse notify the physician of the client's request to assure the wishes of the client will be met. Options #1 and #2 disregard the client's request. Option #4 does attempt to make the staff aware, but does not ensure accountability. By notifying the surgeon of the client's request, and documenting the process, the nurse is covering themself from liability if this request is not met.

16.102 ① The client's concern about her husband's feelings indicates that he may not be able to support her emotionally at this time. Option #2 reflects a reality-based concern. Option #3 indicates an economic concern. Option #4 indicates she needs to talk about her current feelings. It does not give any indication of level of emotional support.

16.103 ④ Assessing the basis for the client's fears and encouraging discussion about those fears are the first positive steps. Option #1 jumps to solutions without adequately defining the problem. Option #2 is an empathetic response but does not gain any more information, or encourage the client to continue. Option #3 provides false reassurance.

16.104 ④ Option #4 is correct. The formula for mean arterial pressure (MAP) is SBP + 2 DBP divided by 3. The blood pressure with mean arterial pressure between 65 and 75 is 105/60 (MAP = 75).

16.105 ③ An objective description of the client's mood and documentation of what actually occurred is the most appropriate nursing action. Options #1, #2, and #4 interpret the behavior, or make assumptions regarding the behavior, rather than describing the behavior.

16.106 ④ Option #4 is correct. Due to the action of this drug which produces smooth muscle relaxation of the corpus cavernosum, this drug should be given with caution in clients with a history of CHF or hypotension. The other options are not correct for this medication.

16.107 ④ Giving away prized possessions is an indication that he does not intend to be using them in the future and is considered a sign of suicidal intentions. Option #1 is of concern, but does not imply active suicidal ideation at the present time. Option #2 may be true but is not a sign of suicidal intent. Option #3 is a normal expression of grief.

16.108 ④ ⑤ Options #4 and #5 are correct. Nasogastric losses are isotonic, containing both sodium and potassium. Option #4 would be a finding from hypokalemia, and option #5 would be from hyponatremia due to hypotension. Option #1 is incorrect since this would occur from hyperkalemia, option #2 would occur from hypernatremia. Option #3 is a finding from hypocalcemia which is not a complication from the NG suctioning.

16.109 ④ Option #4 is correct. Desmopressin Acetate (DDAVP) is an antidiuretic replacement agent. This is used as a synthetic posterior pituitary hormone that causes an increase in water absorption from the kidneys and a decrease in the urine output. This option clearly evaluates this outcome. Option #1 is incorrect. This BP has actually decreased, but still remains elevated. This is not the desired outcome of this treatment. Actually, one of the side effects of this medication could be excessive fluid retention. Option #2 is inaccurate for this medication. Option #3 is not a desired outcome.

16.110 ④ Option #4 is correct. Following a choleycystectomy, it is important to get the client up ambulating in order to decrease risk for pneumonia, DVT, etc. This question is not just evaluating your understanding of the standard of practice for this client, but also the scope of practice for the UAP. UAPs can ambulate clients. Option #1 is incorrect because they must evaluate the characteristics of the drainage when the bag is emptied, and this is not within the scope of practice for the UAP. Option #2 is incorrect because teaching is not within their scope of practice. Option #3 is incorrect because it reads that the UAP would be monitoring for changes in the vital signs, and this is not within their scope of practice.

16.111 ② Option #2 is correct. The LPN demonstrates an understanding of appropriate positioning to facilitate an increase venous return due to the hypotension. Option #1 is incorrect. During this time, the majority of the meds will be administered through the IV. Option #3 is incorrect since the client will require a large amount of fluid replacement, so the fluid administered will be isotonic crystalloid solutions, such as 0.9% Sodium Chloride, or Lactated Ringer's solution. Option #4 is incorrect since this will facilitate arterial perfusion, and may result in a further decrease in the blood pressure.

16.112 ② A side effect of Haldol is hypotension. Moving slowly to a standing position will decrease the problem with orthostatic hypotension. Option #1 would be appropriate for a monoamine oxidase inhibitor (MAO). Option #3 is incorrect because this side effect of a dry mouth, from the anticholinergic effect, is not a priority to safety which could result in a fall. Option #4 is incorrect because salt does not have any effect on the medication.

16.113 ③ Option #3 is the correct answer. Out of 23 points, this client scored 21 which was excellent and requires prevention to continue to be the priority of care. There are six subscales rates factors within the schema from 1 (least favorable) to 4 (most favorable), for a total of 23 points. A score of 16 points or less is the critical cutoff for predicting risk. The six subscales include: sensory perception, moisture, activity, mobility, nutrition, and friction and shear. Each of these scales goes from 1 to 4; with the exception of friction and shear, and it goes from 1 to 3. Option #2 is a correct statement about the Stage II pressure sore, but it is not correct for this client who is not high risk. Option #4 is incorrect since there are 5 other subscales that are evaluated to determine the risk factor. This option also does not address the score of 21 in the question.

16.114 ④ The correct answer is Option #4. Silace is a stool softener that is used to treat occasional constipation. Some of the undesirable effects include abdominal cramps, diarrhea or a sore throat. Option #1 is incorrect. In Option #2, client could have urinary retention or may be distended from the use of opioid medications or an accumulation of gas in the GI tract; however, bowel sounds should not be absent. Option #3, HR of 72, is within the normal range of 60–80 beats per minute.

16.115 ③ Option #3 is correct. Because of the risk of inaccuracy in SpO_2 assessment, an abnormal SpO_2 should always be validated with a second reading. Once this is accomplished, the client should be assessed for other causes of hypoxemia such as airway congestion or narrowing that can be seen in bronchitis. Option #1 is incorrect. It is true that an oxygen delivery of 7 liters per minute is too high for a client with chronic bronchitis because of the risk for respiratory depression, but simply reducing the delivery to 2 liters does not address the client's hypoxemia. Option #2 is incorrect. This practice must be authorized by the provider and does not appropriately address the client's hypoxemia. Option #4 is incorrect. It is likely that the delivery of 7 liters per minute is an error, but this act is low priority in this clinical circumstance.

16.116 ③ After the surgery, swelling can occur which causes respiratory distress. Option #1 is not as specific to this surgery. Option #2 is for monitoring a post-operative tonsillectomy. Option #4 is unsafe. The head of bed should be elevated.

16.117

③ Assume tripod position at the top of the stairs.
① Shift weight to the unaffected leg.
④ Move crutches and the affected leg down onto the next step.
② Transfer weight to the crutches and move the unaffected leg to that step.

16.118 ② Option #2 is correct. This does not follow the standard of care for nasopharyngeal suctioning. The client should be allowed 20 to 30 seconds for recovery between sessions. The LPN needs to review the standard in order to improve the care delivered to clients. Options #1, #3, and #4 are correct and do not require intervention by the charge nurse.

16.119 ① Option #1 is correct. Option #2 is incorrect. Part of this statement about the gauze dressing is correct for the initial dressing, but this should be changed and replaced with a transparent dressing within 24 hours. Option #3 is incorrect. The insertion port should be cleaned with alcohol for 3 seconds and allowed to dry completely prior to accessing it. Option #4 is incorrect. The client should be advised not to immerse arm in water. When taking a shower, cover dressing site to avoid water exposure.

16.120 The fetal heart rate with the LOA position would be ausculated at point A. LOP-point B; ROA-point C; ROP-point D.

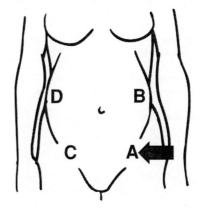

Normal Reference Ranges for Lab Tests Used in Questions

Lab Test	Reference Range
Hematology	
White Blood Cells (WBCs)	5,000–10,000 mm³ (5 x 10⁹/L–10 x 10⁹/L)
Red Blood Cells (RBCs)	4,200,000–5,400,000 mm³ (4.2 x 10¹²/L– 5.4 x 10¹²/L)
Hemoglobin (HGB)	12–16 g/dL (7.45–9.93 mmol/L)
Glycosylated Hemoglobin (HbA1c)	6% or less
HCT	37%–47%
MCV	81–89 μm³
MCH	26–35 pg/cell
MCHC	31–37 g/dL
Platelets	150,000–400,000 mm³ (150 x 10⁹/L–400 x 10⁹/L)
Neutrophils	37%–75%
Lymphocytes	19%–48%
Monocytes	0%–10%
Eosinophils	1%–3%
Basophils	0.0%–1.5%
Urinalysis	
Color	Clear Yellow
Appearance	Clear
Glucose	Negative
Bilirubin	Negative
Ketones	Negative
Specific Gravity	1.015–1.025
Blood	Negative
Ph	4.5–8.0
Protein	Negative
Nitrates	Negative
ABGs	
pH	7.35–7.45
PCO₂	35–45 mm Hg
PO₂	80–100 mm Hg
HCO₃	22–26 mEq/L (22–26 mmol/L)
O₂ Sat	> 95%
Anion Gap	3–10 mEq/L
Cardiac Enzymes	
Myoglobin	25 – 72 ng/mL (1.28 – 3.67 nmol/L)
CK-MB	3 to 5% (percentage of total CK) (30 – 170 units/L)
Troponin I Value	< 0.04 ng/mL
BNP	< 100 pg/mL

Lab Test	Reference Range
Chemistry	
Sodium	135–145 mEq/L (135–145 mmol/L)
Potassium	3.5–5.0 mEq/L (3.5–5.0 mmol/L)
Chloride	98–107 mEq/L (98–107 mmol/L)
Glucose-serum	70–110 mg/dL (3.9–6.1 mmol/L)
Magnesium	1.3–2.1 mEq/L (0.65–1.05 mmol/L)
BUN	10–20 mg/dL (3.57–7.14 mmol/L)
Creatinine	0.6–1.2 mg/dL (53.05–106.1 μmol/L)
Calcium	9.0–10.5 mg/dL (2.25–2.62 mmol/L)
Protein	6.0–8.0 mg/dL
Albumin	3.5–5.4 g/dL (35 g/L–54 g/L)
A/G Ratio	1.5:1.0–2.5:1.0
Serum Osmolality	285–295 mOsm/Kg
Lactic Acid	0.35–1.25 mmol/L
Total Bilirubin	0.1–1.0 mg/dL (1.71–17.1 μmol/L)
Direct Bilirubin	0.1–0.3 mg/dL (1.71–5.13 μmol/L)
Indirect Bilirubin	0.1–1.0 mg/dL (1.71 - 17.1 μmol/L)
ALT, SGPT	7–56 Units/L
AST, SGOT	5–40 Units/L
Ammonia	15–45 mcg/dL (8.81–26.42 μmol/L)
LDH–Serum	140–280 Units/L
Alk Phos	44–147 Units/L
Uric Acid	2.0–7.0 mg/dL
Phosphorus	3.0–4.5 mg/dL
Total Cholesterol	< 200 mg/dL
LDL age > 20	100–125 mg/dL (optimal) < 100 mg/dL (with CAD)
HDL	> 60 mg/dL
Triglyceride	< 150 mg/dL
Medication Levels	
Digoxin	0.5–2.0 ng/mL
Dilantin	10–20 μg/mL
Lithium	0.4–1.0 mEq/L maintenance
Pt (normal) without Anticoagulants	11–12.5 seconds; Therapeutic range for anticoagulant therapy is 1.5 to 2.5 times the normal or control value
Therapeutic INR	2.0–3.0 (with Anticoagulants) 0.8–1.0 (without Anticoagulants)
Ptt	30–40 seconds; Therapeutic range for anticoagulant therapy is 1.5 to 2.5 times the normal or control value
Amylase	40–140 Units/L
Thyroid Hormones	
Thyroxine (T₄)	4.0–12.0 μg/dL
Thyroid stimulating hormone (TSH)	0.4–4.0 mU/L

REFERENCES

Dickison, P., Haerling, K., & Lasater, K. (2019). *Integrating the National Council State Boards of Nursing—Clinical Judgment Model (NCSBN-CJM) into Nursing Educational Frameworks.* [Manuscript submitted for publication].

Lewis, S., Bucher, L., Heitkemper, M., Harding, M, Kwong, J., & Roberts, D. (2017). *Medical-surgical nursing assessment and management of clinical problems* (10th ed.), St. Louis, MO: Elsevier.

Manning, L. (2020). *Maternal newborn nursing made insanely easy.* (1st ed.). I CAN Publishing®, Inc.

Manning, L., & Rayfield, S. (2016). *Nursing made insanely easy* (8th ed.). Duluth, GA: I CAN Publishing®, Inc.

Manning, L., & Rayfield, S. (2017). *Pharmacology made insanely easy* (5th ed.). Duluth, GA: I CAN Publishing®, Inc.

Manning, L., Zager, L. (2019). *Medical surgical nursing concepts made insanely easy.* Duluth, GA: I CAN Publishing®, Inc.

Manning, L., Akins, P., Brocato, C. (2022). *A step-by-step approach to developing clinical judgment for the next generation NCLEX® and clinical success.* Duluth, Georgia: I CAN Publishing®, Inc.

Muntean, W.J. (2015). *Evaluating clinical judgment in licensure tests. Application of decision theory.* Paper presented at the annual meeting of the American Educational Research Association, Chicago, Il.

© National Council of State Boards of Nursing, Inc. (NCSBN). (2022). 2021 *RN Practice Analysis: Linking the NCLEX-RN® Examination to Practice.* Chicago: Author.

Other Books Published by I CAN Publishing®, Inc.

A Step-by-Step Approach to Developing Clinical Judgment for the Next Generation NCLEX® and Clinical Success!
The Eight-Step Approach for Student Clinical Success
Medical Surgical Nursing Concepts Made Insanely Easy!
Concepts Made Insanely Easy for Clinical Nursing!
Maternal Newborn Nursing Made Insanely Easy!
Pharmacology Made Insanely Easy!
Nursing Made Insanely Easy!

Teaching Books & Tools for Nursing Educators

A Step-by-Step Approach to Developing Clinical Judgment for the Next Generation NCLEX® and Clinical Success!
The Teaching Books & Tools for Nursing Educators
The Eight-Step Approach to Teaching Clinical Nursing
Medical Surgical Nursing Made Insanely Easy! Digital Images
Pharmacology Made Insanely Easy! Digital Images
Nursing Made Insanely Easy! Digital Images
Pathways to Teaching Nursing: Keeping It Real!

Student Programs

Next Generation NCLEX® Reviews for students.

Pharmacology NCLEX® Review—A one-day, live interactive program brought to your school to transform learning of pharmacology! Strategies designed to help you master pharmacology recall, prioritization, clinical decision-making, and judgment. You will be on the road to NCLEX® SUCCESS! You will have FUN and experience an increased confidence in your ability to perform successfully both on the Next Generation NCLEX® and in clinical practice.

Medical Surgical Nursing Concepts Made Insanely Easy Review—A one-day review designed to make learning Medical Surgical Nursing Concepts Insanely Easy! Tools and illustrations are integrated throughout the workshop to facilitate both nursing school and NCLEX® SUCCESS.

Tailored Workshops and Presentations designed by you and the authors to meet your specific needs.

Scholarship Fundraisers: Learn while you Earn! Call for details on how your class can earn money while learning how to master Pharmacology, Medical Surgical Nursing Concepts, Maternal Newborn Nursing, Pathophysiology, and/or a tailored program for your class.

 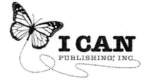

Contact I CAN Publishing®, Inc. today to schedule your program.

770.495.2488

www.icanpublishing.com